European Federation of National Associations
of Orthopaedics and Traumatology

European Instructional Lectures

Volume 13, 2013

European Federation of National Associations of Orthopaedics and Traumatology

Committees and Task Forces

EFORT Executive Committee

Executive Board

Prof. Dr. Pierre Hoffmeyer, *President*
Dr. Manuel Cassiano Neves, *Vice President*
Ass. Prof. Dr. Per Kjaersgaard-Andersen, *Secretary General*
Prof. Dr. Miklós Szendröi, *Immediate Past President*
Mr. Stephen R. Cannon, *Treasurer*
Prof. Dr. Enric Cáceres Palou, *Member at Large*
Dr. George Macheras, *Member at Large*
Prof. Dr. Philippe Neyret, *Member at Large*

Co-Opted Members

Mr. John Albert
Prof. Dr. Thierry Bégué
Prof. Dr. George Bentley, *Past President*
Prof. Dr. Nikolaus Böhler, *Past President*
Dr. Marino Delmi
Prof. Dr. Karsten Dreinhöfer
Prof. Dr. Pavel Dungl
Prof. Dr. Klaus-Peter Günther
Prof. Dr. Norbert Haas
Prof. Dr. Karl Knahr
Prof. Dr. Maurilio Marcacci
Prof. Dr. Jean Puget
Prof. Dr. Wolfhart Puhl, *Past President*
Prof. Dr. Nejat Hakki Sur
Prof. Dr. Karl-Göran Thorngren, *Past President*

Scientific Coordination 14th EFORT Congress, Istanbul 2013

Chairman

Prof. Dr. Nejat Hakki Sur

Standing Committees

EAR Committee

Prof. Dr. Nikolaus Böhler

Education Committee

Prof. Dr. Maurilio Marcacci

Ethics Committee

Prof. Dr. Jean Puget

EA & L Committee

Prof. Dr. Wolfhart Puhl

Finance Committee

Mr. Stephen R. Cannon

Health Service Research Committee

Prof. Dr. Karsten Dreinhöfer

Portal Steering Committee

Prof. Dr. Klaus-Peter Günther

Publications Committee

Prof. Dr. George Bentley

Scientific Congress Committee

Prof. Dr. Enric Cáceres Palou

Speciality Society Standing Committee

Dr. Marino Delmi
Prof. Dr. Pierre Hoffmeyer

Task Forces and Ad Hoc Committees

Awards & Prizes Committee

Prof. Dr. George Bentley

Fora

Prof. Dr. Thierry Bégué

Travelling & Visiting Fellowships

Prof. Dr. Philippe Neyret

Musculoskeletal Trauma Task Force

Prof. Dr. Norbert Haas

EFORT Foundation Committee

Prof. Dr. Karl-Göran Thorngren

European Federation of National Associations
of Orthopaedics and Traumatology

European Instructional Lectures

Volume 13, 2013
14th EFORT Congress, Istanbul, Turkey

Edited by

George Bentley

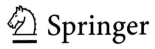

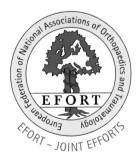

Editor
George Bentley
Royal National Orthopaedic Hospital Trust
Stanmore
Middlesex
United Kingdom

EFORT Central Office
Technoparkstrasse 1
8005 Zürich
Switzerland

ISBN 978-3-642-36148-7   ISBN 978-3-642-36149-4   (eBook)
DOI 10.1007/978-3-642-36149-4
Springer Heidelberg New York Dordrecht London

Library of Congress Control Number: 2013936740

© EFORT 2013

This work is subject to copyright. All rights are reserved by the Publisher, whether the whole or part of the material is concerned, specifically the rights of translation, reprinting, reuse of illustrations, recitation, broadcasting, reproduction on microfilms or in any other physical way, and transmission or information storage and retrieval, electronic adaptation, computer software, or by similar or dissimilar methodology now known or hereafter developed. Exempted from this legal reservation are brief excerpts in connection with reviews or scholarly analysis or material supplied specifically for the purpose of being entered and executed on a computer system, for exclusive use by the purchaser of the work. Duplication of this publication or parts thereof is permitted only under the provisions of the Copyright Law of the Publisher's location, in its current version, and permission for use must always be obtained from Springer. Permissions for use may be obtained through RightsLink at the Copyright Clearance Center. Violations are liable to prosecution under the respective Copyright Law.

The use of general descriptive names, registered names, trademarks, service marks, etc. in this publication does not imply, even in the absence of a specific statement, that such names are exempt from the relevant protective laws and regulations and therefore free for general use.

While the advice and information in this book are believed to be true and accurate at the date of publication, neither the authors nor the editors nor the publisher can accept any legal responsibility for any errors or omissions that may be made. The publisher makes no warranty, express or implied, with respect to the material contained herein.

Printed on acid-free paper

Springer is part of Springer Science+Business Media (www.springer.com)

Foreword

One day, when I was a young resident, I remember my chief resident telling me, quite disparagingly, as we were leaving our chairman's office, "Did you notice all those Journals unpacked on his desk? He never has time to read them!"

But as we had entered the office a few minutes earlier, he was fully concentrating on reading an Instructional Course Lecture Book.

This memory has, ever since then, taught me that an Instructional Course Book is not meant only for beginners but also for the most experienced people.

As a representative of the local organizing committee, it is an honour and a pleasure to present this Instructional Lecture Book for the 14th EFORT Congress, to be held in Istanbul in 2013. These instructional lectures are once again built on the thematic highlights of our meeting.

Many experts with great clinical and scientific experience present their philosophies for dealing with different issues and current debates in Orthopaedics and Traumatology.

As one of the major scientific resources of EFORT, the chapters of this Instructional Lecture series will cover most of the presentations given during the Istanbul Congress. It is presented free to all congress participants. It will therefore be possible to read and study these state-of-the-art presentations given during the Congress in detail when you are back home.

As the local chairman of the EFORT Congress 2013 in Istanbul, I would like to express my gratitude to all of our lecturers for providing their presentations for publication in this volume. Professor George Bentley has once again expertly organized and edited this Instructional Lecture Book.

Istanbul, Turkey

Nejat Hakki Sur
Chairman LOC, Berlin

Preface

This 13th volume of the EFORT *European Instructional Lectures* is a collection of all the Instructional Lectures to be presented at the 14th Congress in Istanbul from June 5–8, 2013.

As previously, the topics were selected to reflect important aspects of current Orthopaedic and Traumatology thinking and practice by a group of specialists who also represent a wide range of expertise which is unique to Europe.

Particular thanks go to the authors, not only for preparing and presenting their lectures but also for other activities such as paper reviewing and chairing of Symposia and Specialist sessions, participating in courses and demonstrations etc., which are vital for the rich totality of the Congress programme.

EFORT is constantly looking for new topics and authors and if you know of suitable lecturers and authors please contact Central Office.

Preparation of this print volume has been by Gabriele Schroeder and her colleagues in the Internationally-recognised Springer Company to whom we are very grateful.

My personal thanks go to, particularly, Larissa Welti and the EFORT Central office staff for their expert and unfailing support, as always.

This volume is dedicated to all those who have contributed, as lecturers, presenters, chairmen and exhibitors, to the ever-expanding educational and scientific development of EFORT, resulting in the greatest Orthopaedic and Traumatology fellowship in Europe.

Stanmore, UK
George Bentley
Editor-in-Chief

Contents

General Orthopaedics

Evidence for Medical Treatment for Tertiary Prophylaxis of Osteoporosis 3
    Kim Brixen, Søren Overgaard, Jeppe Gram, Jesper Ryg, Mette Rothmann, Claire Gudex, and Jan Sørensen

Surgical Site Infections (SSIs): Risk Factors and Prevention Strategies 15
    Olivier Borens, Erlangga Yusuf, and Andrej Trampuz

Exercise Therapy as Treatment for Patients with Osteoarthritis of the Knee 25
    Ewa M. Roos

Tumours

New Trends Based on Experimental Results in the Treatment of Sarcoma 37
    Nicola Baldini and Katsuyuki Kusuzaki

Surgery for Soft Tissue Sarcomas 49
    Rodolfo Capanna and Filippo Frenos

Trauma

Biologics in Open Fractures 73
    Christian Kleber and Norbert P. Haas

Classification and Algorithm of Treatment of Proximal Humerus Fractures 83
    Herbert Resch and C. Hirzinger

Management of Proximal Tibial Fractures 89
    Christos Garnavos

Surgical Treatment of Pelvic Ring Injuries 117
    Jan Lindahl

Paediatrics

Anatomical Reconstruction of the Hip with SCFE, Justified by Pathophysiological Findings 131
    Reinhold Ganz, Kai Ziebarth, Michael Leunig,
    Theddy Slongo, and Young-Jo Kim

Spine

Treatment of the Aging Spine 141
    Max Aebi

Shoulder and Elbow

New Trends in Shoulder Arthroplasty 159
    Anders Ekelund

Surgery of the Elbow: Evolution of Successful Management 173
    Bernard F. Morrey

Forearm

The Forearm Joint 181
    Christian Dumontier and Marc Soubeyrand

Hip

Current Evidence on Designs and Surfaces in Total Hip Arthroplasty 197
    Theofilos Karachalios

Risk Factors and Treatment of Dislocations of Total Hip Arthroplasty 209
    Ullmark Gösta

Treatment of Early and Late Infection Following THA 217
    José Cordero-Ampuero

Knee

Prevention and Management of Cartilage Injury and Osteoarthritis from Sports 227
    Hideki Takeda and Lars Engebretsen

Meniscal Lesions Today: Evidence for Treatment 237
    Philippe Beaufils, Nicola Pujol, and Philippe Boisrenoult

Modern Indications for High Tibial Osteotomy 253
    Matteo Denti, Piero Volpi, and Giancarlo Puddu

Unicompartment Knee Arthroplasty: From Primary to Revision Surgery 259
    Francesco Benazzo and Stefano Marco Paolo Rossi

Foot and Ankle

Osteotomies Around the Ankle 271
    Markus Knupp and Beat Hintermann

Part I
General Orthopaedics

Evidence for Medical Treatment for Tertiary Prophylaxis of Osteoporosis

Kim Brixen, Søren Overgaard, Jeppe Gram,
Jesper Ryg, Mette Rothmann, Claire Gudex,
and Jan Sørensen

Introduction

Hip, forearm and vertebral compression fractures and other low-energy fractures affect a large proportion of the elderly population. Approximately 11–23 % of women and 3–10 % of men will suffer a hip fracture after the age of 50 years [1–4]. Similarly, approximately 3–16 % of women and 1–8 % of men will suffer a clinical vertebral fracture, and approximately 13–21 % of women and 3–5 % of men will experience a forearm fracture [5].

Low-energy fractures are in part caused by osteoporosis, *i.e.* low bone mass resulting from a combination of low peak bone mass, age-related bone loss and (in women) post-menopausal bone loss. Osteoporosis is very prevalent in the elderly. Based on the distribution of bone mineral density (BMD) in the Danish population, approximately 40 % of women and 18 % of men above the age of 50 years have osteoporosis [6]. Both prior fractures and low BMD increase the risk of future fractures [7–10]. Among patients presenting with a hip fracture for example, approximately 9 % will suffer a new hip fracture within 1 year and approximately 20 % within 5 years [11].

An array of drugs including calcium plus vitamin D, oestrogen plus progestin, bisphosphonates (*e.g.* alendronate, risedronate, ibandronate, zoledronic acid), strontium ranelate, denosumab, teriparatide and parathyroid hormone (1-84) reduce the risk of fractures [12–27].

It is thus straightforward to suggest that anti-osteoporosis therapy should be considered in all patients over 50 years old presenting with low-energy fracture, *i.e.* to implement programmes for tertiary prevention (Fig. 1) of further fractures in patients presenting with low-energy fracture. Several reports have documented, however, that patients with fractures – and hip fractures in particular – are rarely offered diagnostic work-up

K. Brixen (✉) • M. Rothmann
Department of Endocrinology, Odense University Hospital, University of Southern Denmark,
DK-5000, Odense C, Denmark
e-mail: kbrixen@health.sdu.dk;
mette.rothmann@ouh.regionsyddanmark.dk

S. Overgaard
Department of Orthopaedic Surgery and Traumatology, Odense University Hospital, University of Southern Denmark, DK-5000, Odense C, Denmark
e-mail: soeren.overgaard@ouh.regionsyddanmark.dk

J. Gram
Department of Endocrinology, Hospital of Southwest Denmark, DK-6700, Esbjerg, Denmark
email: jeppe.gram@svs.regionsyddanmark.dk

J. Ryg
Department of Geriatrics, Odense University Hospital, University of Southern Denmark,
DK-5000 Odense C, Denmark
e-mail: jesper.ryg@ouh.regionsyddanmark.dk

C. Gudex
Department of Endocrinology, Odense University Hospital, DK-5000, Odense C, Denmark
e-mail: claire.gudex@ouh.regionsyddanmark.dk

J. Sørensen
Centre for Applied Health Services Research and Technology Assessment, University of Southern Denmark, DK-5000, Odense C, Denmark
e-mail: jas@cast.sdu.dk

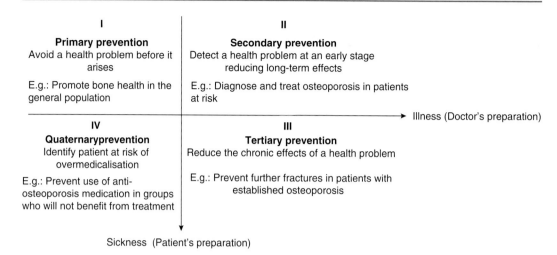

Fig. 1 Definition of primary, secondary, tertiary and quaternary prevention. In the current paper, we use the term "tertiary prevention" to describe interventions to prevent further complications in patients with fractures (*i.e.* established osteoporosis). The term "secondary prevention" is frequently used in the same meaning (Modified from Jamoulle [28, 29])

and treatment for osteoporosis [30–46]. It seems that obvious opportunities to prevent further fractures are neglected.

This paper reviews some of the key issues that need to be considered when designing and implementing questions tertiary prevention of osteoporosis, in particular systematic programmes for fracture prevention.

Osteoporosis

Osteoporosis is *"a disease characterized by low bone mass and deterioration of bone architecture leading to decreased bone strength and increased risk of fractures"* [47]. Methods for evaluating bone architecture such as MRI and high-resolution peripheral quantitative CT have recently become available [48], but these are not yet in routine clinical use. Thus, dual-energy X-ray absorptiometry (DEXA), *i.e.* measurement of bone mass, remains the preferred method for diagnosis of osteoporosis.

Because the prevalence of conditions that introduce artefacts in spinal bone measurements, such as osteoarthritis and aortic calcifications and increases with age, the hip is the preferred site for DXA in the elderly. Results are expressed in T-score units,[1] where osteoporosis is defined by a T-score < −2.5. Severe (or established) osteoporosis is defined by one or more low-energy fractures in addition to a T-score < −2.5. Both BMD and prior fractures are independent predictors of future fractures [7–10]. Assessment of prior fractures (including evaluation of vertebral compression fractures that may not be clinically apparent) is thus important in grading the severity of osteoporosis and in choosing the most appropriate treatment. Lateral spinal X-ray is often useful in this respect. Protocols for lateral spinal imaging – so-called *instant vertebral assessment* or *vertebral fracture assessment* – have recently become standard in modern DEXA-machines (Fig. 2) [49]. A standard set of blood tests is usually performed to exclude conditions predisposing to osteoporosis but needs special attention, such as vitamin-D deficiency, primary hyperparathyroidism and multiple myeloma.

---

[1] T-score is calculated from the patient's bone mineral density ($BMD_{patient}$), the mean BMD of young persons of the same sex ($BMD_{young-normal}$) and the standard deviation of BMD in the normal population (SD), using the formula: $T-score = (BMD_{patient} - BMD_{young-normal})/SD$.

Fig. 2 Protocols for *instant vertebral assessment* or *vertebral fracture assessment* are now standard in modern DEXA-machines and allow diagnosis and quantification of vertebral compression fractures to be performed in the same procedure as measurement of bone mineral density. The *left image* shows a normal spine while the *right image* shows an X-ray in a patient with compression fracture of L2

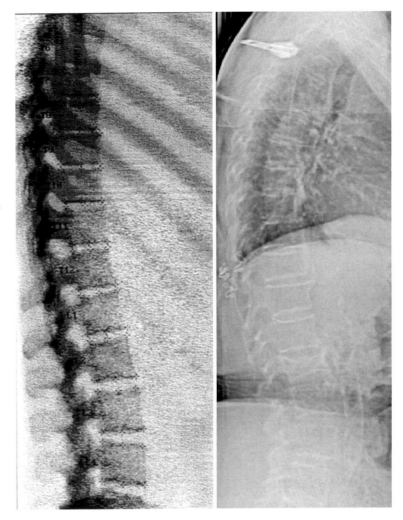

Osteoporosis in Patients Presenting with Fracture

In Denmark, approximately 40 % of women and 18 % of men above the age of 50 years have osteoporosis [6]. The prevalence of osteoporosis is higher in patients with recent low-energy fractures. Different studies have found that 54–88 % of patients with hip fracture have a T-score < −2.5 [40, 50–54]. Prevalent vertebral fractures are also very common (31–74 %) in patients presenting with hip fracture [53, 55–59]. Approximately 45 % of patients with morphometric vertebral compression fractures have a T-score < −2.5 [60], while this is the case in approximately 74 % of patients with clinical vertebral fractures [61]. In patients with forearm fracture, the prevalence of T-score < −2.5 has been reported as 24–50 % [54, 62–66], increases with age and is infrequent before the age of 65 years [62].

Osteoporosis is a silent disease and by itself does not cause any symptoms, but fractures complicating the disease are associated with both morbidity (*e.g.* chronic pain, disability and reduced level of activity) and mortality. Hip fractures are associated with increased mortality rates in both women and men. In Denmark, 1-year mortality is approximately 24 % in women and 33 % in men with hip fracture, while 5-year mortality is 56 % in women and 63 % in men [67]. The increased mortality immediately following the fracture seems to be associated with complications of the fracture, while late excess mortality seems to be explained by co-morbidity [67–70]. Vertebral fractures are also associated with a significant excess mortality rate (4.4; 95 % CI = 1.85–10.6) [71].

Large prospective studies have demonstrated that health-related quality of life is considerably affected by fractures [72, 73]. An American study [72] followed a cohort of 86,128 participants suffering 320 hip fractures, 445 vertebral fractures and 835 forearm fractures. The mean SF-12 score in participants without fractures was 46 (just under the norm of 50 for the general population), while mean scores were 42, 40 and 45 in patients with hip, vertebral and forearm fractures, respectively. Similar results were found in a Canadian study [73]. Health-related quality of life remains decreased 18 months after hip and vertebral fractures but returns to baseline in patients with forearm fractures [74].

Risk of New Fractures

Both prior fractures and low BMD increase the risk of future fractures [7–10]. In a meta-analysis of prospective studies, Klotzbuecher et al. [9] included 6 studies on hip fracture, 15 studies on vertebral fractures and 9 studies on wrist fractures. Women with hip fracture had a relative risk of 2.5 (95 % CI = 1.8–3.5) of subsequent vertebral fractures and 2.3 (95 % CI = 1.5–3.7) of hip fractures. Similarly, women with vertebral fractures had a relative risk of 1.7 (95 % CI = 1.4–2.1) of subsequent vertebral fractures, 1.9 (95 % CI = 1.6–2.2) of hip fractures and 3.3 (95 % CI = 2.0–5.3) of wrist fractures. Among patients with hip fracture, approximately 20 % will suffer a further hip fracture within 5 years [11], and 57 % will suffer a non-hip fracture within the same time frame [75]. Initiation of anti-osteoporosis treatment can thus be effective in preventing subsequent fractures.

Low BMD is also an independent risk factor for future fractures. In a meta-analysis comprising 11 prospective cohort-studies with a total of more than 2,000 fractures during follow-up, Marshall et al. [8] found that a decrease in BMD of 1 SD at the hip increased the relative risk of hip fracture to 2.6 (95 % CI = 2.0–3.5), of vertebral fractures to 1.8 (95 % CI = 1.1–2.7) and of wrist fractures to 1.4 (95 % CI = 1.4–1.6). Recent prospective cohort studies support these findings [76, 77].

Treatment of Osteoporosis

During the last two decades, several drugs to treat osteoporosis have been developed and more are currently under development. These drugs may be categorized as anti-resorptive, anabolic or dual-action (Table 1). Randomized, placebo-controlled clinical trials have demonstrated that pharmaceutical therapy decreases the risk of fractures. In these trials, the outcome has been assessed for vertebral compression fractures (clinical or morphometric), peripheral fractures and hip fractures. Participants have been selected on the basis of low BMD and/or the presence of vertebral fractures. Thus, several bisphosphonates (alendronate [78], risedronate [79], ibandronate [80] and zoledronate [19]), raloxifene [21], strontium ranelate [81], denosumab [22], teriparatide [25] and parathyroid hormone (1-84) decrease the risk of vertebral fractures.

In patients with osteoporosis, the risk of hip fractures was significantly reduced by 26–53 %

Table 1 Drugs approved for treatment of osteoporosis categorized according to their mode of action

Anti-resorptive	Anabolic	Dual-action
Bisphosphonates	Teriparatide (PTH 1-34)	Strontium ranelate
Alendronate	Parathyroid Hormone (1-84)	
Risedronate		
Ibandronate		
Zoledronic acid		
Raloxifene		
Denosumab		

following treatment with alendronate [78], risedronate [79], strontium ranelate [81], zoledronate [19] and denosumab [22]. In contrast, no significant reduction in the occurrence of hip fractures was demonstrated in studies on pamidronate [82], etidronate [83], ibandronate [80], raloxifene [21] or teriparatide [25], and no data are available regarding parathyroid hormone (1-84).

Alendronate [78], risedronate [79], strontium ranelate [81], zoledronate [19], denosumab [22] and teriparatide [25] also decrease the risk of peripheral fractures.

In a recent randomized, placebo-controlled trial including patients with recent hip fracture irrespective of BMD, zoledronate significantly decreased the risk of all fractures (HR 0.65; 95 % CI = 0.50–0.84). The risk of new hip fractures was not significantly decreased but a trend towards reduction was observed (HR 0.70; 95 % CI 0.41–1.19) [20]. As only 41 % of the patients had T-score < −2.5, the results suggest that patients without osteoporosis also benefit from therapy.

Several studies have reported that patients with fractures – and hip fractures in particular – are rarely offered diagnostic work-up and treatment for osteoporosis [30–41]. In Austria, for example, 85 % of the general practitioners included in a study [37] regarded assessment of fracture risk and treatment of osteoporosis in patients with recent low-energy fractures to be their responsibility; they referred only very few patients (7 %) for DEXA, however. Lack of knowledge about osteoporosis and the efficacy of pharmaceutical therapy, low priority and ill-defined clinical obligations have been proposed as barriers for improving the service to fracture patients [84–88]. Moreover, many elderly patients suffer from co-morbidity and already take multiple drugs. Initiating additional therapy may thus seem unrealistic for patients and professionals [39, 89]. The increased risk of further fractures and the availability of efficacious therapy in combination with low rates of DEXA and treatment suggest that a systematic approach to diagnose and treat osteoporosis in patients with recent fractures may be needed.

Fracture Prevention Programmes

McLellan and co-workers pioneered the idea of *Fracture Prevention Programmes* by establishing a successful liaison service in Glasgow [54]. A variety of Fracture Prevention Programmes aiming to provide systematic diagnosis and treatment of osteoporosis in patients with prior fractures have now been tested and reviewed [84, 90]. The programmes represent a continuum from simple to very ambitious programmes and have varying degree of focus on patients, patients' families, general practitioners, hospital staff and the health service system as a whole (Table 2). At one end

Table 2 Fracture Prevention Programmes categorized according to person responsible for initiating action and complexity

Patient
Self-referral for DXA etc.
Information leaflets and/or questions to pose to the general practitioner given to patient
Health care system
Decision support systems for general practitioners
Quality control systems
General practitioners
Information to the general practitioner from the emergency room
Information and guidelines to the general practitioner
Orthopaedic surgeon
DXA performed by department of Orthopaedic surgery – follow-up by general practitioner
Orthopaedic surgeon refers for DXA and initiates therapy if appropriate
Co-ordinator
Dedicated nurse informs, teaches and refers to general practitioner
Dedicated nurse informs, teaches, screens and refers to general practitioner or bone clinic
Dedicated nurse informs, teaches and co-ordinates programme including DEXA and therapy; follow-up by the general practitioner
Dedicated nurse informs, teaches and co-ordinates programme including DEXA and therapy and follow-up
Multi-disciplinary team
Consultation by specialist in internal medicine during hospital stay
Consultation by an ortho-geriatric team during hospital stay

Modified from Marsh et al. [91]

of the continuum are programmes that allow patient self-referral for DXA [92–95] or involve mailing of information to the general practitioner after the patient's visit to the emergency room in order to facilitate decision-making [96–99]. At the other end of the continuum are comprehensive programmes in which a dedicated nurse identifies and teaches patients, and co-ordinates diagnostic work-up, medical consultation and follow-up [54, 100] and programmes with multidisciplinary teams including *e.g.* Orthopaedic surgeons and geriatricians [36, 40].

Fracture Prevention Programmes increase both the number of patients undertaking DEXA and the uptake of pharmaceutical therapy [36, 101–104]. Guidelines or educational programmes aimed at doctors, other health personnel or patients are alone ineffective in reducing the risk of future fractures. In a Dutch cohort study, the incidence of fractures decreased significantly from 9.9 to 6.7 % during 2 years of follow-up after implementing a nurse-led Fracture Prevention Programme [86]. None of the randomized studies on Fracture Prevention Programmes had fracture as primary outcome; however, it seems likely that such programmes may reduce fracture incidence. Recently, the American Society for Bone and Mineral Research published a report on *Making the First Fracture the Last Fracture* [105], recommending increased efforts to prevent further fractures in patients with low-energy fractures and describing the necessary framework. The report includes a toolkit for professionals involved in this challenge.

Health Economics

Hip fractures in particular incur significant health care costs related to hospital stay, surgical treatment and rehabilitation and are the main driver in cost-effectiveness analyses regarding Fracture Prevention Programmes. Health economics analyses are context-specific (*e.g.* costs of hospital services and follow-up, cost of medication and economic environment). Based upon analyses from Scandinavia, costs associated with a hip fracture range between approximately €12,664 and €41,292 during the first year [106–108]. A German study found that the costs of surgical treatment, rehabilitation and care following a hip fracture was €14,000 in the first 6 months and €48,000 in the 20 years following the fracture [109].

In a cost-effectiveness analysis, McLellan et al. [110] found that implementation of the Glasgow Fracture Prevention Programme would incur an additional cost of €105 and €260 for diagnostic procedures and therapy, respectively, for each patient and would lead to a net saving. In similar analysis, a Canadian study found that a co-ordinator-based Fracture Prevention Programme aimed at all patients with fragility fractures dominated in the economic modelling (*i.e.* was cost-saving) compared with standard care [111]. We found similar results modelling the effect of a Fracture Prevention Programme aimed specifically at patients with hip fracture [112]. An Australian study [113] of a Fracture Prevention Program identified an average gain of 0.089 quality-adjusted life-years and additional costs of €1,210 per patient. This programme was considered to be cost-effective.

Conclusions

Low-energy fractures are very frequent in the elderly population and are in part caused by osteoporosis. Both previous fractures and low BMD increase the risk of further fractures. Although randomized placebo-controlled trials have documented that several drugs decrease occurrence of fractures, these drugs are still infrequently used in patients with recent fractures. A variety of Fracture Prevention Programmes in different settings have been shown to increase both the number of patients offered bone scans and the uptake of pharmaceutical therapy, thus potentially reducing the number of further fractures. Cost-effectiveness analyses suggest that such programmes may be net cost-saving. We recommend that Fracture Prevention Programmes be developed and implemented to ensure that patients presenting with fractures are offered diagnosis and treatment for osteoporosis. Moreover, we suggest that performance of such programmes is continuously monitored

References

1. van Staa TP, Dennison EM, Leufkens HG, Cooper C (2001) Epidemiology of fractures in England and Wales. Bone 29(6):517–522. Epub 2001/12/01
2. Cummings SR, Black DM, Rubin SM (1989) Lifetime risks of hip, Colles', or vertebral fracture and coronary heart disease among white postmenopausal women. Arch Intern Med 149(11):2445–2448. Epub 1989/11/01
3. Kanis JA, Johnell O, Oden A, Sembo I, Redlund-Johnell I, Dawson A et al (2000) Long-term risk of osteoporotic fracture in Malmo. Osteoporos Int 11(8):669–674. Epub 2000/11/30
4. Melton LJ 3rd, Chrischilles EA, Cooper C, Lane AW, Riggs BL (1992) Perspective. How many women have osteoporosis? J Bone Miner Res 7(9):1005–1010. Epub 1992/09/01
5. Johnell O, Kanis J (2005) Epidemiology of osteoporotic fractures. Osteoporos Int 16(Suppl 2):S3–S7. Epub 2004/09/15
6. Vestergaard P, Rejnmark L, Mosekilde L (2005) Osteoporosis is markedly underdiagnosed: a nationwide study from Denmark. Osteoporos Int 16(2):134–141. Epub 2004/06/16
7. Johnell O, Kanis JA, Oden A, Johansson H, De Laet C, Delmas P et al (2005) Predictive value of BMD for hip and other fractures. J Bone Miner Res 20(7):1185–1194. Epub 2005/06/09
8. Marshall D, Johnell O, Wedel H (1996) Meta-analysis of how well measures of bone mineral density predict occurrence of osteoporotic fractures. BMJ 312(7041):1254–1259. Epub 1996/05/18
9. Klotzbuecher CM, Ross PD, Landsman PB, Abbott TA 3rd, Berger M (2000) Patients with prior fractures have an increased risk of future fractures: a summary of the literature and statistical synthesis. J Bone Miner Res 15(4):721–739. Epub 2000/04/26
10. Gehlbach S, Saag KG, Adachi JD, Hooven FH, Flahive J, Boonen S et al (2012) Previous fractures at multiple sites increase the risk for subsequent fractures: the Global Longitudinal Study of Osteoporosis in Women. J Bone Miner Res 27(3):645–653. Epub 2011/11/25
11. Ryg J, Rejnmark L, Overgaard S, Brixen K, Vestergaard P (2009) Hip fracture patients at risk of second hip fracture: a nationwide population-based cohort study of 169,145 cases during 1977–2001. J Bone Miner Res 24(7):1299–1307. Epub 2009/03/05
12. DIPART (Vitamin D Individual Patient Analysis of Randomized Trials) Group (2010) Patient level pooled analysis of 68,500 patients from seven major vitamin D fracture trials in US and Europe. BMJ 340:b5463. Epub 2010/01/14
13. Black DM, Cummings SR, Karpf DB, Cauley JA, Thompson DE, Nevitt MC et al (1996) Randomised trial of effect of alendronate on risk of fracture in women with existing vertebral fractures. Fracture Intervention Trial Research Group. Lancet 348(9041):1535–1541. Epub 1996/12/07
14. Cummings SR, Black DM, Thompson DE, Applegate WB, Barrett-Connor E, Musliner TA et al (1998) Effect of alendronate on risk of fracture in women with low bone density but without vertebral fractures: results from the Fracture Intervention Trial. JAMA 280(24):2077–2082. Epub 1999/01/06
15. Reginster J, Minne HW, Sorensen OH, Hooper M, Roux C, Brandi ML et al (2000) Randomized trial of the effects of risedronate on vertebral fractures in women with established postmenopausal osteoporosis. Vertebral Efficacy with Risedronate Therapy (VERT) Study Group. Osteoporos Int 11(1):83–91. Epub 2000/02/09
16. Harris ST, Watts NB, Genant HK, McKeever CD, Hangartner T, Keller M et al (1999) Effects of risedronate treatment on vertebral and nonvertebral fractures in women with postmenopausal osteoporosis: a randomized controlled trial. Vertebral Efficacy With Risedronate Therapy (VERT) Study Group. JAMA 282(14):1344–1352. Epub 1999/10/20
17. McClung MR, Geusens P, Miller PD, Zippel H, Bensen WG, Roux C et al (2001) Effect of risedronate on the risk of hip fracture in elderly women. Hip Intervention Program Study Group. N Engl J Med 344(5):333–340. Epub 2001/02/15
18. Chesnut IC, Skag A, Christiansen C, Recker R, Stakkestad JA, Hoiseth A et al (2004) Effects of oral ibandronate administered daily or intermittently on fracture risk in postmenopausal osteoporosis. J Bone Miner Res 19(8):1241–1249. Epub 2004/07/03
19. Black DM, Delmas PD, Eastell R, Reid IR, Boonen S, Cauley JA et al (2007) Once-yearly zoledronic acid for treatment of postmenopausal osteoporosis. N Engl J Med 356(18):1809–1822. Epub 2007/05/04
20. Lyles KW, Colon-Emeric CS, Magaziner JS, Adachi JD, Pieper CF, Mautalen C et al (2007) Zoledronic acid and clinical fractures and mortality after hip fracture. N Engl J Med 357(18):1799–1809. Epub 2007/09/20
21. Ettinger B, Black DM, Mitlak BH, Knickerbocker RK, Nickelsen T, Genant HK et al (1999) Reduction of vertebral fracture risk in postmenopausal women with osteoporosis treated with raloxifene: results from a 3-year randomized clinical trial. Multiple Outcomes of Raloxifene Evaluation (MORE) Investigators. JAMA 282(7):637–645. Epub 1999/10/12
22. Cummings SR, San Martin J, McClung MR, Siris ES, Eastell R, Reid IR et al (2009) Denosumab for prevention of fractures in postmenopausal women with osteoporosis. N Engl J Med 361(8):756–765. Epub 2009/08/13
23. Reginster JY, Seeman E, De Vernejoul MC, Adami S, Compston J, Phenekos C et al (2005) Strontium ranelate reduces the risk of nonvertebral fractures in postmenopausal women with osteoporosis: Treatment of Peripheral Osteoporosis (TROPOS) study. J Clin Endocrinol Metab 90(5):2816–2822. Epub 2005/02/25
24. Meunier PJ, Roux C, Seeman E, Ortolani S, Badurski JE, Spector TD et al (2004) The effects of

strontium ranelate on the risk of vertebral fracture in women with postmenopausal osteoporosis. N Engl J Med 350(5):459–468. Epub 2004/01/30
25. Neer RM, Arnaud CD, Zanchetta JR, Prince R, Gaich GA, Reginster JY et al (2001) Effect of parathyroid hormone (1-34) on fractures and bone mineral density in postmenopausal women with osteoporosis. N Engl J Med 344(19):1434–1441. Epub 2001/05/11
26. Greenspan SL, Bone HG, Ettinger MP, Hanley DA, Lindsay R, Zanchetta JR et al (2007) Effect of recombinant human parathyroid hormone (1-84) on vertebral fracture and bone mineral density in postmenopausal women with osteoporosis: a randomized trial. Ann Intern Med 146(5):326–339. Epub 2007/03/07
27. Cauley JA, Robbins J, Chen Z, Cummings SR, Jackson RD, LaCroix AZ et al (2003) Effects of estrogen plus progestin on risk of fracture and bone mineral density: the Women's Health Initiative randomized trial. JAMA 290(13):1729–1738. Epub 2003/10/02
28. Jamoulle M (1986) Information et informtisation en médecine générale. In: Berleur J, Labet-Maris CL, Poswick RF, Valenduc G, Van Bastelaer P (eds) Les informagiciens. Presses Universitaires de Namur, Namur, pp 193–209
29. Jamoulle M (2012) Quaternary prevention – prevention as you never heard before. Available from http://www.ulb.ac.be/esp/mfsp/quat-en.html. Accessed 01 Jan 2013
30. Bahl S, Coates PS, Greenspan SL (2003) The management of osteoporosis following hip fracture: have we improved our care? Osteoporos Int 14(11):884–888. Epub 2003/10/22
31. Feldstein A, Elmer PJ, Orwoll E, Herson M, Hillier T (2003) Bone mineral density measurement and treatment for osteoporosis in older individuals with fractures: a gap in evidence-based practice guideline implementation. Arch Intern Med 163(18):2165–2172. Epub 2003/10/15
32. Juby AG, De Geus-Wenceslau CM (2002) Evaluation of osteoporosis treatment in seniors after hip fracture. Osteoporos Int 13(3):205–210. Epub 2002/05/07
33. Gregersen M, Morch MM, Hougaard K, Damsgaard EM (2012) Geriatric intervention in elderly patients with hip fracture in an orthopedic ward. J Inj Violence Res 4(2):45–51. Epub 2011/04/20
34. Murray AW, McQuillan C, Kennon B, Gallacher SJ (2005) Osteoporosis risk assessment and treatment intervention after hip or shoulder fracture. Injury 36(9):1080–1084. Epub 2005/07/30
35. Harrington JT, Lease J (2007) Osteoporosis disease management for fragility fracture patients: new understandings based on three years' experience with an osteoporosis care service. Arthritis Rheum 57(8):1502–1506. Epub 2007/12/01
36. Wallace I, Callachand F, Elliott J, Gardiner P (2011) An evaluation of an enhanced fracture liaison service as the optimal model for secondary prevention of osteoporosis. JRSM Short Rep 2(2):8. Epub 2011/03/04
37. Inderjeeth CA, Glennon DA, Poland KE, Ingram KV, Prince RL, Van VR et al (2010) A multimodal intervention to improve fragility fracture management in patients presenting to emergency departments. Med J Aust 193(3):149–153. Epub 2010/08/04
38. Gardner MJ, Flik KR, Mooar P, Lane JM (2002) Improvement in the undertreatment of osteoporosis following hip fracture. J Bone Joint Surg Am 84-A(8):1342–1348. Epub 2002/08/15
39. Jachna CM, Whittle J, Lukert B, Graves L, Bhargava T (2003) Effect of hospitalist consultation on treatment of osteoporosis in hip fracture patients. Osteoporos Int 14(8):665–671. Epub 2003/07/25
40. Sidwell AI, Wilkinson TJ, Hanger HC (2004) Secondary prevention of fractures in older people: evaluation of a protocol for the investigation and treatment of osteoporosis. Intern Med J 34(3):129–132. Epub 2004/03/20
41. Che M, Ettinger B, Liang J, Pressman AR, Johnston J (2006) Outcomes of a disease-management program for patients with recent osteoporotic fracture. Osteoporos Int 17(6):847–854. Epub 2006/03/30
42. Jacobsen IB, Wiboe L, Mogensen CB (2002) [Osteoporosis prevention in patients with low energy hip fractures hospitalized in the orthopedic department]. Ugeskr Laeger 164(27):3541–3544. Epub 2002/07/16. Osteoporoseprofylakse hos patienter indlagt med hoftenaere lavenergifrakturer pa ortopaedkirurgisk afdeling
43. Wiboe L, Jacobsen IB, Mogensen CB (2002) [Osteoporosis prevention in general practice after hospitalization for hip fracture]. Ugeskr Laeger 164(20):2610–2613. Epub 2002/06/05. Osteoporoseprofylakse i almen praksis efter indlaeggelse for hoftenaer fraktur
44. Sheehan J, Mohamed F, Reilly M, Perry IJ (2000) Secondary prevention following fractured neck of femur: a survey of orthopaedic surgeons practice. Ir Med J 93(4):105–107. Epub 2000/10/19
45. Kamel HK, Hussain MS, Tariq S, Perry HM, Morley JE (2000) Failure to diagnose and treat osteoporosis in elderly patients hospitalized with hip fracture. Am J Med 109(4):326–328. Epub 2000/09/21, PubMed 10996585
46. Staeger P, Burnand B, Santos-Eggimann B, Klay M, Siffert C, Livio JJ et al (2000) Prevention of recurrent hip fracture. Aging (Milano) 12(1):13–21. Epub 2000/04/04
47. Consensus development conference: prophylaxis and treatment of osteoporosis (1991) Am J Med 90(1):107–10. Epub 1991/01/01
48. Krug R, Burghardt AJ, Majumdar S, Link TM (2010) High-resolution imaging techniques for the assessment of osteoporosis. Radiol Clin North Am 48(3):601–621. Epub 2010/07/09
49. Guglielmi G, Muscarella S, Bazzocchi A (2011) Integrated imaging approach to osteoporosis: state-of-the-art review and update. Radiographics 31(5):1343–1364. Epub 2011/09/16
50. Scharla SH, Wolf S, Dull R, Lempert UG (1999) Prevalence of low bone mass and endocrine disorders in hip fracture patients in Southern Germany. Exp

Clin Endocrinol Diabetes 107(8):547–554. Epub 1999/12/28
51. Sharma S, Fraser M, Lovell F, Reece A, McLellan AR (2008) Characteristics of males over 50 years who present with a fracture: epidemiology and underlying risk factors. J Bone Joint Surg Br 90(1):72–77. Epub 2007/12/28
52. Ekman A, Michaelsson K, Petren-Mallmin M, Ljunghall S, Mallmin H (2001) DXA of the hip and heel ultrasound but not densitometry of the fingers can discriminate female hip fracture patients from controls: a comparison between four different methods. Osteoporos Int 12(3):185–191. Epub 2001/04/24
53. Wainwright SA, Marshall LM, Ensrud KE, Cauley JA, Black DM, Hillier TA et al (2005) Hip fracture in women without osteoporosis. J Clin Endocrinol Metab 90(5):2787–2793. Epub 2005/02/25
54. McLellan AR, Gallacher SJ, Fraser M, McQuillian C (2003) The fracture liaison service: success of a program for the evaluation and management of patients with osteoporotic fracture. Osteoporos Int 14(12): 1028–1034. Epub 2003/11/06
55. Hasserius R, Johnell O, Nilsson BE, Thorngren KG, Jonsson K, Mellstrom D et al (2003) Hip fracture patients have more vertebral deformities than subjects in population-based studies. Bone 32(2):180–184. Epub 2003/03/14
56. Takahashi M, Kushida K, Naitou K (1999) The degree of osteoporosis in patients with vertebral fracture and patients with hip fracture: relationship to incidence of vertebral fracture. J Bone Miner Metab 17(3):187–194. Epub 2000/04/11
57. Hutchinson TA, Polansky SM, Feinstein AR (1979) Post-menopausal oestrogens protect against fractures of hip and distal radius. A case-control study. Lancet 2(8145):705–709. Epub 1979/10/06
58. Howat I, Carty D, Harrison J, Fraser M, McLellan AR (2007) Vertebral fracture assessment in patients presenting with incident nonvertebral fractures. Clin Endocrinol (Oxf) 67(6):923–930. Epub 2007/09/07
59. Vega E, Mautalen C, Gomez H, Garrido A, Melo L, Sahores AO (1991) Bone mineral density in patients with cervical and trochanteric fractures of the proximal femur. Osteoporos Int 1(2):81–86. Epub 1991/02/01
60. del Rio L, Peris P, Jover L, Guanabens N, Monegal A, Di Gregorio S (2008) Men suffer vertebral fractures with similar spinal T-scores to women. Clin Exp Rheumatol 26(2):283–287. Epub 2008/06/21
61. Nolla JM, Gomez-Vaquero C, Fiter J, Roig Vilaseca D, Mateo L, Rozadilla A et al (2002) Usefulness of bone densitometry in postmenopausal women with clinically diagnosed vertebral fractures. Ann Rheum Dis 61(1):73–75. Epub 2002/01/10
62. Lashin H, Davie MW (2008) DXA scanning in women over 50 years with distal forearm fracture shows osteoporosis is infrequent until age 65 years. Int J Clin Pract 62(3):388–393. Epub 2007/05/31
63. Jutberger H, Sinclair H, Malmqvist B, Obrant K (2003) [Screening for postmenopausal osteoporosis. Women with distal radius fractures should be evaluated for bone density]. Lakartidningen 100(1–2):31–34. Epub 2003/02/08. Utredning av postmenopausal osteoporos. Kvinnor med distal radiusfraktur bor bentathetsmatas
64. Kanterewicz E, Yanez A, Perez-Pons A, Codony I, Del Rio L, Diez-Perez A (2002) Association between Colles' fracture and low bone mass: age-based differences in postmenopausal women. Osteoporos Int 13(10):824–828. Epub 2002/10/16
65. Tuck SP, Raj N, Summers GD (2002) Is distal forearm fracture in men due to osteoporosis? Osteoporos Int 13(8):630–636. Epub 2002/08/16
66. Ryan PJ (2001) Bone densitometry in the management of Colles' fractures: which site to measure? Br J Radiol 74(888):1137–1141. Epub 2002/01/05
67. Vestergaard P, Rejnmark L, Mosekilde L (2007) Increased mortality in patients with a hip fracture-effect of pre-morbid conditions and post-fracture complications. Osteoporos Int 18(12):1583–1593. Epub 2007/06/15
68. Johnell O, Kanis JA, Oden A, Sernbo I, Redlund-Johnell I, Petterson C et al (2004) Mortality after osteoporotic fractures. Osteoporos Int 15(1):38–42. Epub 2003/11/01
69. Kanis JA, Oden A, Johnell O, De Laet C, Jonsson B, Oglesby AK (2003) The components of excess mortality after hip fracture. Bone 32(5):468–473. Epub 2003/05/20
70. Tosteson AN, Gottlieb DJ, Radley DC, Fisher ES, Melton LJ 3rd (2007) Excess mortality following hip fracture: the role of underlying health status. Osteoporos Int 18(11):1463–1472. Epub 2007/08/30
71. Jalava T, Sarna S, Pylkkanen L, Mawer B, Kanis JA, Selby P et al (2003) Association between vertebral fracture and increased mortality in osteoporotic patients. J Bone Miner Res 18(7):1254–1260. Epub 2003/07/12
72. Brenneman SK, Barrett-Connor E, Sajjan S, Markson LE, Siris ES (2006) Impact of recent fracture on health-related quality of life in postmenopausal women. J Bone Miner Res 21(6):809–816. Epub 2006/06/07
73. Papaioannou A, Kennedy CC, Ioannidis G, Sawka A, Hopman WM, Pickard L et al (2009) The impact of incident fractures on health-related quality of life: 5 years of data from the Canadian Multicentre Osteoporosis Study. Osteoporos Int 20(5):703–714. Epub 2008/09/20
74. Strom O, Borgstrom F, Zethraeus N, Johnell O, Lidgren L, Ponzer S et al (2008) Long-term cost and effect on quality of life of osteoporosis-related fractures in Sweden. Acta Orthop 79(2):269–280. Epub 2008/05/20
75. Ryg J (2009) The frail hip – a study on the risk of second hip fracture, prevalence of osteoporosis and adherence to treatment in patients with recent hip fracture. University of Southern Denmark
76. Fink HA, Harrison SL, Taylor BC, Cummings SR, Schousboe JT, Kuskowski MA et al (2008) Differences

in site-specific fracture risk among older women with discordant results for osteoporosis at hip and spine: study of osteoporotic fractures. J Clin Densitom 11(2):250–259. Epub 2008/02/26
77. Siris ES, Brenneman SK, Barrett-Connor E, Miller PD, Sajjan S, Berger ML et al (2006) The effect of age and bone mineral density on the absolute, excess, and relative risk of fracture in postmenopausal women aged 50–99: results from the National Osteoporosis Risk Assessment (NORA). Osteoporos Int 17(4):565–574. Epub 2006/01/05
78. Wells GA, Cranney A, Peterson J, Boucher M, Shea B, Robinson V et al (2008) Alendronate for the primary and secondary prevention of osteoporotic fractures in postmenopausal women. Cochrane Database Syst Rev (1):CD001155. Epub 2008/02/07
79. Wells G, Cranney A, Peterson J, Boucher M, Shea B, Robinson V et al (2008) Risedronate for the primary and secondary prevention of osteoporotic fractures in postmenopausal women. Cochrane Database Syst Rev (1):CD004523. Epub 2008/02/07
80. Recker R, Stakkestad JA, Chesnut CH 3rd, Christiansen C, Skag A, Hoiseth A et al (2004) Insufficiently dosed intravenous ibandronate injections are associated with suboptimal antifracture efficacy in postmenopausal osteoporosis. Bone 34(5):890–899. Epub 2004/05/04
81. Reginster JY, Felsenberg D, Boonen S, Diez-Perez A, Rizzoli R, Brandi ML et al (2008) Effects of long-term strontium ranelate treatment on the risk of non-vertebral and vertebral fractures in postmenopausal osteoporosis: Results of a five-year, randomized, placebo-controlled trial. Arthritis Rheum 58(6):1687–1695. Epub 2008/06/03
82. Brumsen C, Papapoulos SE, Lips P, Geelhoed-Duijvestijn PH, Hamdy NA, Landman JO et al (2002) Daily oral pamidronate in women and men with osteoporosis: a 3-year randomized placebo-controlled clinical trial with a 2-year open extension. J Bone Miner Res 17(6):1057–1064. Epub 2002/06/11
83. Wells GA, Cranney A, Peterson J, Boucher M, Shea B, Robinson V et al (2008) Etidronate for the primary and secondary prevention of osteoporotic fractures in postmenopausal women. Cochrane Database Syst Rev (1):CD003376. Epub 2008/02/07
84. Sale JE, Beaton D, Posen J, Elliot-Gibson V, Bogoch E (2011) Systematic review on interventions to improve osteoporosis investigation and treatment in fragility fracture patients. Osteoporos Int 22(7):2067–2082. Epub 2011/05/25
85. Andrade SE, Majumdar SR, Chan KA, Buist DS, Go AS, Goodman M et al (2003) Low frequency of treatment of osteoporosis among postmenopausal women following a fracture. Arch Intern Med 163(17):2052–2057. Epub 2003/09/25
86. Huntjens KM, van Geel TC, Geusens PP, Winkens B, Willems P, van den Bergh J et al (2011) Impact of guideline implementation by a fracture nurse on subsequent fractures and mortality in patients presenting with non-vertebral fractures. Injury 42(Suppl 4):S39–S43. Epub 2011/10/05
87. Harrington JT, Broy SB, Derosa AM, Licata AA, Shewmon DA (2002) Hip fracture patients are not treated for osteoporosis: a call to action. Arthritis Rheum 47(6):651–654. Epub 2003/01/11
88. Siris ES, Bilezikian JP, Rubin MR, Black DM, Bockman RS, Bone HG et al (2003) Pins and plaster aren't enough: a call for the evaluation and treatment of patients with osteoporotic fractures. J Clin Endocrinol Metab 88(8):3482–3486. Epub 2003/08/14
89. Bogoch ER, Elliot-Gibson V, Beaton DE, Jamal SA, Josse RG, Murray TM (2006) Effective initiation of osteoporosis diagnosis and treatment for patients with a fragility fracture in an orthopaedic environment. J Bone Joint Surg Am 88(1):25–34. Epub 2006/01/05
90. Little EA, Eccles MP (2010) A systematic review of the effectiveness of interventions to improve post-fracture investigation and management of patients at risk of osteoporosis. Implement Sci 5:80. Epub 2010/10/26
91. Marsh D, Akesson K, Beaton DE, Bogoch ER, Boonen S, Brandi ML et al (2011) Coordinator-based systems for secondary prevention in fragility fracture patients. Osteoporos Int 22(7):2051–2065. Epub 2011/05/25
92. Charalambous CP, Mosey C, Johnstone E, Akimau P, Gullett TK, Siddique I et al (2009) Improving osteoporosis assessment in the fracture clinic. Ann R Coll Surg Engl 91(7):596–598. Epub 2009/06/30
93. Gardner MJ, Brophy RH, Demetrakopoulos D, Koob J, Hong R, Rana A et al (2005) Interventions to improve osteoporosis treatment following hip fracture. A prospective, randomized trial. J Bone Joint Surg Am 87(1):3–7. Epub 2005/01/07
94. Hawker G, Ridout R, Ricupero M, Jaglal S, Bogoch E (2003) The impact of a simple fracture clinic intervention in improving the diagnosis and treatment of osteoporosis in fragility fracture patients. Osteoporos Int 14(2):171–178. Epub 2003/05/06
95. Bliuc D, Eisman JA, Center JR (2006) A randomized study of two different information-based interventions on the management of osteoporosis in minimal and moderate trauma fractures. Osteoporos Int 17(9):1309–1317. Epub 2006/06/29
96. Feldstein A, Elmer PJ, Smith DH, Herson M, Orwoll E, Chen C et al (2006) Electronic medical record reminder improves osteoporosis management after a fracture: a randomized, controlled trial. J Am Geriatr Soc 54(3):450–457. Epub 2006/03/23
97. Majumdar SR, Rowe BH, Folk D, Johnson JA, Holroyd BH, Morrish DW et al (2004) A controlled trial to increase detection and treatment of osteoporosis in older patients with a wrist fracture. Ann Intern Med 141(5):366–373. Epub 2004/09/09
98. Ashe M, Khan K, Guy P, Kruse K, Hughes K, O'Brien P et al (2004) Wristwatch-distal radial fracture as a marker for osteoporosis investigation: a controlled trial of patient education and a physician alerting system. J Hand Ther 17(3):324–328. Epub 2004/07/27

99. Malochet-Guinamand S, Chalard N, Billault C, Breuil N, Ristori JM, Schmidt J (2005) Osteoporosis treatment in postmenopausal women after peripheral fractures: impact of information to general practitioners. Joint Bone Spine 72(6):562–566. Epub 2005/07/06
100. Fraser M, McLellan AR (2004) A fracture liaison service for patients with osteoporotic fractures. Prof Nurse 19(5):286–290. Epub 2004/01/24
101. Feldstein AC, Vollmer WM, Smith DH, Petrik A, Schneider J, Glauber H et al (2007) An outreach program improved osteoporosis management after a fracture. J Am Geriatr Soc 55(9):1464–1469. Epub 2007/10/05
102. Blonk MC, Erdtsieck RJ, Wernekinck MG, Schoon EJ (2007) The fracture and osteoporosis clinic: 1-year results and 3-month compliance. Bone 40(6):1643–1649. Epub 2007/04/17
103. Premaor MO, Pilbrow L, Tonkin C, Adams M, Parker RA, Compston J (2010) Low rates of treatment in postmenopausal women with a history of low trauma fractures: results of audit in a Fracture Liaison Service. QJM 103(1):33–40. Epub 2009/10/30
104. Majumdar SR, Beaupre LA, Harley CH, Hanley DA, Lier DA, Juby AG et al (2007) Use of a case manager to improve osteoporosis treatment after hip fracture: results of a randomized controlled trial. Arch Intern Med 167(19):2110–2115. Epub 2007/10/24
105. Eisman JA, Bogoch ER, Dell R, Harrington JT, McKinney RE Jr, McLellan A et al (2012) Making the first fracture the last fracture: ASBMR task force report on secondary fracture prevention. J Bone Miner Res 27(10):2039–2046. Epub 2012/07/28
106. Ankjaer-Jensen A, Johnell O (1996) Prevention of osteoporosis: cost-effectiveness of different pharmaceutical treatments. Osteoporos Int 6(4):265–275. Epub 1996/01/01
107. Borgstrom F, Zethraeus N, Johnell O, Lidgren L, Ponzer S, Svensson O et al (2006) Costs and quality of life associated with osteoporosis-related fractures in Sweden. Osteoporos Int 17(5):637–650. Epub 2005/11/12
108. Zethraeus N, Stromberg L, Jonsson B, Svensson O, Ohlen G (1997) The cost of a hip fracture estimates for 1,709 patients in Sweden. Acta Orthop Scand 68(1):13–17. Epub 1997/02/01
109. Gandjour A, Weyler EJ (2006) Cost-effectiveness of referrals to high-volume hospitals: an analysis based on a probabilistic Markov model for hip fracture surgeries. Health Care Manag Sci 9(4):359–369. Epub 2006/12/26
110. McLellan AR, Wolowacz SE, Zimovetz EA, Beard SM, Lock S, McCrink L et al (2011) Fracture liaison services for the evaluation and management of patients with osteoporotic fracture: a cost-effectiveness evaluation based on data collected over 8 years of service provision. Osteoporos Int 22(7):2083–2098. Epub 2011/05/25
111. Sander B, Elliot-Gibson V, Beaton DE, Bogoch ER, Maetzel A (2008) A coordinator program in post-fracture osteoporosis management improves outcomes and saves costs. J Bone Joint Surg Am 90(6):1197–1205. Epub 2008/06/04
112. Brixen K, Overgaard S, Gram J, Ryg J, Rothmann M, Gudex C et al (2012) Systematic prevention and treatment of osteoporosis in patients with hip fractures – a health technology assessment (Danish). Danish Health and Medicines Authority, Danish Centre of Health Technology Assessment (DACEHTA), Copenhagen
113. Cooper MS, Palmer AJ, Seibel MJ (2012) Cost-effectiveness of the Concord Minimal Trauma Fracture Liaison service, a prospective, controlled fracture prevention study. Osteoporos Int 23(1): 97–107. Epub 2011/09/29

Surgical Site Infections (SSIs): Risk Factors and Prevention Strategies

Olivier Borens, Erlangga Yusuf, and Andrej Trampuz

Introduction

Surgical site infections (SSIs), formerly called surgical wound infections, are defined as infections occurring at, or near the site of surgery within 30 days after the operation or within 1 year if implant is in place (Fig. 1) [1]. They are the most common nosocomial infection in university hospitals in Switzerland [2]. Their rate varies according to types of procedure, being higher when surgical procedures open the viscera [3]. SSIs are estimated to occur in 1.5 % of all Orthopaedic procedures [4]. The impact of SSIs is substantial on morbidity and mortality. They are associated with 10 extra days spent in hospital [3]; and in Orthopaedic surgery, they are associated with 9 % fatality [4].

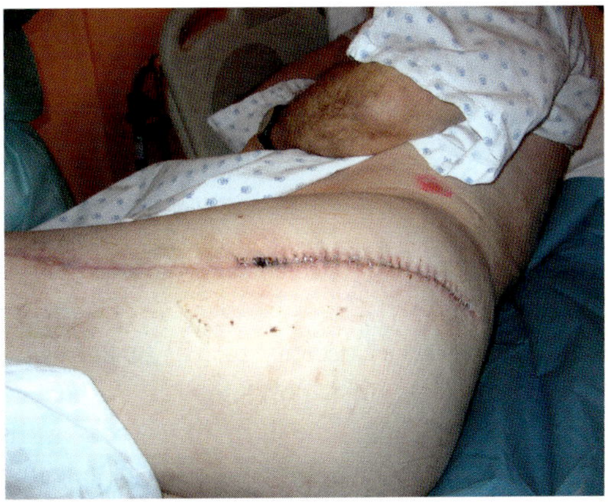

Fig. 1 Surgical site infection in a patient who had a hip arthroplasty recently

O. Borens (✉)
Orthopaedic Septic Surgical Unit, Department of Surgery and Anaesthesiology, Lausanne University Hospital, BH-10 Rue du Bugnon 46, 1011 Lausanne, Switzerland
e-mail: olivier.borens@chuv.ch

E. Yusuf
Infectious Diseases Service, Lausanne University Hospital, Rue du Bugnon 46, 1011 Lausanne, Switzerland
e-mail: angga.yusuf@gmail.com

A. Trampuz
Center for Musculoskeletal Surgery, Charité, University Medicine, Free and Humboldt-University of Berlin, Chariteplatz 1, D-10117 Berlin, Germany
e-mail: andrej.trampuz@gmail.com

Pathophysiology and Microbiology

Although most of the infections are acquired perioperatively, they can also be picked up at distance from the surgery. The source is mostly the patients themselves, but can be also any person present in the operating theatre such as the surgeon, the scrub-nurse and the anesthesiologist.

About 40 % of isolated pathogens in SSI are *Staphylococcus aureus* [5, 6]. According to a study performed between 2004 and 2007, the proportion of methicillin-resistant *Staphylococcus aureus* (MRSA) is increasing, while the proportion of methicillin-susceptible *Staphylococcus*

G. Bentley (ed.), *European Instructional Lectures*, European Instructional Lectures 13,
DOI 10.1007/978-3-642-36149-4_2, © EFORT 2013

Table 1 Factors might be related with surgical site infections

Patients-related	Surgical-related	Operating room-related
Not modifiable	Preoperative patient preparation	(a) Ventilation and laminar flow
(a) Age	(a) Showering	(b) Number of people and traffic
(b) Severity of illness	(b) Nasal colonization	
Modifiable	(c) Hair	
(a) Hyperglycemia (diabetes)	(d) Skin preparation	
(b) Obesity	(e) Surgical and incise drapes	
(c) Malnutrition	Preoperative surgeons preparation	
(d) Smoking	(a) Surgical scrubs	
(e) Immunosuppresive medications	(b) Surgical attire	
	Intraoperative	
	(a) Surgical duration	
	(b) Surgical techniques	

Adapted from Mangram et al. [1], Andersson et al. [7], and Page et al. [8]
These factors have been discussed as possible risks for having SSIs. This list is not exhaustive

aureus (MSSA) is decreasing [6]. In the same study, it is shown that polymicrobial pathogens are found in about one-third of the cases. In around 5 % of these polymicrobial pathogens, MRSA are also found.

Patient-Related Risk Factors

Roughly, risk factors of having SSIs can be divided into patient-related, operation- related and operating room environment-related (Table 1) [5, 7].

Several patient-related risk factors can be modified pre-operatively and several others cannot. Non-modifiable risk factors are advanced age and severity of illness.

Albeit very difficult to modify, these following patient-related risk factors can be corrected pre-operatively: hyperglycemia (diabetes), obesity, malnutrition, smoking, and use of immunosuppressive medications [5, 7, 9]. Several studies have reported the risk of having SSIs when these factors are present. For example regarding hyperglycemia, patients with HbA_{1c} level less than 7 % have a twofold lower infection rate than patients with HbA_{1c} higher than 7 % [10].

Risk Factors Related to Surgery and Strategies to Prevent SSIs

Infection can be related to inadequate patient preparation before incision and to the surgery itself. The environment where the surgery is performed can also play role in SSIs. In contrast to patient-related risk factors, the risk factors related to surgery are mostly modifiable. The following paragraphs will discuss the risk factors related to surgery.

Pre-operative Patient's Preparation

Showering

It has been long recognized that the skin is an important source of micro-organisms for possible cross-contamination [11, 12]. Skin incision can introduce micro-organisms residing on patient's skin to the exposed tissue and can lead to SSIs. Arguably, showering can remove these microorganisms and therefore prevent SSIs. A randomized control trial (RCT) including 1,530 operations, showed that the group of patients showered with chlorhexidine had significant lower risk (risk ratio of 0.4) of having SSIs when it is compared with the group that did not shower pre-operatively [13]. However when this result is pooled in a meta-analysis, no benefit of bathing with chlorhexidine over no bathing is seen [14]. The same meta-analysis also does not show significant difference in SSIs between bathing with chlorhexidine and with bar soap. It could be concluded that bathing might remove the skin micro-organisms but not enough to prevent SSIs. Regarding the timing of showering, it is shown that showering in the evening before and in the morning before the operation gives more reduction of the number of micro-organisms than a single shower, either the evening before or the operation day [15].

Nasal Colonization

Since the majority of isolated pathogens in SSIs are *Staphylococcus aureus*, their eradication is believed to reduce the number of SSIs. One of the main reservoirs of *Staphylococcus aureus* are the nares. The most efficacious agent for their eradication is mupirocin [16]. In a systematic review performed in 2008, mupirocin nasal ointment has been shown to reduce *S. aureus* infection in surgery patients in nasal carriers but not in non-carriers [17]. It should be noted that this conclusion is based on one study only. Moreover, the use of mupirocin can lead to resistance and this warrants careful monitoring [18].

Hair

Traditionally, preparation of the patient for surgery included removal of hair from the incision site. However, a meta-analysis performed in 2011 shows that pre-operative shaving is associated with higher SSIs than no-shaving (9.5 vs. 5.8 %), albeit that this difference is not statistically significant [19]. When it is necessary to remove hair, it should be limited to the incision site only. The existing evidence also suggests that clippers are associated with fewer SSIs than razors. Hair removal by using razor is associated with twofold increase risk of SSIs compared with clippers [19].

Skin Preparation

To reduce the risk of SSIs, the skin of the patients can be prepared by removing soil and other contamination. This step should be followed by application of antiseptic in concentric circles moving toward the periphery to reduce the amount of residing micro-organisms [20]. The usefulness of antiseptic in intact skin is broadly accepted. In the majority of European hospitals, povidone-iodine is the most commonly used antiseptic and its use as skin antiseptic before incision is associated with lower rate for SSIs according to a recently published study [21]. Other widely used antiseptics for skin preparation are: chlorhexidine and alcohol-containing products [22]. A systematic review performed in 2004, showed that there is no evidence that one septic agent is superior than another in preventing SSIs [23]. However, a more recent study in a large group of patient showed that cleansing of the patient's skin with chlorhexidine-alcohol is superior to cleansing with povidone-iodine for preventing surgical-site infection after clean-contaminated surgery [24]. In contaminated surgery, where the wound is already contaminated, antiseptics can also be used. This is contradictory to *in vitro* studies where antiseptics negatively influence the tissue healing [22].

Surgical and Incision Drapes

Surgical drapes should be impermeable to liquids and viruses, and cannot tear [25].

At present, only drapes coated with extra materials such as films or membranes meet the developed standard [26]. It is important to realize that such "liquid-proof" drapes may be uncomfortable because they also inhibit heat loss. Drapes are available in disposable and re-usable form. According to a RCT with 496 participants, no significant difference in SSIs is observed between disposable and re-usable drapes [27].

To keep the surgical drapes in place, transparent sheet adhered to the skin (incision drapes) can be used. A study has shown that the plastic adhesive drapes do not allow bacterial penetration and prevent the skin bacteria from multiplying under the drape [28]. However, a meta-analysis performed in 2007 does not show the benefit of adhesive drapes in reducing SSIs [29]. The present drapes are pliable, have increased water vapor transmission and an aggressive iodophor-incorporated adhesive [11]. Adhesion is important since lifting at the edge of the drapes increased the risk for SSIs [11]. To increase the adhesiveness of drapes, initial alcohol or iodine tincture to the skin can be used [30].

Pre-operative Preparation of Surgical Team

Surgical Hand Scrubs

Surgical hand scrubs is aimed at removal of transient and reduction of resident microorganisms from the nails, hands, and forearms. It also inhibit rapid rebound growth of microorganisms [31]. Surgical hand scrub consists of washing and applying antiseptic. Soap and water are used to remove transient microorganisms. Antiseptics are used to remove resident microorganisms living in hair follicles and to prevent rebound growth of microorganims [31]. Antiseptic should therefore have persistent activity to suppress microorganism. The choice of antiseptic can be alcohol in concentration of 60–95 %, or alcohol 50–95 % in combination with small amounts of chlorhexidine gluconate or hexachlorophene. These formulations have been shown to lower bacterial counts [32]. Povidone iodine is also one of the options. Yet, a recent systematic review without critical assessment of included studies showed that although chlorhexidine and povidone-iodine both reduce bacterial count after scrubbing, the effect of chlorhexidine is both more profound and longer lasting [33]. Scrubbing for 3–5 min should reduce bacterial counts to acceptable levels [34, 35]. Longer duration of scrubbing does not give an added effect and will only increase the risk of skin damage [34, 35].

Surgical Attire

Even a simple movement can liberate microorganisms from the skin and casual clothing [36]. Therefore, surgical scrubs, masks and surgical caps (Fig. 2) are used because they are believed to minimize the introduction of micro-organisms from surgical team to the patients and to the environment. However, there is no scientific evidence that they can prevent SSIs [1].

In the United States, the Association of Operating Room Nurses released recently a

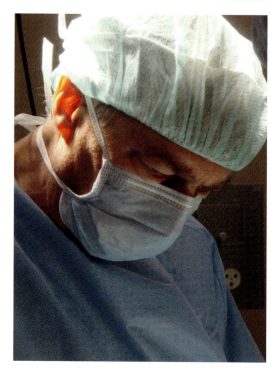

Fig. 2 Surgical masks and surgical caps are used prudently to prevent SSIs

recommendation that surgical scrubs should not be flammable, and should not harbour dust or droplets [37]. The same recommendation also emphasizes the importance of washing surgical scrubs in the health facilities instead of at home. The practice of washing scrubs at home is still done in several countries.

The use of masks is prudent practice. It has been shown that oral flora cannot reach the target within 1 m distance. In an interesting study, volunteers were asked to perform activities to disperse oral microbial flora to a plate placed 1 m away from them. However, these flora failed to grow on the plates [38]. Yet, it is still advisable to wear masks since surgeons stand closer to the patient than 1 m, and to protect the surgeons and operation staffs from contamination from patients.

The only surgical attire that is proven to be associated with lower risk of SSIs are gloves. Procedures in which gloves are perforated are associated with twofold increased risk to develop SSIs [39]. This risk is increased to four times when antibiotic prophylaxis is not used during surgery.

Gloves are perforated quite often: in about one out of five surgeries and in about 9 % of Orthopaedic surgeries [39]. Interestingly, in the majority of the cases, glove perforation is not noticed during the surgery [40]. Therefore, it is advisable to use double gloves to guarantee a sterile barrier between surgeon and patient, even though this will lead to minimal loss of sensitivity [39].

Intra-operative Aspects

Surgical Duration

In total knee arthroplasty, prolonged duration of surgery can increase the risk for SSIs [41]. This observation is also seen in other types of surgery [42]. It is logical to think that the increased risk for SSIs is confounded by other factors that might also increase the risk for SSIs, e.g. obesity and washout of antibiotics given as prophylaxis. If it is possible the duration of surgery should be kept as short as possible.

Surgical Techniques

Aspects such as wound incision, amount of tissue damage, tissue handling, wound closure, drainage, as well as maintaining the patient's temperature, oxygenation and perfusion can influence the SSIs rate [43].

Wound Incision

To make a surgical incision, scalpel or diathermy is used. Diathermy is increasingly used because of the added-advantage of increased haemostasis. The application of diathermy in relation to SSIs is controversial. Although there is no evidence that SSIs risk with diathermy is higher than with scalpel, the National Institute for Health and Clinical Excellence from United Kingdom does recommend avoidance of the use of diathermy in making skin incision [31].

Tissue Damage and Tissue Handling

Intuitively, tissue should be handled gently, devitalized tissue should be removed and dead space should be minimized in order to prevent SSIs. However, it is difficult to investigate the effect of these practices on SSIs because quantifying tissue handling is problematic. Debris can be removed by irrigation. It seems logical that irrigation will remove the micro-organisms introduced into the wound or in the cavity. However, this practice is not shown to be effective in reducing SSIs [31].

Wound Closure

Depended on the expected risk of infection, the surgical wound can be left open or closed [43]. In procedures where the risk of infection is low, wounds should be closed. Like any other foreign material, sutures may promote the growth of micro-organisms. Roughly, sutures can be divided into absorbable and non absorbable. Absorbable sutures are made from catgut, polyglycolic acid (DexonTM), polyglactic acid (VicrylTM), polydioxanone (PDSTM) and polytrimethylene carbonate (MaxonTM). The time for these sutures to be completely absorbed varies between 60 and 210 days [44]. Non-absorbable sutures are used when absorbable sutures are precluded, for example due to infection in the surroundings of the wounds [43]. Examples of non-absorbable sutures are silk, nylon (Ethilon TM), polypropylene (ProlenTM, SurgileneTM), braided polyester (MersileneTM, EthibondTM), and polybutester (NofavilTM) [44]. Absorbable and non-absorbable sutures can be mono- or multi-filamentous. Multi-filamentous sutures allow easy handling at cost of higher risk for infection. According to a study that included 1,000 patients, the rate of SSIs does not differ among suture materials used [45]. To close the wound staples can also be used. Like sutures, they are absorbable (i.e. Insorb®) or non-absorbable (i.e. Proximate®). Contaminated wounds closed with staples are associated with lower SSIs compared when the wounds are closed with suture [46].

Drainage

Drainage is used to evacuate fluid and haematoma from wounds or body spaces. Fluid and haematomata are thought to impair wound healing by increasing pressure that subsequently leads to problems in tissue perfusion [47]. On the other hand, a tube connected to suction can be also a conduit for infection. Several studies have investigated the dilemma on using closed-drain suction in Orthopaedics procedures. Evidence suggests that closed-drain suction is not associated with SSIs in hip fracture surgery [48] and after anterior cruciate ligament reconstruction, though this may depend on the duration [49].

Patient's Temperature, Ocygenation and Perfusion

Maintaining adequate tissue oxygenation seems to be important in preventing SSIs. It is believed that adequate tissue oxygenation has a role in immune function, for example in oxidative killing of micro-organisms by neutrophils. Tissue oxygenation can be guaranteed by maintaining normal temperature [50], giving supplemental oxygenation [51] and by maximizing cardiac output by means of extra colloid administration during the surgery [52]. Indeed, there are evidences that normothermia [50], and supplemental oxygen [51] are associated with lower SSIs compared to hypothermia and no supplemental oxygen, respectively. However, extra colloid administration does not decrease SSIs rate [52].

Operating Room

Ventilation and Laminar Flow

The purpose of ventilation in the operating room is to dilute and remove airborne microorganisms [53]. This can be done by applying positive pressure in the operating theatre with respect to corridors and adjacent area. Positive pressure prevents airflow from less clean into more clean areas [54]. By the same logic, the airflow should go from the ceiling to the floor level [1].

An interesting issue for the Orthopaedic field is the use of laminar airflow. Laminar airflow is thought to be particularly important in joint prosthesis surgery because the prosthesis is a foreign material where micro-organisms can attach [55]. The extra ventilation with laminar flow is aimed to move particle-free air over the aseptic operating field at uniform velocity. The flow can be delivered horizontally (wall-mounted) or vertically (ceiling to floor). The evidence on the use of laminar airflow in Orthopaedic surgery, and surgery in general is still under discussion [55]. While several early studies (for example study from Friberg and co-workers [53]) show that laminar air flow reduce SSIs, the more recent studies does not (for example study from Brandt and co-workers [56]).

Number of People and Traffic in Theatre

In the operating theatre, people with different functions are present. These people could disperse micro-organisms from their hair, skin, and clothes to their environment, including to the patients [36]. The dispersion occurs by simple movement or by talking [36]. The number of persons and their movement in the operating room are associated with higher number of bacterial contaminants [57]. In order to reduce the risk of infection, it might therefore be important to keep the number of people in the operating theater as low as possible [53, 57] and minimize needless talk [58].

Antibiotics

Peri-operative antibiotic prophylaxis in Orthopaedic surgery is a broadly accepted practice, especially in prosthetic surgery. In Germany for example, prophylaxis is given to 98 % of the patients having hip and knee replacements [56]. Important questions related to antibiotics before surgery are: which antibiotics to give, when to give and for how long.

The choice of the antibiotics depends on the micro-organisms expected to cause SSIs. This will be related in some way to the type of surgery. For practical reason and due to better biodisponibility, prophylaxis is given intravenously (iv.). The American Academy of Orthopaedic Surgeons released several recommendations on prophylactic antibiotics in Orthopaedic procedures [59]. According to the present state of knowledge, cefazolin (recommended dose of 1 to 2 g iv) or cefuroxim (1.5 g iv) are the preferred antibiotics (Table 2) [59, 60]. Cefazolin is a first generation cephalosporin, and is active against streptococci and MSSA. Cefuroxim is a second generation cephalosporins and has broader activity against gram- negative bacteria than the first generation [61]. When patients are allergic to beta-lactam antibiotics, clindamycin (600–900 mg) or vancomycin (1 g iv) can be used. A study in

Table 2 Recommendations on prophylactic antibiotics in orthopedic procedures [59]

First option	In case of allergy
Cefazolin (1–2 g iv) or	Clindamycin (600–900 mg)
Cefuroxim (1.5 g iv)	Vancomycin (1 g iv)

28,702 cardiac surgeries procedures showed that the rate of SSIs are comparable between cefuroxim and vancomycin: 2.0 % vs. 2.3 %, respectively [62]. Vancomycin should be used cautiously since its use is associated with vancomycin-resistant Enterococcus colonization and infection [63]. Next to be used in patients with beta-lactam antibiotics allergies; vancomycin should be reserved for patients with known colonization of MRSA and with higher risk with post-operative MRSA infection (e.g. recent hospitalization). It is further important to keep in mind that the recommended dose should be adjusted to patient's weight [59].

A remark should also be made on the situations where contamination is already present before the surgery is performed, for example in open fractures. In our yet unpublished study, we found that tissues biopsies from the wound in Gustilo type III open fractures grow next to coagulase-negative staphylococci and also gram-negative bacilli. Therefore, prophylactic antibiotics in contaminated wounds (pre-emptive antibiotics) should cover gram-positive and negative microorganisms.

When is the best time to give prophylactic antibiotic in clean surgery? Classen and co-workers showed that the post-operative infection rate is at its lowest when antibiotics are given within 2 h before incision [64]. Comparing with giving antibiotics within this time frame, giving antibiotics longer than 2 h before and after incision is associated with higher infection rates. A study from Switzerland elaborated further the question about the timing of prophylactic antibiotics. That study shows that administration of cefuroxime 59–30 min before incision is more effective than during the last half hour [65].

Antibiotic prophylaxis usually involves just a single dose and must be regarded as different to antibiotic treatment that is given for a period of time. However, in several situations, another dose of prophylactic is needed. Some examples of such situations are significant blood loss (more than 1.5 l) and long duration of operation (beyond 3 h). For long duration operations, antibiotics should be re-dosed at intervals of one to two times half-life of the antibiotics. As prophylaxis, cefazolin can be re-dosed every 2–5 h, cefuroxime every 3–4 h, clindamycin ever 3–6 h and vancomycin every 6–12 h [66].

A study from Germany produced a list of the common mistakes in peri-operative antibiotic prophylaxis. Antibiotics are given too early (e.g. on the ward) or too late (e.g. during the operation). Sometimes too broad-spectrum antibiotics are given in order to give false sense of security in covering 'all' potential pathogens. Also a common mistake is giving antibiotics for longer than 24 h [67].

Conclusions

Surgical procedures can lead to post-operative infection. Many risk factors of SSIs have been investigated extensively. Several measures can be taken to modify the risk factors in order to minimize risk of SSIs. There are some traditional surgical measures that have been shown to reduce SSIs. However, some others are not scientifically proven but still prudently performed. A Combination of the measures will perhaps reduce SSIs even further and warrants more studies.

References

1. Mangram AJ, Horan TC, Pearson ML, Silver LC, Jarvis WR (1999) Guideline for prevention of surgical site infection, 1999. Hospital Infection Control Practices Advisory Committee. Infect Control Hosp Epidemiol 20:250–278
2. Pittet D, Harbarth S, Ruef C et al (1999) Prevalence and risk factors for nosocomial infections in four university hospitals in Switzerland. Infect Control Hosp Epidemiol 20:37–42
3. de Lissovoy G, Fraeman K, Hutchins V, Murphy D, Song D, Vaughn BB (2009) Surgical site infection: incidence and impact on hospital utilization and treatment costs. Am J Infect Control 37:387–397
4. Astagneau P, Rioux C, Golliot F, Brucker G (2001) Morbidity and mortality associated with surgical site

infections: results from the 1997–1999 INCISO surveillance. J Hosp Infect 48:267–274
5. Emori TG, Gaynes RP (1993) An overview of nosocomial infections, including the role of the microbiology laboratory. Clin Microbiol Rev 6:428–442
6. Weigelt JA, Lipsky BA, Tabak YP, Derby KG, Kim M, Gupta V (2010) Surgical site infections: causative pathogens and associated outcomes. Am J Infect Control 38:112–120
7. Anderson DJ, Kaye KS, Classen D et al (2008) Strategies to prevent surgical site infections in acute care hospitals. Infect Control Hosp Epidemiol 29(Suppl 1):S51–S61
8. Page CP, Bohnen JM, Fletcher JR, McManus AT, Solomkin JS, Wittmann DH (1993) Antimicrobial prophylaxis for surgical wounds. Guidelines for clinical care. Arch Surg 128:79–88
9. Jamsen E, Nevalainen P, Eskelinen A, Huotari K, Kalliovalkama J, Moilanen T (2012) Obesity, diabetes, and preoperative hyperglycemia as predictors of periprosthetic joint infection: a single-center analysis of 7181 primary hip and knee replacements for osteoarthritis. J Bone Joint Surg Am 94: e1011–e1019
10. Dronge AS, Perkal MF, Kancir S, Concato J, Aslan M, Rosenthal RA (2006) Long-term glycemic control and postoperative infectious complications. Arch Surg 141:375–380
11. Alexander JW, Solomkin JS, Edwards MJ (2011) Updated recommendations for control of surgical site infections. Ann Surg 253:1082–1093
12. Hugonnet S, Pittet D (2000) Hand hygiene-beliefs or science? Clin Microbiol Infect 6:350–356
13. Wihlborg O (1987) The effect of washing with chlorhexidine soap on wound infection rate in general surgery. A controlled clinical study. Ann Chir Gynaecol 76(5):263–265
14. Webster J, Osborne S (2006) Preoperative bathing or showering with skin antiseptics to prevent surgical site infection. Cochrane Database Syst Rev. (2): CD004985
15. Edmiston CE Jr, Krepel CJ, Seabrook GR, Lewis BD, Brown KR, Towne JB (2008) Preoperative shower revisited: can high topical antiseptic levels be achieved on the skin surface before surgical admission? J Am Coll Surg 207:233–239
16. Perl TM, Cullen JJ, Wenzel RP et al (2002) Intranasal mupirocin to prevent postoperative Staphylococcus aureus infections. N Engl J Med 346:1871–1877
17. van Rijen MM, Bonten M, Wenzel RP, Kluytmans JA (2008) Intranasal mupirocin for reduction of Staphylococcus aureus infections in surgical patients with nasal carriage: a systematic review. J Antimicrob Chemother 61:254–261
18. Jones JC, Rogers TJ, Brookmeyer P et al (2007) Mupirocin resistance in patients colonized with methicillin-resistant Staphylococcus aureus in a surgical intensive care unit. Clin Infect Dis 45:541–547
19. Tanner J, Norrie P, Melen K (2011) Preoperative hair removal to reduce surgical site infection. Cochrane Database Syst Rev (2);CD004122
20. Association of Operating Room Nurses (1996) Recommended practices for skin preparation of patients. (abstract) Association of Operating Room Nurses. AORN J 64:813–816
21. Tschudin-Sutter S, Frei R, Egli-Gany D et al (2012) No risk of surgical site infections from residual bacteria after disinfection with povidone-iodine-alcohol in 1014 cases: a prospective observational study. Ann Surg 255:565–569
22. Drosou A, Falabella A, Kirsner R (2012) Antiseptics on wounds: an area of controversy. Wounds 15(5):149–166
23. Edwards PS, Lipp A, Holmes A (2004) Preoperative skin antiseptics for preventing surgical wound infections after clean surgery. Cochrane Database Syst Rev (3):CD003949
24. Darouiche RO, Wall MJ, Jr., Itani KM, et al. Chlorhexidine-Alcohol versus Povidone-Iodine for Surgical-Site Antisepsis. The New England journal of medicine. 2010;362(1):18–26.
25. Werner H (2001) Qualität von OP-Abdeckmaterial und OP-Mäntel. Hyg Med 26:62–75
26. American Society for Testing Materials (1998) Standard test method for resistance of materials used in protective clothing to penetration by synthetic blood. [abstract] American Society for Testing Materials. ASTM. F1670–1698
27. Garibaldi RA, Maglio S, Lerer T, Becker D, Lyons R (1986) Comparison of nonwoven and woven gown and drape fabric to prevent intraoperative wound contamination and postoperative infection. Am J Surg 152:505–509
28. French ML, Eitzen HE, Ritter MA (1976) The plastic surgical adhesive drape: an evaluation of its efficacy as a microbial barrier. Ann Surg 184:46–50
29. Webster J, Alghamdi AA (2007) Use of plastic adhesive drapes during surgery for preventing surgical site infection. Cochrane Database Syst Rev (4): CD006353
30. Jacobson C, Osmon DR, Hanssen A et al (2005) Prevention of wound contamination using DuraPrep solution plus Ioban 2 drapes. Clin Orthop Relat Res 439:32–37
31. National Collaborating Centre for Womens and Childrens Health (2008) Surgical site infection prevention and treatment of surgical site infection. Ref type: Report
32. Centers for Disease Control and Prevention (2002) Guideline for hand hygiene in health-care settings: recommendations of the Healthcare Infection Control Practices Advisory Committee and the HICPAC/

SHEA/APIC/IDSA HandHygiene Task Force. Ref type: Report
33. Jarral OA, McCormack DJ, Ibrahim S et al. Should surgeons scrub with chlorhexidine or iodine prior to surgery? Interactive cardiovascular and thoracic surgery. 2011;12(6):1017–21. Epub 2011/03/03.
34. Hingst V, Juditzki I, Heeg P, Sonntag HG (1992) Evaluation of the efficacy of surgical hand disinfection following a reduced application time of 3 instead of 5 min. J Hosp Infect 20:79–86
35. Chen CF, Han CL, Kan CP, Chen SG, Hung PW (2012) Effect of surgical site infections with waterless and traditional hand scrubbing protocols on bacterial growth. Am J Infect Control 40:e15–e17
36. Duguid JP, Wallace AT (1948) Air infection with dust liberated from clothing. Lancet 2:845–849
37. Braswell ML, Spruce L (2012) Implementing AORN recommended practices for surgical attire. AORN J 95:122–137
38. Mitchell NJ, Hunt S (1991) Surgical face masks in modern operating rooms – a costly and unnecessary ritual? J Hosp Infect 18:239–242
39. Misteli H, Weber WP, Reck S et al (2009) Surgical glove perforation and the risk of surgical site infection. Arch Surg 144:553–558
40. Laine T, Aarnio P (2001) How often does glove perforation occur in surgery? Comparison between single gloves and a double-gloving system. Am J Surg 181:564–566
41. Leong G, Wilson J, Charlett A (2006) Duration of operation as a risk factor for surgical site infection: comparison of English and US data. J Hosp Infect 63:255–262
42. Peersman G, Laskin R, Davis J, Peterson MG, Richart T (2006) Prolonged operative time correlates with increased infection rate after total knee arthroplasty. HSS J 2:70–72
43. McHugh SM, Hill AD, Humphreys H (2011) Intraoperative technique as a factor in the prevention of surgical site infection. J Hosp Infect 78:1–4
44. Tajirian AL, Goldberg DJ (2010) A review of sutures and other skin closure materials. J Cosmet Laser Ther 12:296–302
45. Gabrielli F, Potenza C, Puddu P, Sera F, Masini C, Abeni D (2001) Suture materials and other factors associated with tissue reactivity, infection, and wound dehiscence among plastic surgery outpatients. Plast Reconstr Surg 107:38–45
46. Hochberg J, Meyer KM, Marion MD (2009) Suture choice and other methods of skin closure. Surg Clin North Am 89:627–641
47. Parker MJ, Roberts CP, Hay D (2004) Closed suction drainage for hip and knee arthroplasty. A meta-analysis. J Bone Joint Surg Am 86-A:1146–1152
48. Clifton R, Haleem S, McKee A, Parker MJ (2008) Closed suction surgical wound drainage after hip fracture surgery: a systematic review and meta-analysis of randomised controlled trials. Int Orthop 32:723–727
49. Clifton R, Haleem S, McKee A, Parker MJ (2007) Closed suction surgical wound drainage after anterior cruciate ligament reconstruction: a systematic review of randomised controlled trials. Knee 14:348–351
50. Kurz A, Sessler DI, Lenhardt R (1996) Perioperative normothermia to reduce the incidence of surgical-wound infection and shorten hospitalization. Study of Wound Infection and Temperature Group. N Engl J Med 334:1209–1215
51. Greif R, Sessler DI (2004) Supplemental oxygen and risk of surgical site infection. JAMA 291:1957–1959
52. Kabon B, Akca O, Taguchi A et al (2005) Supplemental intravenous crystalloid administration does not reduce the risk of surgical wound infection. Anesth Analg 101:1546–1553
53. Friberg B (1998) Ultraclean laminar airflow ORs. AORN J 67:841–851
54. Lidwell OM (1986) Clean air at operation and subsequent sepsis in the joint. Clin Orthop Relat Res (211):91–102
55. Anderson D, Sexton D (2012) Controversies in control measures to prevent surgical site infection. www.uptodate.com. Accessed on Sep 13, 2012
56. Brandt C, Hott U, Sohr D, Daschner F, Gastmeier P, Ruden H (2008) Operating room ventilation with laminar airflow shows no protective effect on the surgical site infection rate in orthopedic and abdominal surgery. Ann Surg 248:695–700
57. Lynch RJ, Englesbe MJ, Sturm L et al (2009) Measurement of foot traffic in the operating room: implications for infection control. Am J Med Qual 24:45–52
58. Ayliffe GA (1991) Role of the environment of the operating suite in surgical wound infection. Rev Infect Dis 13(Suppl 10):S800–S804
59. American Academy of Orthopedic Surgeons (2004) Recommendations for the use of intravenous antibiotic prophylaxis in primary total joint arthroplasty. Ref type: Unenacted Bill/Resolution
60. Bratzler DW (2001) Osteopathic manipulative treatment and outcomes for pneumonia. J Am Osteopath Assoc 101:427–428
61. Kalman D, Barriere SL (1990) Review of the pharmacology, pharmacokinetics, and clinical use of cephalosporins. Tex Heart Inst J 17:203–215
62. Koch CG, Nowicki ER, Rajeswaran J, Gordon SM, Sabik JF III, Blackstone EH (2012) When the timing is right: antibiotic timing and infection after cardiac surgery. J Thorac Cardiovasc Surg 144(4):931–937
63. French GL (1998) Enterococci and vancomycin resistance. Clin Infect Dis 27(Suppl 1):S75–S83

64. Classen DC, Evans RS, Pestotnik SL, Horn SD, Menlove RL, Burke JP (1992) The timing of prophylactic administration of antibiotics and the risk of surgical-wound infection. N Engl J Med 326:281–286
65. Weber WP, Marti WR, Zwahlen M et al (2008) The timing of surgical antimicrobial prophylaxis. Ann Surg 247:918–926
66. American Society of Health-System Pharmacists (1999) ASHP therapeutic guidelines on antimicrobial prophylaxis in surgery. Am J Health Syst Pharm 56:1839–1888
67. Dettenkofer M, Forster DH, Ebner W, Gastmeier P, Ruden H, Daschner FD (2002) The practice of perioperative antibiotic prophylaxis in eight German hospitals. Infection 30:164–167

Exercise Therapy as Treatment for Patients with Osteoarthritis of the Knee

Ewa M. Roos

Exercise Is Core Treatment for Knee and Hip OA

Exercise is evidence-based medicine for patients with osteoarthritis (OA) [1]. Twelve supervised sessions of aerobic exercise or strength training reduce pain more effectively than a full dose of acetaminophen or non-steroidal anti-inflammatory drugs (NSAID's.) (Fig. 1). Simultaneously, parallel improvements are seen in physical function and quality of life. As a result, exercise is recommended as core treatment for mild and moderate knee and hip OA in European, North American and global clinical guidelines [3–5].

Exercise in an Orthopaedic Context

In an Orthopaedic context, exercise can be applied as a single non-operative treatment for patients not eligible for surgery, or as an adjunct to surgery in those eligible for surgery. In combination with surgery, exercise can be prescribed prior to surgery or after surgery. In those with mild and moderate OA where an arthroscopic procedure is considered, exercise is a similarly effective, or more effective, treatment [6–8]. In those with severe OA awaiting total joint replacement (TJR), exercise is safe, feasible [9] and effective [10]. The first meta-analysis of pre-operative exercise indicates a possible short-term effect post-operatively in comparison to surgery alone, valuable for those where a fast functional improvement is warranted [11]. Post-operative exercise after total knee replacement is associated with short-term beneficial effects [12] while no effects are seen from exercise following total hip replacement [13]. A general problem is that the quality of many studies is poor and the exercise programmes themselves are of questionable therapeutic effect [14]. If the exercise programme is ineffective in improving aerobic capacity, muscle strength or functional performance, pain relief and functional improvement cannot be expected. This chapter will discuss exercise as a treatment concept and in different contexts relevant from the perspective of the Orthopedic surgeon. Since the knowledge is much greater regarding exercise in patients with knee OA than hip OA, this chapter will focus on knee OA. The emerging evidence for hip OA is, however, in line with the results for knee OA and, thus, most likely the findings from knee OA are relevant also for hip OA.

Why Prescribe Exercise as OA Treatment?

TJR is the preferred treatment of end-stage OA, and a recent review article in the Lancet on TJR points out the need for an increased focus on

E.M. Roos, PT, MSc, PhD
Research Unit for Musculoskeletal
Function and Physiotherapy,
Institute of Sports Science and Clinical Biomechanics
University of Southern Denmark,
Campusvej 55, Odense, Denmark
e-mail: eroos@health.sdu.dk

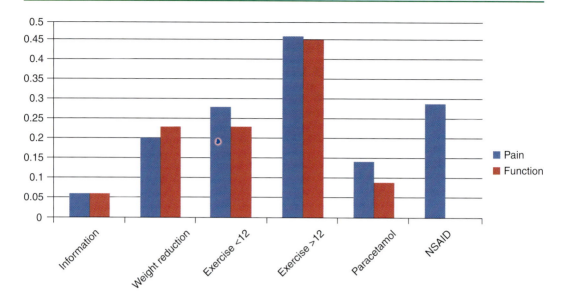

Fig. 1 Pain relief and functional improvements seen from common non-surgical treatments for knee OA measured as Effect Size (ES). ES is defined as score change divided by baseline standard deviation. An ES of <0.2 is considered small, 0.5 moderate and >0.8 large. Exercise <12 refers to the ES of studies of programs with less than 12 exercise sessions while >12 refers to studies of programs with more than 12 exercise sessions (Data has been derived from Zhang et al. [2] and Fransen et al. [1])

interventions in the early stages of the disease that may prevent patients from reaching end-stage OA and surgery [15]. It is therefore proposed that in addition to severe, often nocturnal, pain and major disability that affects work and walking ability, patients must have undergone a sufficiently long period of non-surgical treatment before TJR is indicated [15]. Exercise, information and weight reduction constitute evidence-based first line treatment for OA. There are several reasons for the increasing focus on non-surgical treatment of OA, one being that of those who seek primary care with knee pain, it is a minority who have symptoms that warrant a surgical procedure [15, 16]. There is no absolute indication for TJR and incidence varies widely both within and between countries [17, 18]. The majority of patients with symptoms of knee and hip OA do not reach the final stage of the disease, and there are few treatment options available for patients with mild and moderate OA in today's health care system.

OA Affects the Whole Joint and the Muscles

Today we know that OA is a disease that affects the entire joint and not just the cartilage. Degeneration in the meniscii [19] and ligaments [20] precedes cartilage degeneration and OA. This is new information. Previously we knew that traumatic injury to the meniscus and ligaments was associated with a greatly increased risk of OA [21]. The fact that the menisci and ligaments degenerate without known injury is important information in several ways: first, large groups of patients can be identified before they have developed OA that is visible on radiographs and therefore a 'window of opportunity' exists for prevention, and second, these other structural changes in the joint help to explain the pain and loss of function that are cardinal signs of OA, but have weak correlation with cartilage loss. Previously, we knew that muscle weakness was common in patients with OA [22] and can possibly explain the pain better than radiographic changes [23, 24].

Information, Exercise and Weight Reduction Should Be Offered Early During the Disease Course

There is no causal therapy for OA, and treatment is focussed on relieving the symptoms. Modern evidence-based treatment for OA starts with information, exercise, and if indicated, weight reduction. These interventions form the basis of OA treatment in both international and national clinical guidelines [3–5]. Information, exercise and weight reduction may be the only treatment or be used in combination with pharmacological or surgical treatment. Information, exercise and weight reduction offered early in the disease process increase the likelihood of reduced personal suffering and reduced societal health care costs associated with OA.

The type of treatment patients with OA are offered is largely the consequence of the clinical profession with whom the patient interacts in the health care system. If the patient is referred to a physiotherapist, there is a high likelihood that the patient will be offered an exercise programme. If the patient consults a primary care physician or rheumatologist, there is greater likelihood that the patient will be offered injection therapy or other pharmacological treatment, while a visit to the Orthopaedic surgeon will usually result in the patient's being offered surgery. Clinical guidelines point out that patients with OA usually need a combination of different therapies, and therefore it would be a wise strategy to treat patients with OA using a multi-professional team, as often occurs in patients with rheumatoid arthritis. There is, however, a difference in treatment focus between OA and rheumatoid arthritis. While pharmacological treatment is crucial in the treatment of rheumatoid arthritis, the recommended focus of early osteoarthritis treatment is on information, exercise, and if necessary weight reduction. This highlights the need for a physiotherapist to be a key member of the team around the OA patient. Whether the patient is treated in the primary or the secondary health care sector is dependent on the country's health care system.

The Role of Exercise in the Treatment and Prevention of Pain, Functional Limitations and OA

Exercise is safe and rarely has side effects for the affected joint, even for those with severe OA [9], and after 6–8 weeks gives better analgesia than full dose acetaminophen and NSAID's (Fig. 1). In addition, exercise is the only treatment that leads to measurable improvement in physical capacity, which is equally as important as pain relief for patients with OA [25]. For obese patients, exercise should be adapted so that part of the body weight is supported; training in water and cycling, for example, are good alternatives. Overweight and obese patients should be referred for weight reducing treatment which is best done in parallel with exercise since weight reduction results in a relative loss of muscle strength [26].

Therapeutic exercise is defined as "a subset of physical activity that is planned, structured, and repetitive and has as a final or an intermediate objective, the improvement or maintenance of physical fitness" [27]. Physical fitness is multifaceted and includes aerobic capacity, muscle strength and neuromuscular control. Obviously, it is essential that the type of training is matched to the result you want to achieve; in other words, you improve at what you practice. In OA, exercise has the objectives to reduce pain and improve physical function, and more recently it has also been questioned if exercise can be used to improve cartilage quality, reduce the load on the knee joint or even prevent cartilage loss. There is a role for cardiovascular exercise, strength training and neuromuscular training in patients with OA. While neuromuscular training specifically targets the OA joint, the cardiovascular exercise and strength training provided to patients with OA need not differ from the cardiovascular exercise and strength training recommended for everyone else.

Aerobic (Cardiovascular) Exercise

Aerobic exercise – typically, walking is the activity that has been studied – has been shown to be associated with moderate relief of knee pain and moderate improvement in self-rated physical function [1]. This is in line with results from other groups without OA where increased physical activity has been reported to lead to reduced bodily pain. One can conclude that aerobic exercise is safe and effective for pain relief in patients with OA of the knee, just as it is for people in general. As for everyone else, exercise for patients with OA should be dosed according to current guidelines for good health and be progressed in such a way that it brings improved aerobic capacity. In addition to pain relief and improvement of function, exercise leads to increased physical activity which reduces the risk of cardiovascular disease. This is especially important for patients with OA who have been shown to have an elevated mortality from cardiovascular disease [28].

Strength Training

Patients with knee OA often have reduced muscle strength in the lower extremity, but most significantly in the anterior thigh. The first step in motivating patients to exercise to improve their muscle strength is to investigate if there is a weakness. In the clinic, muscle strength can be evaluated by a simple stair test [29] (Fig. 2). Strength training can have a direct effect on the osteoarthritic joint because strong muscles help to stabilize the joint, and dampen the forces resulting from contact with the ground with every step taken [30]. The goal of strength training is to increase the ability of the muscles to develop force, and training can take place on machines, with rubber bands as resistance, or with the body acting as a load. Strength training leads to pain relief and improvement in function with a magnitude similar to that of aerobic exercise [1].

As with aerobic exercise, it is important that the dosage and progression is sufficient to bring about an increase in strength. It is debated, however, if heavy strength training of individual muscles (anterior thigh) is unquestionably good for the joint [31]. Strength training of the anterior thigh muscles only may be associated with increased compressive forces across the joint, which could contribute to increased progression of the OA disease. The research results are divergent. This has contributed to a shift in focus from strength training of the anterior thigh muscles only to exercising both legs and the trunk muscles.

Neuromuscular Training

Patients with knee OA are analogous to younger patients with knee injury, who experience functional instability and impaired neuromuscular function (such as proprioception). In that younger group, an adaptation of neuromuscular training has been successfully used to both prevent and treat knee injuries. Similarly, neuromuscular training has been used in middle-aged and older patients with OA who often have significantly lower levels of functioning than younger people.

There are some fundamental differences between neuromuscular training and strength training. The goal of neuromuscular training is to improve sensory and motor control, and to achieve functional stabilization of the joint with the help of the surrounding muscles. To this end, weight-bearing exercises are used in starting positions that mimic the demands of daily life and in sports (see Fig. 3 for examples). A complete neuromuscular training program designed for patients with severe hip or knee OA can be downloaded from the Internet (http://www.biomedcentral.com/1471-2474/11/126/additional). The exercises should be adapted to the patient's current level of activity, and to the functional goals that the patient wants to achieve. The focus is on the quality of the movement and progression is allowed when the patient can perform the exercises with appropriate quality. This is different from strength training, where progression is dependent on the weight the patient can lift.

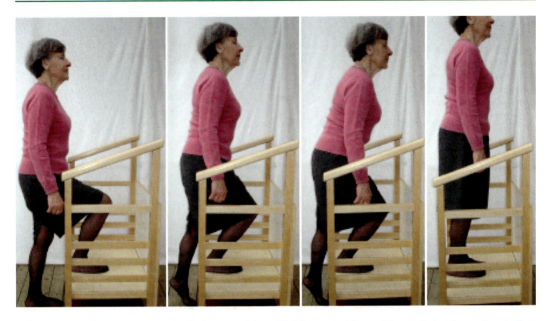

Fig. 2 Stair test. Difference in step height between right and left leg, or problems with completing the test is an indication for prescribing strength training (Reproduced from Nyberg et al. [29])

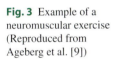

Fig. 3 Example of a neuromuscular exercise (Reproduced from Ageberg et al. [9])

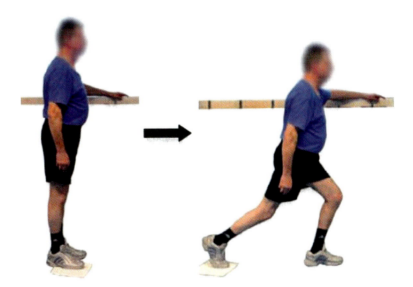

In neuromuscular training, movements should be performed in a well-coordinated manner and with optimal alignment. In this context, alignment refers to the relationship between the hip, knee and ankle. All three joints should be in line with each other, a posture we call 'neutral alignment' (Fig. 4a). Commonly, patients with OA rotate the hip joint inwardly and bear weight on a pronated foot with a lowered medial arch. In the clinic, this is seen as the knee being located medial to the foot and the longitudinal axis of the femur not being parallel to the longitudinal axis of the foot. This can easily be examined in the standing position in the clinic. If the alignment of the patient's knee is medial to (Fig. 4b), or less commonly lateral to the alignment of the foot the patient may benefit from neuromuscular training. Note that patients may have a good or bad

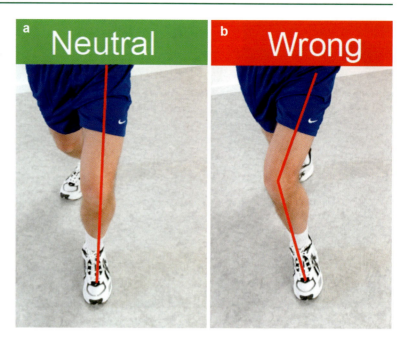

Fig. 4 (**a**, **b**) Neutral (good) alignment can be achieved with neuromuscular exercise. Poor alignment is an indication for prescribing neuromuscular exercise (Authors own pictures)

alignment when examined in motion during weight-bearing (Fig. 4a, b), regardless of the static structural varus-valgus alignment that can be measured on x-rays. These are two different measurements that are not necessarily dependent on each other. The explanation for this is that radiography is a static two-dimensional examination of the skeleton while functional alignment (Fig. 4a, b) examined during a weight-bearing dynamic activity is dependent on the position of the hip, knee and ankle joints and the muscles that work across these joints [32].

Exercise Therapy Can Affect Joint Mechanics and Joint Structures Positively

A few studies have examined whether strength training or neuromuscular training can affect the cartilage of the knee joint or the mechanical stress on the knee joint. These studies show that exercise is not bad for the joint. This type of study is associated with significant design challenges, since conventional imaging requires a total of 300 patients and a follow-up of at least 2.5 years. The only study that has used this approach achieved no increase in strength in the exercise group (suggesting poor adherence or lack of progression in training), but showed that cartilage loss was not increased in the exercise group, in contrast to the control group where cartilage loss increased over time [33]. Due to the insensitivity of radiographs, indirect methods have been used to measure changes related to radiological changes. Two methods used are dGEMRIC (delayed gadolinium-enhanced MRI of the cartilage) for evaluation of the proteoglycan content of the cartilage, and three-dimensional gait analysis in combination with a force platform for calculation of the mechanical load on the knee joint.

The first thing occurring when cartilage is degraded is that proteoglycan is released and the proteoglycan content of the cartilage is reduced. Thereafter follows collagen degradation. It thus seems likely that exercise early in the disease process, before collagen degradation has started, i.e. in stages without cartilage loss as seen on radiographs, would have a greater opportunity to influence the process. It is also here that dGEMRIC can be used as an evaluation method when there is cartilage still left in the joint. A randomized study of 4 months of neuromuscular training in meniscectomized middle-aged patients with a high risk of developing OA showed increased proteoglycan content of the cartilage compared to a control group [34], and thus confirmed previous findings from animal studies. These findings need to be repeated, but do suggest that neuromuscular training can positively affect the viscoelastic properties of the cartilage. The effect of neuromuscular training on knee joint load in patients with early OA has been investigated in a few smaller studies [35, 36]. These results suggest that exercise also may affect the loading of the knee joint positively, but more research is needed to confirm this.

What Can the Orthopaedic Surgeon Do to Increase Compliance with Exercise Therapy?

Today there is good evidence that exercise is safe and also an effective treatment for patients with OA, even for those with severe osteoarthritis. But patients with OA are first and foremost people, and just like the general population, it is difficult to get OA patients to change their behaviour, to exercise and to increase their physical activity level. In addition, patients with arthritic pain from the joints instinctively believe that they should rest for the pain to go away. We now have overwhelming evidence that this is wrong; patients with OA should exercise to relieve their pain. Here Orthopaedic surgeons who see patients with OA in their everyday clinical practice can have a large impact by informing their patients about the pain relief and functional improvement seen from exercise, that exercise is safe for OA patients, with positive side effects such as improved mood, quality of life and improved general health, including reduced risk of other diseases such as cardiovascular disease and diabetes.

Tips During Consultation

- Inform the patient about OA disease and the positive effects of exercise and weight reduction
- Tell the patient that exercise is safe for people with OA
- Advise the patient that pain decreases as the number of training sessions increases
- Ask for the patient's level of physical activity and encourage an exercise regime equivalent to at least 30 min most days of the week to a level where the effort produces sweating
- Evaluate the muscle strength of the legs, for example by using a stair test (Fig. 2), prescribe and encourage strength training if there is a difference in strength between the right and left legs, or if the patient has problems performing the test
- Evaluate the functional alignment of the hip, knee and ankle (Fig. 4a, b), prescribe and encourage neuromuscular training if the patient has difficulty controlling how they load and bear weight on their joints.

References

1. Fransen M, McConnell S (2008) Exercise for osteoarthritis of the knee. Cochrane Database Syst Rev (4):CD004376
2. Zhang W, Nuki G, Moskowitz RW, Abramson S, Altman RD, Arden NK et al (2010) OARSI recommendations for the management of hip and knee osteoarthritis: part III: Changes in evidence following systematic cumulative update of research published through January 2009. Osteoarthritis and cartilage/OARS, Osteoarthritis Research Society 18(4):476–499
3. Zhang W, Doherty M, Arden N, Bannwarth B, Bijlsma J, Gunther KP et al (2005) EULAR evidence based recommendations for the management of hip osteoarthritis: report of a task force of the EULAR Standing Committee for International Clinical Studies Including Therapeutics (ESCISIT). Ann Rheum Dis 64:669–681
4. Zhang W, Moskowitz RW, Nuki G, Abramson S, Altman RD, Arden N et al (2008) OARSI recommendations for the management of hip and knee osteoarthritis, part II: OARSI evidence-based, expert consensus guidelines. Osteoarthritis Cartilage 16:137–162
5. Hochberg MC, Altman RD, April KT, Benkhalti M, Guyatt G, McGowan J et al (2012) American College of Rheumatology 2012 recommendations for the use of nonpharmacologic and pharmacologic therapies in osteoarthritis of the hand, hip, and knee. Arthritis Care Res 64:455–474
6. Kirkley A, Birmingham TB, Litchfield RB, Giffin JR, Willits KR, Wong CJ et al (2008) A randomized trial of arthroscopic surgery for osteoarthritis of the knee. N Engl J Med 359:1097–1107

7. Herrlin S, Hallander M, Wange P, Weidenhielm L, Werner S (2007) Arthroscopic or conservative treatment of degenerative medial meniscal tears: a prospective randomised trial. Knee Surg Sports Traumatol Arthrosc 15:393–401
8. Herrlin SV, Wange PO, Lapidus G, Hallander M, Werner S, Weidenhielm L (2013) Is arthroscopic surgery beneficial in treating non-traumatic, degenerative medial meniscal tears? A five year follow-up. Knee Surg Sports Traumatol Arthrosc 21(2):358–364
9. Ageberg E, Link A, Roos EM (2010) Feasibility of neuromuscular training in patients with severe hip or knee OA: the individualized goal-based NEMEX-TJR training program. BMC Musculoskelet Disord 11:126
10. Villadsen A, Roos EM, Overgaard S, Holsgaard-Larsen A (2011) Neuromuscualr exercise improves functional performance in patients with severe hip osteoarthritis. In: Osteoarthritis Society International (OARSI), Chicago
11. Wallis JA, Taylor NF (2011) Pre-operative interventions (non-surgical and non-pharmacological) for patients with hip or knee osteoarthritis awaiting joint replacement surgery – a systematic review and meta-analysis. Osteoarthritis Cartilage 19:1381–1395
12. Minns Lowe CJ, Barker KL, Dewey M, Sackley CM (2007) Effectiveness of physiotherapy exercise after knee arthroplasty for osteoarthritis: systematic review and meta-analysis of randomised controlled trials. BMJ 335:812
13. Minns Lowe CJ, Barker KL, Dewey ME, Sackley CM (2009) Effectiveness of physiotherapy exercise following hip arthroplasty for osteoarthritis: a systematic review of clinical trials. BMC Musculoskelet Disord 10:98
14. Hoogeboom TJ, Oosting E, Vriezekolk JE, Veenhof C, Siemonsma PC, de Bie RA et al (2012) Therapeutic validity and effectiveness of preoperative exercise on functional recovery after joint replacement: a systematic review and meta-analysis. PLoS One 7:e38031
15. Carr AJ (1999) Beyond disability: measuring the social and personal consequences of osteoarthritis. Osteoarthritis Cartilage 7:230–238
16. Peat G, McCarney R, Croft P (2001) Knee pain and osteoarthritis in older adults: a review of community burden and current use of primary health care. Ann Rheum Dis 60:91–97
17. Dieppe P, Judge A, Williams S, Ikwueke I, Guenther KP, Floeren M et al (2009) Variations in the pre-operative status of patients coming to primary hip replacement for osteoarthritis in European orthopaedic centres. BMC Musculoskelet Disord 10:19
18. Gossec L, Paternotte S, Maillefert JF, Combescure C, Conaghan PG, Davis AM et al (2011) The role of pain and functional impairment in the decision to recommend total joint replacement in hip and knee osteoarthritis: an international cross-sectional study of 1909 patients. Report of the OARSI-OMERACT Task Force on total joint replacement. Osteoarthritis Cartilage 19:147–154
19. Englund M, Guermazi A, Gale D, Hunter DJ, Aliabadi P, Clancy M et al (2008) Incidental meniscal findings on knee MRI in middle-aged and elderly persons. N Engl J Med 359:1108–1115
20. Hasegawa A, Otsuki S, Pauli C, Miyaki S, Patil S, Steklov N et al (2012) Anterior cruciate ligament changes in the human knee joint in aging and osteoarthritis. Arthritis Rheum 64:696–704
21. Lohmander LS, Englund PM, Dahl LL, Roos EM (2007) The long-term consequence of anterior cruciate ligament and meniscus injuries: osteoarthritis. Am J Sports Med 35:1756–1769
22. Roos EM, Herzog W, Block JA, Bennell KL (2011) Muscle weakness, afferent sensory dysfunction and exercise in knee osteoarthritis. Nature reviews. Rheumatology 7:57–63
23. McAlindon TE, Cooper C, Kirwan JR, Dieppe PA (1993) Determinants of disability in osteoarthritis of the knee. Ann Rheum Dis 52:258–262
24. O'Reilly SC, Jones A, Muir KR, Doherty M (1998) Quadriceps weakness in knee osteoarthritis: the effect on pain and disability. Ann Rheum Dis 57:588–594
25. Nilsdotter AK, Toksvig-Larsen S, Roos EM (2009) Knee arthroplasty: are patients' expectations fulfilled? A prospective study of pain and function in 102 patients with 5-year follow-up. Acta Orthop 80:55–61
26. Henriksen M, Christensen R, Danneskiold-Samsoe B, Bliddal H (2012) Changes in lower extremity muscle mass and muscle strength after weight loss in obese patients with knee osteoarthritis: a prospective cohort study. Arthritis Rheum 64:438–442
27. Caspersen CJ, Powell KE, Christenson GM (1985) Physical activity, exercise, and physical fitness: definitions and distinctions for health-related research. Public Health Rep 100:126–131
28. Nuesch E, Dieppe P, Reichenbach S, Williams S, Iff S, Juni P (2011) All cause and disease specific mortality in patients with knee or hip osteoarthritis: population based cohort study. BMJ 342:d1165
29. Nyberg LA, Hellenius ML, Kowalski J, Wandell P, Andersson P, Sundberg CJ (2011) Repeatability and validity of a standardised maximal step-up test for leg function – a diagnostic accuracy study. BMC Musculoskelet Disord 12:191
30. Mikesky AE, Meyer A, Thompson KL (2000) Relationship between quadriceps strength and rate of loading during gait in women. J Orthop Res 18:171–175
31. Bennell KL, Hunt MA, Wrigley TV, Lim BW, Hinman RS (2008) Role of muscle in the genesis and management of knee osteoarthritis. Rheum Dis Clin North Am 34:731–754
32. Ageberg E, Bennell KL, Hunt MA, Simic M, Roos EM, Creaby MW (2010) Validity and inter-rater reliability of medio-lateral knee motion observed during a single-limb mini squat. BMC Musculoskelet Disord 11:265
33. Mikesky AE, Mazzuca SA, Brandt KD, Perkins SM, Damush T, Lane KA (2006) Effects of strength training on the incidence and progression of knee osteoarthritis. Arthritis Rheum 55:690–699

34. Roos EM, Dahlberg L (2005) Positive effects of moderate exercise on knee cartilage glycosaminoglycan content. A four-month randomized controlled trial in patients at risk of osteoarthritis. Arthritis Rheum 52:3507–3514
35. Thorp LE, Wimmer MA, Foucher KC, Sumner DR, Shakoor N, Block JA (2010) The biomechanical effects of focused muscle training on medial knee loads in OA of the knee: a pilot, proof of concept study. J Musculoskelet Neuronal Interact 10: 166–173
36. Thorstensson CA, Henriksson M, von Porat A, Sjodahl C, Roos EM (2007) The effect of eight weeks of exercise on knee adduction moment in early knee osteoarthritis – a pilot study. Osteoarthritis Cartilage 15:1163–1170

Part II

Tumours

New Trends Based on Experimental Results in the Treatment of Sarcoma

Nicola Baldini and Katsuyuki Kusuzaki

Current Status of Sarcoma Treatment and Outcomes

Limited progress has been made over the past three decades in improving the outcome of patients with sarcomas. Based on state-of-the-art imaging [46] and staging systems [55], multi-modal treatment (surgery plus pre- and/or post-operative chemotherapy, brachytherapy, chemotherapy, intra-arterial perfusion, etc.) is effective in controlling local disease with a high rate of limb-salvage. However, the overall survival remains 20 % or less for patients with metastases and even in patients presenting with local disease relapse occurs in over 40 %. Biochemical resistance to anticancer agents is one of the frustrating limits opposing an improvement in survival [6], however endless attempts based on increased or prolonged administration of adjuvant chemotherapy did not translate into significant changes in prognosis, but rather increased the acute and chronic side effects, in keeping with the failure of the popular 'magic bullet' concept in cancer therapy as introduced by Paul Ehrlich more than 100 years ago [47]. Moreover, despite the technical progress and the advantage of adjuvants, in some anatomical sites limb-sparing procedures are not feasible and excisional surgery is the only unfortunate alternative.

Given the complexity of malignant transformation and progression and the heterogeneous phenotype of sarcomas, dissecting the biomolecular events associated with neoplastic change of putative mesenchymal precursors and seeking individualized treatment are reasonable options to improve the prognosis of sarcoma patients. Indeed, the main focus of cancer research for the past years has been based on standard in vitro evaluation of malignant cancer cells, seeking to understand the dominant oncogenes and tumour suppressor genes whose respective activation or loss of function trigger neoplastic transformation and progression. Highly sophisticated genome sequencing and transcriptional profiling have presented incredibly huge amounts of data, with great expectations to be translated into effective therapies. With rare exception, however, therapies for most forms of human cancer remain incompletely effective and transitory, despite knowledge of driving oncogenes and crucial oncogenic signalling pathways amenable to pharmacological intervention with targeted therapies. Also in sarcomas extensive preclinical investigations have led to significant improvements in

---

N. Baldini (✉)
Department of Biomedical and Neuromotor Sciences,
University of Bologna,
Via di Barbiano 1/10,
I-40136 Bologna, Italy

Orthopaedic Pathophysiology Unit,
Istituto Ortopedico Rizzoli,
Bologna, Italy
e-mail: nicola.baldini@ior.it

K. Kusuzaki
Department of Molecular Cell Physiology,
Kyoto Prefectural University of Medicine,
Kyoto, Japan

knowledge of the molecular events of tumorigenesis underlying the clinical behaviour, and this has led to hypothesize the adoption of targeted agents, such as those interfering with the signaling of growth factor receptors [3], in the hope of achieving improved chances of healing. Still, even such tailored approaches have proved unacceptably toxic or unsuccessful in the vast majority of cases [48].

The Tumour Microenvironment

The unfortunate failure of a simplistic approach based on the identification of deranged molecular pathways in isolated cancer cells, and the consequent testing of antibodies or small molecules specifically addressing such mechanisms, has prompted a critical re-appraisal of the problem and the evolution of a new concept taking into primary consideration the complexity of the tumour setting, in particular the concept that cancer cells do not manifest the disease alone, but rather involve and are influenced by a number of normal, reactive cell types, including immune cells, endothelia and cancer-associated fibroblasts and live in a context of multifaceted metabolism (Fig. 1). The tumour microenvironment is therefore emerging as a novel, broad, promising field of investigation [19]. The complexity of the tumour, an entity where interactions of cancer and normal cells give rise to multiple effects, largely unpredictable, based on pre-clinical in vitro and in vivo settings, requires a higher level of study and a critical revision of previous findings and accepted postulates.

Besides the role of individual cell components within the tumour, and, among cancer cells, the role of the stem cell niche, a striking feature of malignant tumours is the fact that cancer cells have an altered metabolism to support chronic proliferation, in particular, a flexible utilization of fuel sources and modes of consuming them to generate energy and products; most notable is the activation of aerobic glycolysis that complements the output of (sometimes reduced) oxidative phosphorylation for such purposes. In 1924, the future Nobel laureate Otto Heinrich Warburg first

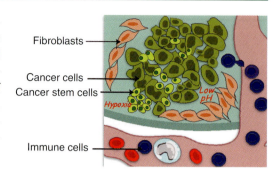

Fig. 1 The microenvironment of sarcoma, in which cancer cells and their notable subset cancer stem cells proliferate, invade surrounding tissues, and metastasize after interaction with reactive fibroblasts and immune cells in a hypoxic and acidic milieu

suggested that the driver of tumorigenesis is an insufficient cellular respiration caused by insult to mitochondria [58]. Warburg hypothesized that cancer cells mainly generate energy (ATP) by non-oxidative breakdown of glucose (glycolysis), in contrast to normal cells which mainly generate energy from oxidative breakdown of pyruvate (Fig. 2). The use of glycolytic metabolism even in the presence of normal oxygen tension is an apparent paradox, since glycolysis is 18-fold less efficient than oxydative phosphorylation in producing energy. This apparent disadvantage is however counterbalanced by the profit that anaerobic metabolism allows the selection of cells that are able to survive in an hypoxic environment and the adaptation of a glycolytic phenotype with generation of lactate.

Indeed, cancer cells metabolize large amounts of glucose in order to fuel energy production and growth. Increased amounts of glucose are needed in order for the cells to become rapidly dividing cancer cells, and this is particularly crucial for sarcoma, a type of cancer with a volume doubling time that may be counted in days. Cancer imaging with [^{18}F] 2-deoxy-2fluoro-D-glucose (FDG) PET has become commonplace in sarcomas, demonstrating that over 90 % of clinical cancers take up glucose several fold more than adjacent normal tissue. This is also the case of bone and soft tissue sarcomas, in which FDG-PET may help differentiating between benign and malignant lesions [2, 7] with a high level of specificity.

Fig. 2 Energy (ATP) production in normal cells (**a**) is different from proliferating and cancer cells (**b**), where aerobic glycolysis (so called Warburg effect) is prevalent

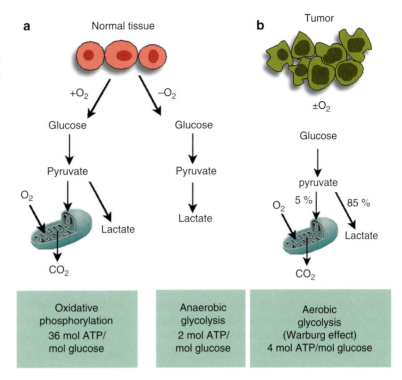

Extracellular Acidity and Tumour Growth

Large variations in vascular supply and viability are common features in sarcomas, and it is likely that significant metabolic variations take place at different areas of the same tumour. Among these, of great interest are the events occurring in the surroundings of cancer stem cells, key elements that are responsible for the clinical occurrence of drug and radiation resistance, local relapse, and metastasis. Activation of such elements is finely tuned by environmental variations of pO_2 and paracrine stimuli by reactive elements.

Warburg also discovered that cancer cells are, unlike normal cells, able to live in the acidic environment that develops also as a consequence of elevated lactic acid production by glycolysis. The diagnostic importance of lactate has been emphasized in studies showing a correlation between high lactate concentration and metastatic incidence [53], and it is known that in sarcomas high serum levels of lactate dehydrogenase, the enzyme modulating the metabolism of lactate, are adverse prognostic factors [4, 5, 8], possibly reflecting the development of a rapidly growing, metabolically active, pathologic entity.

However, lactic acid is not the only source of acid in tumours [45]. The interstitial fluid of several tumour types contains high levels of CO_2, another potential source of acidity [18], as a consequence of abnormal vascularization. Moreover, transmembrane pH regulation is markedly altered in cancer cells. In fact, to prevent acidosis-induced apoptosis by acidification of intracellular pH, glycolytically-produced acid must be extruded by tumour cells. As a consequence, the extracellular pH level (pHe) of different tumour types, including sarcomas, ranges from 6.4 to 7.3, whereas the pHe level of normal tissues is significantly more alkaline (7.2–7.5) [13].

The acidic interstitial micro-environment of the tumour triggers the proliferation and the metastatic potential of cancer cells [17], and promotes tumour-induced angiogenesis [52]. Moreover, in contrast to cancer cells, the acidic extracellular space reduces both the viability and function of most normal cells, including cytotoxic T cells that ordinarily mediate the immune response to tumour antigens. As a result, the tumour becomes a sanctuary in which immune cells are significantly inhibited [16]. The acidic pH of tumour micro-environment also favours the recruitment of immunosuppressive cells, further promoting escape from immune surveillance [10]. The increased tumour-induced proton efflux is also directly responsible for cell adhesion and invasion of the extracellular matrix. Integrin-mediated adhesion to extracellular matrix strongly depends on extracellular pH that is stabilized by the pericellular glycocalyx. If the glycocalyx is removed, the characteristic pH nano-environment is no longer maintained, and the formation of cell-matrix contacts is impaired [22]. On the other hand, extensive hypoxia and high lactate cause an aberrant compartmentalization of lysosome-like activity, and an upregulation of matrix metalloproteinases and of cathepsins B and L [43]. These phenomena have profound effects on tumour metastatic activity, as suggested by the high incidence of metastases associated with hypoxia and acidity [12, 32].

A link between proton dynamics and tumour-induced angiogenesis is suggested by the stabilization of hypoxia-inducible factors (HIF-1α and HIF-2α) induced by poor vascular supply. In cancer, HIF-1α promotes the formation of blood vessels by regulating tumour angiogenesis-related molecules, such as vascular endothelial growth factor-A, interleukin-8, basic fibroblast growth factor, platelet derived growth factor, and angiopoietin-2. Interestingly, under hypoxia, HIF also modulates proliferation and differentiation of various normal as well as cancer stem cells, maintaining their undifferentiated status [39]. In highly aggressive tumours that harbour cancer stem cell populations, the inhibition of HIF-2α prevents in vivo tumorigenesis. Stabilization of HIFs, in turn, promotes the expression of glycolitic enzymes and causes a reduction of pHe [54]. An increased rate of aerobic glycolysis, as suggested by HIF-1α nuclear overexpression, is present in over 60 % of osteosarcomas and is recognized as an adverse prognostic factor [38, 60]. Expression of both HIF-1α and HIF-2α has also been reported in chondrosarcoma, and correlated with a reduced survival rate. Moreover, high serum levels of VEGF, a HIF target gene, are prognostic in Ewing's sarcoma, and the EWS-FLI1 product is upregulated by hypoxia in a HIF-1α-dependent manner. Notably, the IGFs that are key factors for survival, tumourigenesis, and metastatic ability of sarcomas, potently modulate HIF-1 activity. IGF-1 induces both HIFs at the translation level through the PI-3-kinase and the MAPK cascades. As a result, blocking the IGF1R diminishes the accumulation of HIFs. In turn, HIF-1α is required for the expression of genes encoding IGF-2, IGF-binding protein (IGFBP)-2, and IGFBP-3 [15].

The abnormal pH gradient characterizing tumour cells is finely tuned by a number of ion/proton pumps (Fig. 3). The V-ATPase is associated with tumour invasion/metastases [29], and in multidrug resistant tumour cells V-ATPase activity is also enhanced [42]. Owing to their positive electric charge at weak pH, most anticancer drugs accumulate in their protonated form on the side of the membrane at which the pH is lower. This suggests that cationic molecules become "acid-trapped" in acidic vesicles [59]. This sequestration affects drug accumulation by its acidic degradation or extrusion from the cells through the secretory pathway, and intracellular drug cannot reach intranuclear critical effective concentrations. This phenomenon has been observed both in cells overexpressing or not overexpressing multidrug efflux transporters, such as P-glycoprotein. Indeed, in animal models, extracellular alkalinization leads to substantial improvement in the therapeutic effectiveness of antitumour drugs [11, 40]. Another proton pump, the Na^+/H^+ exchanger (NHE), is associated with cell proliferation, survival, malignant transformation, and tumour progression, as well as with changes in cellular morphology, adhesion and migration. The carbonic anhydrases (CA) II, IX and XII, which catalyze the production of H^+ and HCO_3^- ions, are overexpressed in some cancers and are functionally related to oncogenesis [49]. The proton-linked monocarboxylate transporters play a central role for the transport of monocarboxylates, such as lactate, across the plasma membrane, and are often expressed in cancer

Fig. 3 In cancer cells overexpressing the proton pump V-ATPase at the cell and vacuolar membrane protons are actively transported from the cytoplasm to the extracellular space or inside vacuoles respectively (**a**). Inhibition of V-ATPase by proton pump inhibitors triggers apoptotic signalling pathways, inhibits tumour growth, and reverts drug resistance (**b**)

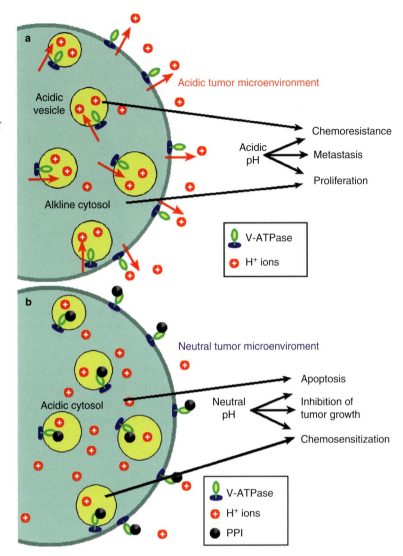

cells. The Cl⁻/HCO3⁻ anion exchangers and the ATP synthase have also been related to proton efflux in tumours. All these proton transporters can be located on acidic vesicle membranes, or on the plasma membrane, to compartmentalize or to directly pump excessive cytosolic H$^+$ into the extracellular nano-environment.

Increased extracellular acidification as a result of overexpression and/or increased activity of proton transporters may not be apparent under conventional in vitro conditions due to the presence of artificial and strong buffering solutions in culture media, such as HEPES. When cultured under unbuffered conditions, however, sarcoma cells are able to significantly decrease pHe. Interestingly, sarcoma cells are also able to survive up to a pH around 6.0. The pHi of sarcoma cells contains abundant acidic lysosomes, as revealed by acridine orange staining, in contrast to normal fibroblasts. The active extrusion of protons from these acidic vacuoles to the extracellular environment is mediated by an increased expression of V-ATPase and CA IX proton transporters.

Recent studies have shown that when cancer cells are co-cultured with fibroblasts, their mitochondrial mass increases, while fibroblasts lose their mitochondria. Moreover, it has been found that aerobic glycolysis also occurs in the stromal cells and not just in cancer cells. Based on these data, a new tumour growth theory has recently been proposed, and named "Reverse Warburg Effect" [51]. In particular, cancer cells induce oxidative stress in the neighbouring fibroblasts, mimicking hypoxia, where over-production of reactive oxygen species (ROS) triggers transcription factors like HIF1α and NFkB [31]. These events signal fibroblasts mitochondria to break down, and induce the Warburg effect. Thus, oxidative stress causes autophagy and mitophagy, producing recycled cell nutrients through glycolysis, like pyruvate, lactate and ketone bodies (3-hydroxy-butyrate) [50]. Epithelial cancer cells are able to take up the above-mentioned energy metabolites and use them in the mitochondrial TCA cycle, promoting energy production and generating ATP via oxidative phosphorylation. Secretion and re-uptake of lactate or pyruvate would be mediated by the monocarboxylate family of transporters, such as MCT1/4. This mechanism may explain how cancer cells are able to survive without blood vessels as a food source, given they can simply extract nutrients from the surrounding stromal cells after induction of oxidative stress. Importantly, fibroblast oxidative stress leads to increased DNA damage and random mutagenesis in cancer cells [30]. The final result is a higher proliferative capacity causing tumour growth and metastasis formation [9]. Such phenomena have been detected also in osteosarcoma cells, suggesting that circulating fibroblast-like cells are recruited at the site of the primary and secondary lesions and activate metabolic pathways in cancer cells, promoting their proliferation and possibly activating the stem cell component.

Systemic Therapies Targeting Sarcoma Micro-Environment

Molecular silencing and pharmacological inhibitors of proton pumps, such as bafilomycin A1 for V-ATPase, can delay cancer cell growth, but such approaches inevitably results in severe toxicity and are unfeasible. Other drugs, however,

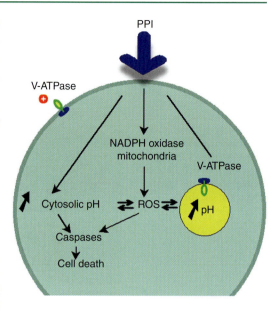

Fig. 4 Effects of pharmacological inhibition of V-ATPase by proton pump inhibitors (PPI)

including the proton pump inhibitors that are largely used for the treatment of peptic disease (omeprazole and derivatives), have sparked great interest because of their minimal side effects even when administered at high doses. An attractive feature of these compounds is that they are recruited by the acidic compartments, including the acidic tumour microenvironment, and require acidic conditions to be converted into their active form, therefore providing the possibility of tumour-specific selection. These drugs have been shown to cause cancer cell death through the induction of acidification and caspase-dependent apoptosis, both in vitro and in vivo [14] (Fig. 4). Physiological concentrations of proton pump inhibitors significantly increase the pH of acidic intracellular vesicles and the extracellular pH, inducing dysfunction accumulation of acidic vesicles in the cells, and, in turn, cell death by apoptosis.

Also in sarcoma cells, harvested under unbuffered conditions, the administration of V-ATPase inhibitors is followed by a significant decrease in viability via apoptosis, suggesting the potential usefulness of these agents, in addition to conventional therapy, for the treatment of sarcomas. Nanotechnology data have also identified peptides able to selectively insert into the membrane of cancer cells only at acidic pH, thus providing another interesting tool for the selective delivery of therapeutic agents to the acidic compartments of the tumour [1, 56]. Among new drugs targeting oxidative stress in cancer-associated fibroblasts are anti-oxidant, such as N-acetyl-cystein, metformin, and quercetin, and lysosomal inhibitors, including chloroquine. Most of these agents are available as dietary supplements and/or are approved drugs.

All these drugs specifically target the tumour acidic microenvironment and spare the normal tissues. They may be conveniently associated to conventional chemotherapy and open new perspectives for the systemic treatment of sarcomas, to prevent or cure lung metastases.

Photodynamic Therapy for Local Tumour Control

An alternative approach to target sarcoma acidic microenvironment is the use of acridine orange (AO). This is a fluorescent cationic molecule that rapidly diffuses into the cytoplasm, and in the past century it has been used as a dye specific for DNA and RNA, as a pH indicator, as a photosensitizer, and as an antitumour and antiprotozoal drug. Although mutagenic in bacteria [37], AO is not tumourigenic in mice, rats or rabbits, and in particular does not show evidence of carcinogenicity in humans [57]. The International Agency for Research on Cancer of the World Health Organization reports this agent as non-carcinogenic for humans [21]. In living cells, monomeric AO binds to acidic DNA and RNA to give a green fluorescence. AO also concentrates within lysosomes and other acidic organelles, and in these acidic compartments AO protonation causes the formation of di- and oligomeric aggregates that appear as bright orange fluorescent granules [23, 28, 62] (Fig. 5a). Tumour cells with an acidic pHe and a high number of lysosomes selectively uptake orange-emitting AO, as extensively demonstrated in different musculoskeletal sarcomas [33] (Fig. 5b), and on this basis AO has been tested as a tumour targeted drug. After continuous exposure to AO, mouse osteosarcoma

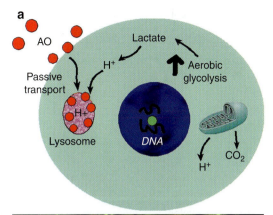

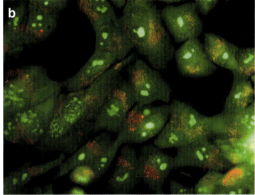

Fig. 5 Mechanism of acridine orange accumulation in cancer cells with selective uptake by acidic vacuoli (**a**); acridine orange staining in living osteosarcoma cells (**b**), showing drug accumulation in lysosomes (red fluorescence) (**b**)

cells show a dose-dependent inhibition of cell growth [25], possibly related to AO binding to RNA and impairment of protein synthesis [63]. Thanks to its ability to generate singlet oxygen in AO-loaded cells illuminated with blue light [61], AO can be used for photodynamic therapy targeting tumor acidic microenvironment. Both in vitro and in vivo, the photoactivation of AO causes a disruption of AO-containing vesicles and plasma membrane damage through blebbing in osteosarcoma cells, whereas normal fibroblasts are not affected [24, 25, 61, 63].

Limb salvage surgery for the treatment of sarcomas has advanced remarkably over the last 40 years. However, function recovery is often unsatisfactory and such disability may markedly interfere with the quality of life of the patients,

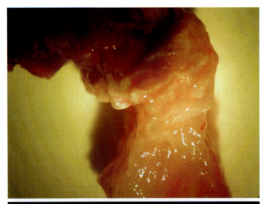

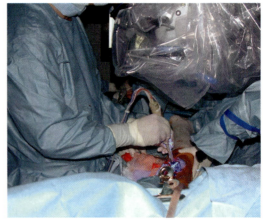

Fig. 7 Intralesional curettage under photodynamic visualization of the tumor mass (photodynamic surgery)

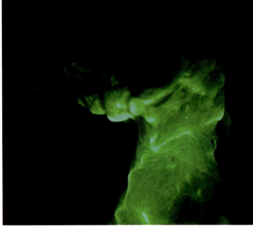

Fig. 6 Selective visualization of a leiomyosarcoma after acridine orange staining and blue light excitation, in sharp contrast to the surrounding normal tissue

especially in children and adolescents. Moreover, in some instances conservative procedures cannot be performed and either excisonal or palliative surgery are the alternative. In such instances, AO therapy (AOT), consisting of three procedures of photodynamic surgery (PDS), photodynamic therapy (PDT) and radiodynamic therapy (RDT) may provide a valuable alternative with minimal damage of normal tissues.

Under blue light excitation and exposure to AO solution, sarcoma specimens emit intense green fluorescence from the tumour area but not from the surrounding normal tissues (Fig. 6), indicating that these tumours are acid [26]. In fact, in a prospective series analyzed by using a needle type pH-meter, the pH is 6.78 was in sarcomas (n = 35), 7.16 in benign tumours (n = 27), 7.26 in normal muscle and 7.43 in normal adipose tissue. The fluorescence intensity of AO increases in a manner dependent on acidity of those tissues. Staining with AO is therefore useful to visually detect tumour localization during surgery under fluorescence operative microscope, which makes it easy for surgeons to excise only tumour tissue with minimal damage of normal tissue (Photodynamic surgery: PDS) (Fig. 7).

Interestingly, low-dose X-ray irradiation of osteosarcoma after exposure to AO has a similar strong cytocidal effect, both in vitro and in vivo [20, 41] (Radiodynamic Therapy, RDT). X-ray irradiation has an advantage of reaching deeper areas of the human body than a light beam. Indeed, AO itself also invades deeper tissues quickly at the rate of 5 mm per 30 min.

The procedure for clinical application of AOT is as follows:
1. macroscopic curettage of the tumour;
2. additional microscopic curettage with ultrasonic surgical knife under tumour visualization with green fluorescence after local administration of 1 μg/ml AO solution for 5 min, followed by excitation with blue light using fluorescence surgical microscope (PDT);
3. AO-PDS to the tumour curettage area for 10 min using the surgical microscope;
4. after closure of the surgical wound without washing-out of AO solution, 5 Gy of X-ray irradiation to the resected area for AO-RDT (Fig. 8).

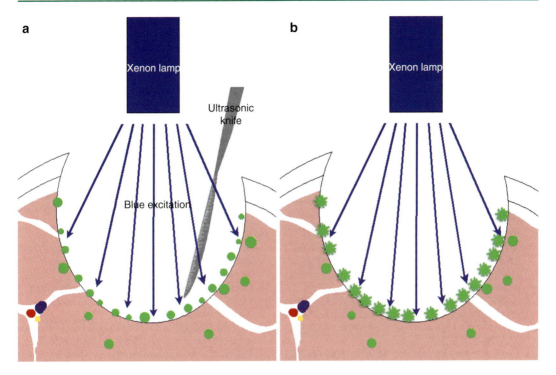

Fig. 8 Photodynamic therapy (**b**) after photodynamic surgery (**a**)

So far, AOT has been applied to a total of 67 patients with high grade malignant musculoskeletal sarcomas. The 5-year survival rate was 68 % and the 5-year local recurrence-free survival rate was 71 % in soft tissue lesions. The 5-year survival rate was 86 % and the local recurrence-free rate was 94 % in bone sarcomas. The local control rate of AO-PDT is not superior to that of conventional wide resection surgery, but the resulting limb function after surgery appear to be far superior [27, 34–36, 44] due to the possibility to limit damage to the surrounding normal tissues.

Conclusions

Progress in sarcoma treatment may only occur as a result of a continuous research effort dissecting the molecular and biochemical features underlying the clinical behaviour and the response to current therapies. The enduring impasse in the success rate of conventional treatment may only be overcome by a critical re-appraisal of the methods of investigation and the therapeutic tools. Standard in vitro culture of cancer cells does not reproduce the hypoxic, acidic conditions at the tumor site. Consistent evidence shows that sarcoma microenvironment is a complex stage where different players, including cancer cells and their stem cell component, reactive fibroblasts, and immune cells, mutually exert paracrine activities, more or less dependent on the vascular supply. A peculiar feature of these interactions is an increased acidity of the extracellular environment as a result of metabolic imbalances of cancer and reactive cells and the increased activity of proton transporters from the inside of cellular compartments. These peculiar features can be exploited for pharmacological therapies based on the inhibition of proton extrusion and the consequent selective cytotoxic effects on cancer cells and aimed at the control of systemic disease. Moreover, on the same basis, the increased acidity of tumour microenvironment can be exploited by using acridine orange photodynamic and radiodynamic therapy, combining very conservative surgery with the local cytotoxic effect of this fluorescent dye. This method has already been successfully applied for the treatment of musculoskeletal sarcomas in order to preserve a satisfactory limb function with a negligible risk of local relapse.

Acknowledgment Grant support: Ministry of Health (Grant RBAP10447J_004 to N. Baldini), Italian Association for Cancer Research (Grant 11426 to N. Baldini), IOR "5 per mille".

References

1. Andreev OA, Dupuy AD, Segala M et al (2007) Mechanism and uses of a membrane peptide that targets tumors and other acidic tissues in vivo. Proc Natl Acad Sci USA 104:7893–7898
2. Aoki J, Watanabe H, Shinozaki T (2001) FDG-PET of primary benign and malignant bone tumours: standardized uptake value in 52 lesions. Radiology 219:774–777
3. Avnet S, Sciacca L, Salerno M et al (2009) Insulin receptor isoform a and insulin-like growth factor II as additional treatment targets in human osteosarcoma. Cancer Res 69:2443–2452
4. Bacci G, Ferrari S, Longhi A et al (1988) Prognostic significance of serum LDH in Ewing's sarcoma of bone. Oncol Rep 6:807–811
5. Bacci G, Longhi A, Ferrari S et al (2004) Prognostic significance of serum lactate dehydrogenase in osteosarcoma of the extremity: experience at Rizzoli in 1421 patients treated over the last 30 years. Tumori 90:478–484
6. Baldini N, Scotlandi K, Barbanti-Brodano G et al (1995) Expression of P-glycoprotein in high-grade osteosarcomas in relation to clinical outcome. N Engl J Med 333:1380–1385
7. Bastiaannett E, Groen H, Jager PL (2004) The value of FDG-PET in the detection, grading and response to therapy of soft tissue and bone sarcomas; a systematic review and meta-analysis. Cancer Treat Rev 30:83–101
8. Bien E, Rapala M, Krazczyk M et al (2010) The serum levels of soluble interleukin-2 receptor alpha and lactate dehydrogenase but not B2-microglobulin correlate with selected clinico-pathological prognostic factors and response to therapy in childhood soft tissue sarcomas. J Cancer Res Clin Oncol 136:293–305
9. Bonuccelli G, Tisirigos A, Whitaker-Menezes D et al (2010) Ketones and lactate "fuel" tumor growth and metastasis: evidence that epithelial cancer cells use oxidative mitochondrial metabolism. Cell Cycle 9:3506–3514
10. Calcinotto A, Filipazzi P, Grioni M et al (2012) Modulation of microenvironment acidity reverses anergy in human and murine tumor-infiltrating T lymphocytes. Cancer Res 72:2746–2756
11. De Milito A, Canese R, Marinio ML et al (2010) pH-dependent antitumor activity of proton pump inhibitors against human melanoma is mediated by inhibition of tumor acidity. Int J Cancer 127:207–219
12. DeClerck K, Elble RC (2010) The role of hypoxia and acidosis in promoting metastasis and resistance to chemotherapy. Front Biosci 15:213–225
13. Engin K, Leeper DB, Cater JR et al (1995) Extracellular pH distribution in human tumours. Int J Hyperthermia 11:211–216
14. Fais S, De Milito A, You H et al (2007) Targeting vacuolar H+-ATPases as a new strategy against cancer. Cancer Res 67:10627–10630
15. Feldser D, Agani F, Iyer NV et al (1999) Reciprocal positive regulation of hypoxia-inducible factor 1alpha and insulin-like growth factor 2. Cancer Res 59:3915–3918
16. Gabrilovich DI, Nagaraj S (2009) Myeloid-derived suppressor cells as regulators of the immune system. Nat Rev Immunol 9:162–174
17. Gatenby RA, Gillies RJ (2008) A microenvironmental model of carcinogenesis. Nat Rev Cancer 8:56–61
18. Gullino PM, Grantham FH, Smith SH et al (1965) Modifications of the acid–base status of the internal milieu of tumors. J Natl Cancer Inst 34:857–869
19. Hanahan D, Coussens LM (2012) Accessories to the crime: functions of cells recruited to the tumor microenvironment. Cancer Cell 21:309–322
20. Hashiguchi S, Kusuzaki K, Murata H et al (2002) Acridine orange excited by low-dose radiation has a strong cytocidal effect on mouse osteosarcoma. Oncology 62:85–93
21. International Agency for Research on Cancer (1978) Acridine orange. In: IARC monographs program on the evaluation of carcinogenic risks to humans, vol 16. IARC Press, Lyon, p 145
22. Krähling H, Mally S, Eble JA et al (2009) The glycocalyx maintains a cell surface pH nanoenvironment crucial for integrin-mediated migration of human melanoma cells. Pflugers Arch 458:1069–1083
23. Krolenko SA, Adamyan SY, Belyaeva TN et al (2006) Acridine orange accumulation in acid organelles of normal and vacuolated frog skeletal muscle fibres. Cell Biol Int 30:933–939
24. Kusuzaki K, Aomori K, Suginoshita T et al (2000) Total tumor cell elimination with minimum damage to normal tissues in musculoskeletal sarcomas by photodynamic reaction with acridine orange. Oncology 59:174–180
25. Kusuzaki K, Minami G, Takeshita H et al (2000) Photodynamic inactivation with acridine orange on a multi-drug-resistant mouse osteosarcoma cell line. Jpn J Cancer Res 91:439–445
26. Kusuzaki K, Murata H, Matsubara T et al (2005) Clinical outcome of a new photodynamic therapy with acridine orange for synovial sarcomas. Photochem Photobiol 81:705–709

27. Kusuzaki K, Murata H, Matsubara T et al (2005) Clinical trial of photodynamic therapy using acridine orange with/without low dose radiation as new limb salvage modality in musculoskeletal sarcomas. Anticancer Res 25:1225–1236
28. Kusuzaki K, Murata H, Takeshita H et al (2000) Intracellular binding sites of acridine orange in living osteosarcoma cells. Anticancer Res 20:971–976
29. Lu X, Qin W, Li J et al (2005) The growth of metastasis of human hepatocellular carcinoma xenografts are inhibited by small interfering RNA targeting to the subunit ATP6L of proton pump. Cancer Res 65:6843–6849
30. Martinez-Outschoorn UE, Balliet RM, Rivadeneira DB et al (2010) Oxidative stress in cancer associated fibroblasts drives tumor-stroma co-evolution: a new paradigm for understanding tumor metabolism, the field effect and genomic instability in cancer cells. Cell Cycle 9:3256–3276
31. Martinez-Outschoorn UE, Lin Z, Whitaker-Menezes D et al (2010) Autophagy in cancer associated fibroblasts promotes tumor cell survival: role of hypoxia, HIF1 induction and NFkB activation in the tumor stromal microenvironment. Cell Cycle 9:3515–3533
32. Martinez-Zaguilan R, Seftor EA et al (1996) Acidic pH enhances the invasive behavior of human melanoma cells. Clin Exp Metastasis 14:176–186
33. Matsubara T, Kusuzaki K, Matsumine A et al (2006) Acridine orange used for photodynamic therapy accumulates in malignant musculoskeletal tumors depending on pH gradient. Anticancer Res 26:187–194
34. Matsubara T, Kusuzaki K, Matsumine A et al (2009) A new therapeutic modality involving acridine orange excitation by photon energy used during reduction surgery for rhabdomyosarcomas. Oncol Rep 21:89–94
35. Matsubara T, Kusuzaki K, Matsumine A et al (2010) Clinical outcomes of minimally invasive surgery using acridine orange for musculoskeletal sarcomas around the forearm, compared with conventional limb salvage surgery after wide resection. J Surg Oncol 102:271–275
36. Matsubara T, Kusuzaki K, Matsumine A et al (2010) Photodynamic therapy with acridine orange in musculoskeletal sarcomas. J Bone Joint Surg Br 92:760–762
37. McCann J, Ames BN (1976) Detection of carcinogens as mutagens in the Salmonella/microsome test: assay of 300 chemicals: discussion. Proc Natl Acad Sci USA 73:950–954
38. Mizobuchi H, Garcia-Castellano JM, Philip S et al (2008) Hypoxia markers in human osteosarcoma: an exploratory study. Clin Orthop Relat Res 466:2052–2059
39. Mohyeldin A, Garzòn-Muvdi T, Quiñones-Hinolojosa A (2010) Oxygen in stem cell biology: a critical component of the stem cell niche. Cell Stem Cell 7:150–161
40. Morimura T, Fujita K, Akita M et al (2008) The proton pump inhibitor inhibits cell growth and induces apoptosis in human hepatoblastoma. Pediatr Surg Int 24:1087–1094
41. Moussavi-Harami F, Mollano A, Martin JA et al (2006) Intrinsic radiation resistance in human chondrosarcoma. Biochem Biophys Res Commun 346:379–385
42. Murakami T, Shibuya I, Ise T et al (2001) Elevated expression of vacuolar proton pump genes and cellular pHin cisplatin resistance. Int J Cancer 93:869–874
43. Nagaraj NS, Vigneswaran N, Zacharias W (2007) Hypoxia inhibits TRAIL-induced tumor cell apoptosis: involvement of lysosomal cathepsins. Apoptosis 12:125–139
44. Nakamura T, Kusuzaki K, Matsubara T et al (2008) A new limb salvage surgery in cases of high-grade soft tissue sarcoma using photodynamic surgery, followed by photo- and radio- dynamic therapy with acridine orange. J Surg Oncol 97:523–528
45. Newell K, Franchi A, Pouyssegur J et al (1993) Studies with glycolysis-deficient cells suggest that production of lactic acid is not the only cause of tumor acidity. Proc Natl Acad Sci USA 90:1127–1131
46. Noebauer-Huhmann IM, Panotopoulos J, Kotz RI (2010) Bone tumours: work up 2009. In: Bentley G (ed) European instructional lectures, vol 10. Springer, Berlin, pp 23–36
47. Nygren P, Larsson R (2003) Overview of the clinical efficacy of investigational anticancer drugs. J Intern Med 253:46–75
48. Ocana A, Pandiella A, Siu LL et al (2011) Preclinical development of molecular-targeted agents for cancer. Nat Rev Clin Oncol 8:200–209
49. Parks SK, Chiche J, Poyssegur J (2011) pH control mechanisms of tumor survival and growth. J Cell Physiol 226:299–308
50. Pavlides S, Tsirigos A, Migneco G et al (2010) The autophagic tumor stroma model of cancer: role of oxidative stress and ketone production in fueling tumor cell metabolism. Cell Cycle 9:3485–3505
51. Pavlides S, Whitaker-Menezes D, Castello-Cros R et al (2009) The reverse Warburg effect: aerobic glycolysis in cancer associated fibroblasts and the tumor stroma. Cell Cycle 8:3984–4001
52. Rofstad EK, Mathiesen N, Kindem K et al (2006) Acidic extracellular pH promotes experimental metastasis of human melanoma cells in athymic nude mice. Cancer Res 66:6699–6707
53. Schwickert G, Walenta S, Sundfør K et al (1995) Correlation of high lactate levels in human cervical cancer with incidence of metastasis. Cancer Res 55:4757–4759
54. Swietach P, Patiar S, Supuran C et al (2009) The role of carbonic anhydrase 9 in regulating extracellular and intracellular pH in three-dimensional tumor cell growth. J Biol Chem 284:20299–20310
55. Szendröi M, Sápi Z, Karlinger K et al (2010) Diagnosis and treatment of soft tissue sarcomas. In: Bentley G

(ed) European instructional lectures, vol 10. Springer, Berlin, pp 37–50
56. Tian L, Bae YH (2012) Cancer nanomedicine targeting tumor extracellular pH. Colloids Surf B Biointerfaces 99:116–126
57. Van Duuren BL, Sivak A, Katz C et al (1969) Tumorigenicity of acridine orange. Br J Cancer 23:587–590
58. Warburg O, Posener K, Negelein E (1924) Über den Stoffwechsel der Tumoren. Biochem Zeitschrift 152:319–344
59. Warren L, Jardillier JC, Malarska A et al (1992) Increased accumulation of drugs in multidrug-resistant cells induced by liposomes. Cancer Res 52:3241–3245
60. Yang QC, Zeng BF, Dong Y et al (2007) Overexpression of hypoxia-inducible factor-1(alpha) in human osteosarcoma: correlation with clinicopathological parameters and survival outcome. Jpn J Clin Oncol 37: 127–134
61. Zdolsek JM (1993) Acridine orange-mediated photodamage to cultured cells. APMIS 101:127–132
62. Zelenin AV (1966) Fluorescence microscopy of lysosomes and related structures in living cells. Nature 212:425–426
63. Zelenin AV, Liapunova EA (1964) Inhibition of protein synthesis by acridine orange. Nature 204:45–46

Surgery for Soft Tissue Sarcomas

Rodolfo Capanna and Filippo Frenos

Introduction

Conservative surgery in soft tissue sarcomas is possible in more than 90 % of the patients. In the past amputations were sometimes performed or several tumours were removed with inadequate margins, not because the tumour was "unresectable" but because the surgeon was reluctant or unable to undertake major and often multidisciplinary reconstructive procedures that were necessary if several anatomical structures had been removed to obtain wide surgical margin. Today the increased experience with reconstructive techniques allow more aggressive surgery as well as an extension of conservative surgery and the current indications for amputation are rare. This paper is focussed mainly on surgical indications (resection vs. amputation) and provides general and specific guidelines for surgical removal and reconstructive techniques and an overall strategy for local control.

Incidence

The annual incidence of soft tissues sarcomas is low (17.5 cases per million inhabitants) with a slight predominance of male sex (57 %). The most common histotypes are: Malignant Fibrous Hystiocytome (41 %), Leiomyosarcoma (13 %), Liposarcoma (10 %) and Synovial Sarcoma (7 %). All these tumours most often affect the elderly (over 60 years), except the Synovial Sarcoma which is most common in young adults. Preferential localization is in the lower limb (63 %), followed by the upper limb (24 %) and trunk (13 %). In the extremities, proximal tumours are more frequent than distal ones (2:1 in upper and 3:1 in the lower limb). The only exception is the synovial sarcoma with more distal locations, especially at the level of hand and wrist. The location of the sarcoma is subcutaneous in 30 % of cases and deep sub-fascial in 70 % of cases. Superficial tumours have significantly lower average dimensions (about 5 cm) to those of deep-seated tumours (about 9 cm). More detailed information on epidemiology, basic science, classification, adjuvant treatment and outcome of soft tissue sarcoma may be found in the recent review of Szendroi et al. [40].

Classification and Staging

Histological classification of sarcoma of soft parts is extremely complex. There are indeed more than 400 entities separate, benign or malignant.

Sim et al. [36] proposed a classification of sarcomas in three groups:

Type I: sarcomas that can be graded histologically from low (grade 1 or 2) to high (grade 3 or 4) malignancy: Malignant Fibrous Hystiocytoma, Liposarcoma, Fibrosarcoma, Leiomyosarcoma, Neurofibrosarcoma.

R. Capanna, MD (✉) • F. Frenos, MD
Department of Orthopaedic and Traumatology,
Referring Centre for Orthopaedic Oncology and
Reconstructive Surgery, Policlinico di Careggi,
Largo Palagi 1, Florence, Italy
e-mail: rodolfo.capanna@gmail.com;
capannar@aou-careggi.toscana.it

Type II: sarcomas that cannot be graded histologically, but generally regarded as of high grade: Synovial Sarcoma, Epithelioid Sarcoma, Clear Cell Sarcoma, Alveolar Sarcoma and Mesenchymal Chondrosarcoma.

Type III: Sarcoma in small cells that cannot be graded, but considered by definition as highly malignant and very radio – and chemosensitive (Soft Tissue Ewing's Sarcoma; Rabdomyosarcome; Neuroblastoma; Small Cell Undifferentiated Sarcoma).

The staging of these neoplasms is performed according to the *Surgical Staging System of Muscolo-Skeletal Tumor Society* (Table 1), either according to the criteria of the *American Joint Committee on Cancer* for sarcomas of adult (Table 2) or child (Table 3). Recently, other systems, based on prognostic factors, have been proposed.

Table 1 Classification of muscolo-skeletal tumor society

Grade of malignancy	Anatomical compartment		
	Intra	Extra	Metastasis
I = low[a]	IA	IB	III
II = high[a]	IIA	IIB	

[a]According to the classification of Broder: low (=grade 1–2); high (=grade 3–4)

Table 2 Classification of American Joint Committee on Cancer (GTNM) for soft tissue sarcomas of the adult

Grade of malignancy (G)	Size (T)		Lymph node metastases	Metastasis
	≤5 cm	>5 cm		
I = low[a]	Ia	Ib		
II = intermed[a]	IIa	IIb	IVa[b]	IVb[b]
III = high[a]	IIIa	IIIb		

[a]According to the classification of Broder: low (=grade 1); intermediate (=grade 2); high (=grade 3–4)
[b]Any grade or tumor size

Table 3 Classification of American Joint Committee for soft tissue sarcomas of the children

Stage	Tumor	Lymph node	Metastasis
I	T1a	N0	M0
II	T1b	N0	M0
	T2a	N0	M0
	T2b	N0	M0
III	All T	N1	M0
IV	All T	N0/M1	M1

T1: tumor confined to the organ or tissue of origin (a ≤ 5 cm; b ≥ 5 cm)
T2: tumor invades adjacent organs or tissues (a ≤ 5 cm; b ≥ 5 cm)

General Prognostic Factors

Several negative prognostic factors have been highlighted: age, male sex, proximal site, deep location, tumour size, inadequate surgery, absence of radiation, presence of a local recurrence, histological aspects (grading, mitotic index, intratumoural necrosis, vascular invasion, DNA aneuploid, specific histotypes) [19, 22, 24, 33]. Later, some of these factors (male sex, advanced age, tumour histotype, absence of radiation) have not been confirmed. A multivariate analysis showed that other negative factors (proximal or deep location, adequate local treatment) were correlated with the simultaneous presence of another prognostic factor of greater importance (e.g. the size of the neoplasm). Finally, various histological prognostic factors (mitotic index, DNA aneuploid, etc.) are only a reflection of biological aggressiveness of the tumour and may be better represented by other objective parameters which are easier to analyze (tumour necrosis, vascular invasion). Currently, five factors have prognostic significance.

1. *Tumour size*: it is perhaps the more important and universally recognized factor even if there is not yet consensus on the precise value (5 or 10 cm). Of 471 operated cases, Gustafson reported a 5 years metastases-free rate of 80 % for tumours less than 5 cm, 60 % between 5 and 10 cm, 50 % between 10 and 15 cm and 40 % more than 15 cm [19].

2. *Depth*: superficial tumours (above the fascia) have better prognosis than those deeply located. Superficial tumours that invade through the fascia to deeper muscle have worse prognosis.

3. *Grading*: is an important prognostic factor, which is however considered by some as too subjective. Gustafson [19] reported a 5 years disease-free survival of 100 % for grade 1, 90 % for grade 2, 70 % for grade 3 and 50 % for grade 4. Some authors have recently replaced this parameter by others (tumour necrosis, vascular invasion).

4. *Tumour necrosis*: is an important factor. It is observed in 50 % of sarcomas of the soft parts [15]. There is no consensus on how to assess it: some authors use microscopic criteria (necrosis absent, <15 %, >15 %), other macroscopic criteria (presence or absence of a zone of necrosis of more than 4 mm in diameter) [19, 22, 24]. Five-year metastasis-free survival is 80 %, while 50 % in presence of tumour necrosis [19].
5. *Neoplastic invasion of vessels*: it is important and easily determinable. It is observed in about 26 % of cases [19]. Survival at 5 years without metastasis is 80 % in absence, while 40 % in the presence of vascular invasion [19].

Recently [33], a few new adverse prognostic parameters have been identified: high rates of urokinase plasminogen activator (an enzyme that regulates the proteolysis of the extracellular matrix) in tumour tissue, a high density of nucleolus organizer regions of the kernel (DNA segments with ribosomal genes important for mitosis), a fraction of phase S elevated, high cellular expression of nuclear antigen of cell proliferation and elevated Ki-67 (two proteins associated with the proliferative phase of the mitotic cycle) and cytogenetic abnormalities.

Prognostic Factors and Local Recurrence

Local recurrences are relatively frequent: from 6 to 30 %. Factors correlated [19, 43] with the risk of local recurrence are: greater than 10 cm tumour size (×5), spontaneous necrosis (×3), some histotypes like the Leiomyosarcoma Epithelioid Sarcoma (×3), inadequate surgical margin (×3), the absence of adjuvant irradiation (×2) and distal localization at the level of senior members (×3). Choong et al. [8] recently introduced the concept of GRI (*growth rate index*), defined by the quotient between the dimensions (in cm) of local recurrence and the number of months between the resection of the primary tumour and the discovery of local recurrence. The percentage of 2 years survival without metastasis in patients with a greater than 0.4 GRI was 80 % compared to 30 % in patients with the GRI less than 0.4. Combining the characteristics of the primary tumour (necrosis) and the GRI, Choong et al. have identified four prognostic groups [9]: the percentage of 5 years metastasis-free survival in patients without necrosis and with a <0.4 GRI was 90 %, while almost all of the patients with necrosis and a high GRI showed a negative outcome. Other authors showed correlation of surgical margins with local recurrence but not with survival [45, 47].

Prognostic Factors and Outcome

About 30–50 % of patients with high grade soft tissue sarcoma develop distant metastases. They occur in the first 3 years in 90 % of cases and involve the lung (62 %), soft tissue (10 %; particularly Liposarcoma), lymphnodes (8 %; in particular Synovial Sarcoma, Angiosarcoma and Rabdomyosarcome), skeleton (5 %) and sometimes are multiple (15 %). Metastatic risk factors are, in order of importance: tumours exceeding 10 cm (×3.5), the occurrence of local recurrences (×3.4), the presence of spontaneous necrosis (×3) and vascular (×2.2) invasion [14]. Local recurrences and metastases are the expression of the intrinsic biology of tumour: sarcomas that more easily give metastases also tend to locally recur more easily because of the likely presence of skip lesion *in situ*. Some of these parameters were chosen to select groups of patients with a poor prognosis for therapeutic purposes. A system with four parameters has been selected by the *National Cancer Institute* [18] (diameter >5 cm, local infiltration, spontaneous necrosis, high grade), and by Abbatucci et al. [1] (diameter >5 cm, infiltration, necrosis, inadequate treatment). Gustafson [18, 19] system, based on three parameters (diameter >10 cm, areas of necrosis >4 mm, vascular invasion) is particularly interesting. None or only one of these negative factors were observed in 70 % of patients with sarcoma of soft tissues. In this group of favorable prognosis, disease-free survival at 5 years was 80 %. On the other hand two or three negative factors were found in 30 % of the remaining patients: in this second group of poor prognosis, survival was only 30 %. This method has a limit: the spontaneous tumour necrosis and vascular invasion assessment requires careful examination of the tumour and it is therefore difficult in cases treated with chemo – or radiotherapy pre-operatively. For pulmonary metastases, the effectiveness of the surgical resection, which provides approximately 25 % of long term survivals, has already been demonstrated. From the study of 214 patients treated surgically for lung metastasis, Choong et al. [7] highlighted the following risk factors: diameter of metastases >2 cm, number of metastases >2, interval free <18 months. In patients without risk factor, the 5-year survival was 60 % and among those who had 1, 2 or 3 risk factors, it was 30, 20 and 0 % respectively.

Surgery of Soft Tissue Sarcoma

Anatomical Compartments and Natural Barriers

A surgical compartment is an anatomical structure bounded by natural barriers to limit tumor growth (Enneking 1980, 1983). Tumours that are confined in one compartment are "intracompartmental" while those that break a natural barrier and invade another compartment are defined as "extracompartmental". A tumour may be classified as intracompartmental (T1) and extracompartmental (T2) according site and extension. Natural barriers may be subdivided into **strong** (articular cartilage, growth-plate, cortical bone, fascia and fascial septa, joint capsule, tendons) **relative** because they are thin (periosteum, synovial membrane, sheath of major nerves -perinervium -tendon sheath) and **weak** (or at risk: bone marrow, fat and epidural space, muscle, fat and interstitial areolar tissue around neurovascular bundles, tendon and capsular insertions, areas of vascular perforations of strong natural barriers). Perhaps only the joint cartilage is a reliable barrier because it has no vascular perforations and probably has an intrinsic resistance to tumour. Anyway an intra-articular soft tissue sarcoma may invade the bone growing along epiphyseal insertion of the capsule, ligaments, or synovial membrane or after a joint fracture. Ulceration and consequent bleeding of the synovial membrane may produce also a haemarthrosis containing tumour cells and consequent joint contamination. Epiphyseal and metaphyseal areas are at risk for tumour erosion, the cortex being very thin with several vascular perforations at this level. Cortical bone, fascia and fascial septa are considered strong barriers and they really are: however they may also be invaded through their vascular perforations.

Excision and Surgical Margins

Surgery is the treatment of choice for soft-tissue sarcomas. Either in conservative resections or amputations, surgical margins are evaluated according to the classification of the Musculo-Skeletal Tumour Society and are divided into radical, wide, marginal and intralesional.

Radical surgery consist of an total en block neoplasm ablation with removal from proximal to distal insertion of all compartmental muscles dissecting outside the compartmental boundaries (i.e. removal of the entire quadriceps, fascia and both medial and lateral fascial septa and periosteum for tumour included in the anterior thigh compartment). This procedure has low risk of local recurrence (2 %) and it does not require further loco-regional adjuvant treatment to improve local control [34]. However it often requires advanced surgical reconstructions (free flaps, megaprosthesis, motor unit transplant, nerve or vascular grafts etc.) to recover a functional limb.

Wide surgery is an en block tumour removal surrounded by a layer of a healthy, non-reactive tissue, dissecting inside the anatomical compartmental boundaries. It is not yet determined what the ideal thickness of muscle coverage is to define a "wide" margin. If a limited amount of healthy tissue (2/3 mm) covering the pseudocapsule ("minimal wide") may be sufficient to prevent residual tumour at this level, of course this may prove to be totally inadequate to prevent local recurrence from skip metastases. However the incidence of skip lesion in high and low grade sarcoma, as well their average (and maximal) distance from main tumour mass are still unknown. A cuff of 2 cm of normal muscle is usually accepted as a satisfactory "wide" margin. Kawaguchi et al. [21] has divided this type of margins according to the thickness and quality of the removed tissue. Quality of the margin is more important than quantity: 1 mm. of fascial layer is more effective than 2 cm of muscle or fat. This doubt regarding the accuracy of surgical removal of residual skip lesions is the rationale for adjuvant radiation therapy. The procedure can leave skip lesions on-site, especially in high grade sarcomas: the risk of local recurrence is about 15–30 %. Radiotherapy (pre-, intra-, or post-operative) may decrease the local recurrence rate to 9–18 %.

Marginal surgery (with a plane of dissection in contact with the tumour pseudocapsule) leaves behind satellite tumour (skip lesions) and the peritumour capsule in which neoplastic cells can be disseminated. The procedure may be adopted in benign lesions. This enucleation (shell out technique) should be rejected in high grade tumours because it risks a high percentage of local recurrences (40–60 %) [19, 37]. It is only in selected cases that we can intentionally accept marginal margins of resection for limited extension and, usually, in an attempt to save major neuro-vascular structures. In these cases, the dissection must include vascular adventitia and the perinervium. In the body there are several areas (axilla, elbow, hand, groin, popliteal fossa, foot, peri-articular areas) that have not clear and effective fascial boundaries and are crossed by major neuro-vascular structures (so call extra-compartmental sites). In these instances a general opinion is that any conservative surgery results automatically in marginal (or even less) procedures and thus a wide amputation is suggested as treatment of choice in case of high grade sarcoma located in these areas. Even in these areas, in untouched patients, it is possible to achieve wide surgical margins and perform a conservative procedures but the surgeon should be prepared to perform very aggressive surgery and multiple, difficult reconstructions.

Intralesional surgery means an intratumoural dissection that is unacceptable leaving macroscopic residual areas of disease and exposing to a high rate of local recurrence (90 %), both in benign and malignant tumour even after post-operative radiation therapy (60 %).

Any excision that incidentally resulted in marginal or intralesional procedures should be re-operated (radicalization) if better margins can be achieved without jeopardizing the final functional outcome. Surgery is also judged by its closest margin (for instance a wide resection that shows an exposed pseudocapsule – even in a limited area- will be defined as marginal). Any of the previous procedures are considered "**contaminated**" if the surgeon inadvertently enters the lesion (even for a limited zone and even if subsequently is able to widen the margins in normal tissue).

Surgical Planning and Techniques

General Concepts

Ten fundamental rules should be respected in order to properly treat soft tissue sarcomas:

1. **Concept of "custom-made" "preoperative planning"**. Plan mentally the tri-dimensional configuration of the tumour (based on pre-operative work-up), select the more appropriate plane of dissection and draw it on a printed MRI image. Doing this planning takes into account prognostic factors for local recurrence.
2. **Concept of "custom-made" resection**. Be more generous in muscle removal around areas of higher contrast medium uptake in MRI or PET scan, particularly in patient who had pre-operative treatment because possible residual areas of living chemo/radio-resistant cells [27].
3. **Strategy of "surgical barriers"**. If you cannot improve the quantity of your surgical margins try to improve the quality, including in the specimen effective anatomical barriers (bone cortex, periosteum, fascia, capsule joint, tendons and ligaments, tendon sheath, perinervium).
4. **Concept of "custom-made" reconstruction**. Based on the planned resection, establish the appropriate reconstruction to maximize the functional results.

5. **Strategy of widest excision for same function**. When dealing with "expendable" tissues not included in any compartmental barrier (muscle, fat) try to maximize the amount of tissue removed around the tumour, that still allows the same selected reconstructive procedure or the same planned functional outcome. If excision of a tumour located in the centre of rectus femuris requires its interruption, it is preferable to remove the muscle from insertion to insertion (giving the same functional outcome but potential better control of skip lesion).
6. **"Feeling" technique**. Try not to expose the tumour pseudocapsule and feel tumour edges only by gentle palpation, avoiding excessive traction that may break the pseudocapsule allowing spillage of tumour (particularly if mucoid, mixoid or colliquated areas are present) ending in a contaminated procedure.
7. **Flexibility**. Promptly change plane of dissection and increase your surgical margins if the reactive-degenerated-oedematous area around the tumour is visualized or entered.
8. **"Doubt"resolution**. If you have any doubt on the type of tissue (normal, reactive, pathological) you are crossing, make histological evaluation by frozen section.
9. **"Double check" control**. At the end of the excision and before the reconstruction, make multiple frozen sections to check intra-operatively surgical margins. If inadequate try to improve them; if impossible mark the areas at risk with metallic clips to better address post-operative radiotherapy.
10. **Pluridisciplinary approach**. If a more extensive resection than it was planned is required, the surgeon should be prepared intra-operatively to modify or switch to a different reconstructive method and a pluridisciplinary team should be available (general surgeon, vascular surgeon, microsurgical team).

These rules are fundamental when:
1. the tumour is of high grade malignancy;
2. shows a permeative growth pattern;
3. is known to have frequent occult and extracapsular extension (Ewing's sarcoma, osteosarcoma, malignant fibrous hystiocytoma, leiomyosarcoma);
4. a poor response to pre-operative treatment is observed.
5. it is located in extracompartmental sites or in contact with viscera or major neurovascular bundles.

How to Deal with Single Tissues

Skin

In superficial sarcoma, all the skin overlying the tumour as well the surrounding red, oedematous area with congested superficial vessels has to be removed with a peripheral margin of at least 2.5 cm of normal-looking skin. The extension of the inflammatory area, the pathological network of superficial vessels and the extension of superficial oedema is better evaluated in the MRI. Pre-operative evaluation with echography may be helpful to identify and to mark over the skin unexpected areas or skip lesion to be included in the specimen. The fascia is transected immediately under the skin section and sutured to the skin edges. The dissection is then extended below the deep surface of the fascia (used as an effective barrier) cutting the muscular fibres here attached at 1 cm.

In deeply-located sarcoma, the dissection should include the biopsy tract and scar from previous surgery, removing a wide elliptical area of normal skin around it. The subcutaneous tissue may be split outwards in an oblique way and removed more widely than the overlying skin (technique of oblique section). If necessary the dissection may be extended faraway between the subcutaneous tissue and fascia, subtotally or totally removing the fascia. Then the fascia is transected leaving this structure as an effective anatomical barrier covering the tumour. Although oncologically effective, this approach may impair the blood supply of the cutaneous flap with a higher incidence of wound complications: thus it is recommended only for selected tumours protruding prominently under the skin.

In large superficial soft tissue tumours or after erroneous biopsies or surgical approaches (with multiple, parallel or even transverse incisions or displaced drainage tracts) the extensive skin loss may prevent primary closure. In these cases if the surgical bed is just represented by muscle, no reconstruction is required, the skin edges are simply sutured onto the muscle and repaired in a second step (usually after 2–3 weeks) with the Thiersch technique. Sometimes the same techniques used after conventional fasciotomy (crossed streams) or the VAC system are applied to save time. If in the surgical bed important structures (bone, vessels, nerve or implants) are exposed a coverage flap is requested. Often the problem may be solved with local pedicled fascio-cutaneous or muscle flaps; sometimes a free microvascular cutaneous or musculo-cutaneous transplant is required. Selection of the flap is made according to the size of the gap, location, weight-bearing situation, structures to be covered, the need for post-operative radiation therapy. Fascio-cutaneous rotational local flaps are preferred by plastic surgeons because they are more cosmetic, faster, and have no need of micro-anastomoses (and its complications). However these are less favoured by the Orthopaedic Oncologist because they are usually limited in size (which is a potential psychological bias limiting the aggressiveness of the surgery) and, in case of local recurrence, the local area considered as a "contaminated" field is widely increased. In cases of exposure of implants (prostheses or bone transplants) musculo-cutaneous flaps (free or peduncolated) afford better protection against infection. In patients requiring simultaneous repair of skin and vessel by-pass, the Chinese forearm free flap may be a good option. In patients in which repair of skin and simultaneous recovery of muscle function is required, motor unit transplantation plus Thiersch technique may be a solution. In soft tissue sarcoma widely involving a foot or a long bone (tibia. radius, ulna, humerus) and the overlying skin, a free osteocutaneus microvascular fibular or iliac crest transplant can solve both problems. When a free flap is planned a long pedicle should be taken in order to place the anastomosis distant from the edges of the planned post-operative irradiation field. Furthermore, if brachytherapy is used, the micro-anastomosis should be at least 3 cm away from the catheter for brachytherapy. Moreover brachytherapy should start 14 days (instead of 7 days) after surgery in order to allow normal healing of the anastomosis. When a reconstructive muscular free flap, nerve graft, or vessels by-pass is planned, pre-operative instead of post-operative radiotherapy is preferred in order to not damage the grafted tissue (see strategy).

Muscle

Tumour located within a muscle is excised with the surrounding reactive and oedematous zone plus a cuff of normal muscle around it -ideally 2 cm- (intramuscular wide excision). When the tumour arises in an expandable muscle or it involves the full muscle belly, a longitudinal en block excision (total myectomy) with removal of its fascial coverage is the treatment of choice. If the tumour on the contrary is located in the interfascial areolar tissue between several muscles the surgical margins often are marginal or minimally wide (the surrounding cuff being of areolar fat tissue and of a few mm. width). In these cases the quality of margins may be increased if the dissection removes also the fascia and a small amount of adjacent peripheral muscles (extramuscolar wide excision) (Table 4). In the first three clinical settings (intramuscular wide excision, total myectomy, and extramuscular wide resection of an expendable muscle) reconstruction is not required (Tables 5 and 6). In huge tumours sometimes a

Table 4 Intra-extra compartment according to Enneking-MSTS classification

Intracompartmental (T1)	Extracompartmental (T2)
Intraosseous	*Soft tissue extension*
Intra-articular	*Soft tissue extension*
Superficial to fascia	*Deep extension to fascia*
Para-osseous	*Intra-osseous or extrafascial extension*
Intrafascial compartments	*Extrafascial planes or spaces*
Ray of hand or foot	Midfoot and hindfoot
Sura	Popliteal space
Anterolateral leg	Inguino-femoral triangle
Anterior thigh	Intrapelvic
Medial thigh	Midhand
Posterior thigh	Antecubital fossa
Buttock	Axilla
Anterior forearm	Periclavicular
Posterior forearm	Paraspinal
Anterior arm	Head and neck
Posterior arm	
Periscapular	

Table 5 Expendable muscles of upper limb

Expendable muscle upper limb	Function afforded by
Pectoralis major	Minor disability
Dorsalis major	" "
Deltoid	Rotator cuff if intact
Elbow flexors (biceps)	If epitroclear muscle saved
Triceps	Extension provided by gravity
Epitroclear superficial flexor muscles	Function by flexors deep layer

Table 6 Expendable muscle of lower limb

Expendable muscle lower limb	Function afforded by
Gluteus medius and minor	Gluteus maximus
Gluteus maximus	Trendelenburg only
Ileo-psoas	Abdominal muscle
Rectus femoris	Remaining quadriceps
Vastus medialis and intermedius	Remaining vastus lateralis
Vastus lateralis and intermedius	Remaining vastus medialis
Adductors	Minor disability
Medial or lateral Knee flexors	Compensation by gastrocnemius activity
Medial or lateral gastrocnemius	If soleus intact
Soleus	If gastrocnemius intact
Tibialis posterior	Minor disability
Peroneal muscle	Minor disability
Tibialis anterior	Orthosis

complete removal of a major muscle or a radical excision of an entire compartment is required. In this situation and in selected patients reconstruction is required using a tendon transfer technique, or a motor unit transplantation has to be considered. After a radical resection of a muscle, its function can be restored by transplantation of a motor unit. The dorsalis muscle may be detached from the trunk and rotated 180° on his nervous and vascular pedicle (technique of Ito) to restore elther deltoid or biceps or triceps function according to the new given position (anterior, lateral, or posterior). The quadriceps, the sural triceps or the gluteus maximus may be also reconstructed by microsurgical transplantation of the greater dorsalis with neurorraphy of its motor branch on a terminal branch of the femoral nerve or posterior tibial nerve or superior/inferior gluteal nerve. The Group of muscles (flexor or extensor) of the wrist and the hand may be replaced by transplantation of gracilis muscle with neurorraphy on the median nerve (or the motor branch of the radial nerve). Reconstructive techniques that we use most frequently are summarized in Tables 7 and 8.

Adjacent Bone

If a soft tissue tumour is adjacent to a bone, a decision should be taken whether the latter has to be removed en bloc with the lesion or not (Fig. 1). The following criteria are useful:
1. if the mass is clinically freely movable over the underlying cortex separated by a layer of normal muscle and the imaging studies are negatives, no bone removal is required and periosteum may be saved;
2. if the tumour is clinically fixed but bone scan and imaging studies are still negative, en bloc removal with periosteal stripping is recommended. When an extensive stripping of the periosteum is performed, there is an increased risk of pathological fracture particularly if adjuvant radiation therapy is scheduled as part of the treatment: Helmstadter et al. 1998 reported no pathological fracture in the absence of periosteal stripping, 9 % in limited extension (<20 cm), and 36 % in extended (>20 cm) stripping. In this case a prophylactic osteosynthesis should be considered; however still now there is not a consensus whether to use an intramedullary rod or a plate with angular stability.
3. if an increased isotope uptake of the adjacent bone is observed without cortical changes on C.T. scan examination, a partial tangential removal of the bony shaft is required, the periosteum being involved in the tumoral pseudocapsule. In this case bone grafting procedures with internal osteosynthesis are necessary to avoid fracture.
4. if the bone scan uptake is associated with periosteal reaction, superficial cortical erosion, oedema inside the medullary canal or a skip intramedullary lesion a complete segmental en bloc removal of the bone is required. Periosteal reaction and cortical erosion are best assessed by C.T. scan, while medullary oedema or intramedullary skip lesions by M.R.I.

Table 7 Reconstruction after soft tissue sarcoma excision: upper extremities

Deltoid	Total myectomy	Rotational flap of dorsalis major on its neuro-vascular bundle (Ito technique)
	Deltoid and rotator cuff	Scapulo-Humeral arthrodesis
Periscapular muscle and scapula	Radical excision+scapulectomy…(rotator cuff present)	Prosthesis "inversa" with massive scapular allograft. The affected scapula, if intact, may be re-implanted after freezing, autoclaving or irradiation
	+ scapulectomy…(rotator cuff absent) or scapular Tikhof Linberg	Scapular suspended to the clavicle
Axillary space+plexus+ vessels	Forequarter amputation	None
	+ rib resection	Marlex mash+cement
	+ skin	Free microvascular fascio-cutaneous or muscular flap taken from the amputated leg
Anterior arm	Removal of biceps+brachialis anterior	None (epitroclear and epicondilar muscle may allow active elbow flexion) anterior transfer dorsalis major (Ito technique) for heavy worker
	+ humeral vessels	By-pass
	+ median or ulnar nerve	Nerve grafting (young/no or pre-op.Rxtherapy) tendon transposition (elderly/post-op.Rxtherapy)
	+ bone	Massive allograft or Masquelet technique or vascularized fibula
Elbow	Large skin removal	Free or peduncolatedi skin flap (Chinese anterior forearm)
	Extra-articular elbow resection	Total elbow massive allograft or composite allo- prosthesis (±dorsalis major myocutaneous flap)
Anterior forearm	Large skin removal (only)	Thiersh technique
	Large skin+epitroclear (superficial flexor) muscle	Wrist tendon transposition (extensor pro flexor)+counter lateral free transfer (Chinese anterior forearm)
	Large skin+superficial and deep flexor muscles	Motor unit transfer (gracilis pro flexors digitalis longus)+tendon transfer (extensor radialis longus carpi pro flexor longus pollicis+extensor ulnaris to flexor ulnaris carpi or wrist arthrodesis in heavy worker)
	+ median and/or ulnar nerve	Autogenous nerve grafting
	+ radial and/or ulnar artery	None if one artery saved and hand anasthomosis present microsurgical by-pass of at least one artery if both resected with hand anasthomosis present (otherwise double by-pass is required). If a Chinese free flap from counterlateral fore arm is done, the radial artery may be used as by-pass.
	+ bone (either radius or ulna)	Masquelet technique or vascularised fibula (the peroneal artery may be used as by-pass
Dorsal forearm	Total excision of extensor muscle (finger and wrist)	Classical tendon transposition (flexor pro extensor)±wrist arthrodesis (elderly/post-op.Rxtherapy/heavy worker)
	+ skin	Peduncolated Chinese flap from anterior forearm or motor unit transfer (gracilis pro extensor)+Thiersh (young/preop. Rxtherapy)
	+ bone (either radius or ulna)	see before
Palmar wrist and hand	Skin	Axial inverted local flap (radial, interosseous posterior, ulnaris)
	+ ulnar or median nerve	Nerve autogenous grafting
	+ flexor tendons	Tendon grafting or transposition
	+ extra-articular wrist resection	Distal radius allograft arthroplasty or wrist arthrodesis with vascular fibula (if osteocutaneous contemporary treatment of skin loss; peroneal as by-pass) artery may serve
	Interdigitorum space	Longitudinal amputation
Dorsal wrist and hand	Skin and extensor tendons	Free flap dorsalis pedis or free flap fascio-cutaneous lateralis brachii or inverted radial local flap plus tendon transfer (flexors digitorum superficial is on extensor digitorum)
Thumb	Amputation	Transposition two or three finger to thumb or WAF microsurgical transfer

Table 8 Reconstruction after soft tissue sarcoma excision: lower extremities

Buttocks	Medius and minimal gluteus	None (slight trendelemburg)
	Gluteus maximus	None (moderate trendelemburg)
	All glutei	None (severe trendelemburg) or motor unit transplant (dorsalis major on gluteal nerve)
	+ Iliac wing	Allograft or the affected ilium may be re-implanted after freezing, autoclaving or irradiation
	Extra-articular hip resection	Arthrodesis with intercalary allograft and delayed lengthening (child) massive pelvic allograft + megaprosthesis
Quadriceps	Rectus femoris or sartorius	None
	Vastus lateralis (VL) + intermedius	None or biceps transfer pro VL
	Vastus medialis (VM) + intermedius	None or sartorius transfer pro VM
	Total quadriceps	Motor unit transplant (dorsalis major on femoral nerve)
	Femoral vessels	By-pass
	Femur	Massive allograft or Masquelet technique (diaphysis) megaprosthesis (proximal or distal femur) cemented
Adductors	Total removal	None (minor deficit)
Posterior thigh	Removal medial and lateral flexors	None (moderate deficit) active flexion provided by gastrocnemii
	Sciatic nerve	Salvaged if possible using perineural dissection resection and orthosis or autogenous grafting (partial) or nerve frozen allograft grafting (experimental) or foot tendon transposition
Periarticular knee	Large skin removal	Rotational pedicled gastrocnemius flaps or free flap Dorsalis major to cover major reconstruction
	Extensor apparatus removal	Both rotated gastrocnemii or fascia lata allograft or transplant of the entire extensor apparatus
	Periarticular medial or lateral condyle or	Hemi-articular femoral allograft
	medial or lateral plateau	Hemi-articular tibial allograft
	Extraarticular knee removal	Allograft arthrodesis or distal femur megaprosthesis + proximal tibia composite prosthesis with the entire quadriceps mechanism
Popliteal fossa	Large skin	Rotated gastrocnemius flap or free dorsalis major miocutaneous flap
	+ popliteal vessels	By-pass
	+ nerve (SPE and SPI)	Salvaged (perineural dissection) no reconstruction resected: orthosis or autogenous grafting (partial) or nerve frozen allograft grafting (experimental) or foot tendon transposition.
Anterolateral leg compartment	Skin removal	Free flap
	Bone removal (diaphysis)	Masquelet or vascularized fibula.
	Radical compartmental muscle removal	Transfer tibialis posterior to tibialis anterior or ankle arthrodesis
	Skin + muscle	Motor unit transplantation (dorsalis major pro extensors to SPE)
Posterior leg compartment	Gastrocnemius	None if soleus present
	Soleus	None if gastrocnemius present
	Skin + distal Achille's tendon	Free flap + tendon reconstruction with fascia lata or artificial ligament
	Total triceps removal ± skin	Transposition peroneous longus and tibialis posterior to calcaneous or free flap of coverage (dorsalis major) plus ankle arthrodesis or motor unit transplant (dorsalis major).
Ankle joint	Extra-articular ankle resection ± skin	Ankle arthrodesis (Masquelet or vascularised fibula) ± free flap
Dorsal foot	En block resection skin, tendons and bone	Free flap dorsalis major or antero-lateral of thigh + tendon graft for tibialis anterior
Plantar foot	En block resection skin, tendons and bone	Free flap dorsalis major or antero-lateral of thigh

Surgery for Soft Tissue Sarcomas

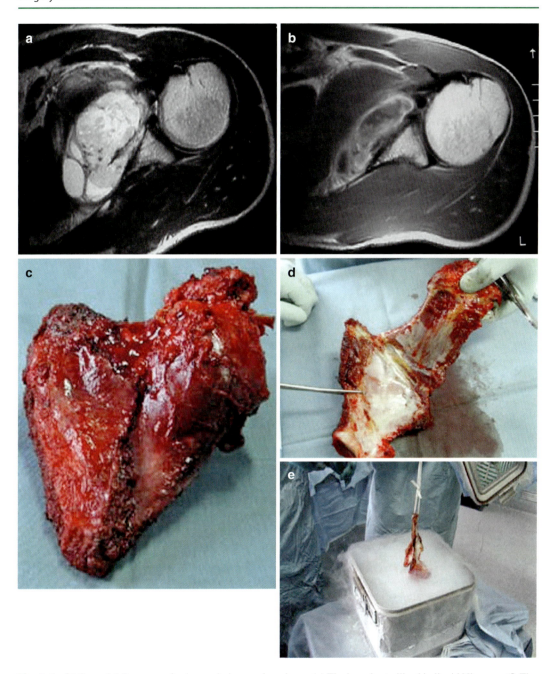

Fig. 1 (**a**, **b**) Synovial Sarcoma of subscapularis muscle attached to the bone. A shrinkage is observed after chemotherapy. (**c**) The subscapularis muscle was resected en bloc with the scapula. (**d**) The tumour is removed from the bone. (**e**) The bone is sterilized in liquid Nitrogen. (**f**) The scapula was re-implanted. (**g**) Xray result. (**h**) Clinical and functional result

5. finally, even if all others studies (X-rays, C.T., M.R.I.) are negative, an en bloc removal of the entire bone is also required when the tumour surrounds the shaft completely. Patients with segmental resection may require reconstruction with a conventional megaprosthesis or a composite allo-prosthesis for better soft tissue anchorage in case of peri-articular lesion. If the resected bone is not destroyed by the tumour, it may be cleaned on a separate table and re-implanted (usually as a composite prosthesis) after an adequate "tumour cell

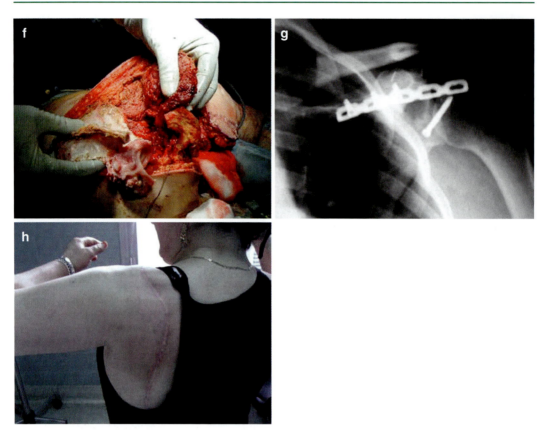

Fig. 1 (continued)

sterilization". Our preferred method is the freezing–thawing technique by immersion three times in liquid nitrogen. This method:

(a) better preserves the biomechanical properties of the bone and tendon structures because there is less damage to the collagen fibres compared with autoclaving and/or irradiation techniques,

(b) it is faster (30 min) in preparation compared with alcohol treatment (36 h) and

(c) it is more practical than irradiation. Because with radiation therapy (either pre, intra, or post-operative) the prosthesis always needs cementing.

Vessels

Pre-operatively echo-doppler, or angio-CT or -M.R.I. should be used to assess involvement of major vessels. When a by-pass is scheduled, the classical angiography, although more invasive, is still requested to better evaluate size of vessels and site of anastomosis. Sometime a popliteal mass investigated by CT or MRI with the leg in full extension may give a false impression of vessels compression (in this case further studies with the leg in lateral position and in flexion or dynamic Doppler are needed) When a deep vessel by-pass is planned, great care should be taken in preserving the superficial major vein and peripheral circle while performing skin incision and tumour approach.

If the vessels are compressed by the tumour, these should be identified proximally and/or distally and prepared over a vase loop. The vessels then are gently retracted ligating the collateral branches. If a "blunt dissection" is feasible the vessels may be retained and isolated from proximally to distally. When the artery is free but dissection of the major vein is troublesome, or tumour clots within collateral vein branches are observed, the latter can be removed without need for reconstruction if the superficial circulation is preserved.

However when the vascular adventitia is involved with the tumour pseudocapsule, dissociation is difficult and a "sharp dissection" using scissors will be required: in such instance the vessels have to be resected en bloc. When performing a vessels by-pass several authors suggest reconstructing only the artery, because the vein is often rapidly obstructed by thrombus: in our opinion it is best to reconstruct both (artery and vein) for the beneficial (although temporary) effect of the venous by-pass decreasing resistance to blood circulation in the immediate and more critical post-operative period. We prefer biological reconstruction (saphenous vein autograft): artificial prostheses are used only in case of post-operative radiation therapy for their supposed better resistance to shrinkage of irradiated connective tissues [35]. In the past the success rate of conventional by-pass distally to the elbow or the knee was discouraging. Recently good results on by-pass of very peripheral vessels have been obtained using more accurate microsurgical techniques.

Viscera

The same criteria ("blunt" versus "sharp" dissection) is used to decide intra-operatively if to remove en bloc with the tumour, a segment of an adjacent adherent viscera (for instance bladder or bowel in pelvic tumour).

Neoplastic Thrombi in the Venous Branches

Fortunately this rarely occurs, usually when large tumours are pushing or compressing the main vascular bundle. Unfortunately, such an event is rarely detected pre-operatively even with the most advanced imaging techniques, particularly if major vessels are not involved and the phenomenon is limited to the peripheral branches. A wide area of oedema or contrast medium uptake surrounding the tumour ("inflammatory area") in MRI or PET investigation is worrisome. The suspicion of clotted vessels (hard in consistency, when ligating or cutting) should warn the surgeon and a frozen section is mandatory. Neoplastic thrombi clotting venous branches running from the tumour and confluent into the major vessels sometimes produce an obstruction extending for a long distance within the principal vein. If neoplastic thrombi are confirmed, a wider dissection (possibly with major vessel removal) or an amputation should be considered instead of relying on post-operative adjuvant treatment (chemo-radiation therapy).

Nerves

Nerve compression and dislocation is often observed but rarely does the nerve have strong adherence with the pseudocapsule of a sarcoma. Paradoxically this situation is more often observed in dysplastic lesions (fibromatosis, myositis ossificans). The epineurium is considered an effective anatomical barrier, although thin, to tumour infiltration. For this reason the nerve is usually approached and exposed proximally (where the anatomy is normal) and the epineurium is longitudinally split and peeled off, extracting the nerve. The epineurium covering the surface of the lesion is removed en bloc with the tumour. This is easy to perform in an untouched lesion but may be difficult or impossible in recurrent tumours when post-surgical or post-irradiation scar tissue and fibrosis surround the nerve and/or a previous neurolysis has been done.

When the nerve is not lying over the exposed surface of the tumour but it is deeply displaced and not visible to the surgeon, it is recommended to detect and gently retract the nerve both proximally and distally (in normal anatomical areas). Then the muscles enveloping the tumour are cut again proximally and distally at a safe level: thus the surgical specimen becomes freely movable and, rotating it 180°, it is possible to expose the nerve with its tumour-free surface facing the surgeon. The neurolysis is then easy performed as previously described.

If the nerve, instead, is completely surrounded by the tumour, or involved, a segmental nerve resection should be considered. When major or multiple nerve sacrifice are required the expected functional results of limb salvage versus amputation should be compared taking also in account of the different oncological safety of the two surgical procedures. This may push the surgeon towards a much more conservative approach in the upper than in lower extremities. However even sciatic nerve involvement it is not any more considered an absolute indication for amputation. The patient with complete nerve sciatic palsy may have a paralysed foot but still keep active knee motion, he may stabilize the ankle with an external orthotic device or an arthrodesis while the major complaint is the lack of sensibility and trophic complications. The functional loss of a major nerve may be compensated by several reconstructive methods such as: autogenous or homologous nerve grafting, motor unit transplantation, tendon transfers, joint arthrodesis or their combination. The choice is made according to the age of the patient, the anatomical location, the entity of muscle removal, the size of the nerve, the length of the gap, the number of nerves involved and finally the need for further adjuvant treatment.

Autogenous nerve grafts are chosen as a reconstructive method at young ages (faster recovery), usually when only one nerve and a short gap repair is required and no postoperative radiation therapy is scheduled. Before cutting the nerve it may be useful to map by electrical stimulation the nerve in order to recognize motor and sensitive fibres: this will help in selecting priorities on grafting (often limited availability of autogenous grafts allows only partial anatomical restoration in extensive resection of major nerves) and thus greatly improve accuracy and quality of reconstruction. Functional loss of the radial nerve may be also repaired by classical tendon transposition (flexors-to- extensors sometimes combined with a wrist arthrodesis) that seems to be adequate or even preferable particularly in the elderly or when radiotherapy is applied. On the contrary, when feasible, it is preferable to reconstruct always the median and the ulnar nerve because tendon transfer (extensor-to-flexors) is a less effective procedure, with permanent impairment of intrinsic hand muscles. It is possible to repair both nerves of the forearm (median and ulnar nerve) for a gap of 10 cm using a bilateral autogenous saphenous nerve transplant; if reconstruction of both nerves is impossible, the preference is for the ulnar nerve for its prevalent role in hand control. Sacrifice of SPE may be occasionally repaired by nerve grafting; more often the foot is stabilized by a tenodesis of the tibialis anterior, or an anterior transfer of the tibialis posterior through the interosseous membrane or an ankle arthrodesis or, more simply, with an external orthosis. Sacrifice of SPI is often left unrepaired. In case of major nerve resection (sciatic trunk, brachial plexus, multiple removals) often no or only partial reconstruction are feasible. Recently there is an increasing interest in homologous cryopreserved major nerve grafting procedures but these are still experimental procedures. When a major nerve and its muscle group is en bloc resected, a transplant motor unit should be considered.

Joint Invasion

Joint invasion by a peri-articular soft tissue tumour is a quite rare event. Sometimes this is related to a jatrogenic complication such as misdiagnosis (bursitis, infection, peri-articular haematoma) and erroneous procedures (infiltration, surgical debridement, incorrect biopsy tract). Moreover the surgeon should aware that some tumours (such as synovial sarcoma) may occasionally arise inside a joint. When an intra-articular bump is suspected, an accurate pre-operative MRI examination with contrast medium should be done in order to study densitometric aspects and vascularity of the lesion: in case of suspicion, a pre-operative PET scan is recommended. When a doubtful malignancy is present any arthroscopic investigation should be avoided and a conventional (minimally-open) incisional biopsy or, even better, a echo or CT-guided needle biopsy has to be done in order to decrease joint space contamination.

In case of joint involvement, it is necessary to perform an extra-articular resection. A real extra-articular resection is obtained when:
1. the joint space is removed en block with its capsular and ligament structures left intact and synovial pouches left closed;

2. the two articular bone extremities are transected leaving capsular and synovial insertions attached to the surgical specimen;
3. any articular hiatus is removed closed. When a joint is removed restoration may be achieved by massive allograft, megaprostheses or their combination (composite prostheses). Arthrodesis with allo- or autograft are still preferred in particular sites (ankle.) or used when hard work is expected (wrist) or in children (hip, shoulder, knee) as intercalary graft after extra-articular resection. An osteo-articular allograft of the entire joint is used in elbow, wrist or scapula The hip may be reconstructed with a pelvic allograft and a proximal femur megaprosthesis. A mobile knee can be expected using a distal femur megaprosthesis and a composite proximal tibial prosthesis with its full extensor apparatus.

Skip Lesions

Separated nodules from the main tumour mass may be observed usually inside the same anatomical muscular compartment. More rarely these skip lesions are in the adjacent bone, or inside the joint (in peri-articular tumours) or outside the joint (for intra-articular ones): it seems that this extension happens through vascular perforation of the cortical bone or joint capsule. MRI or PET scan may be useful in their detection. These lesion should be en bloc included in the resected specimen. In these patients the prognosis become worse both for local and distal control.

Amputation

Major criteria for amputation are:
1. A patient whose precarious general status does not allow complex interventions.
2. Simultaneous involvement of multiple nervous and vascular structures, whose removal would result in a functionless extremity even after repair (i.e. sarcomas massively involving the axillary or brachial plexus and the vascular axis). In selected cases, some authors proposed amputations-resection with proximal replantation of the member or rotationplasty.
3. Sarcomas with multiple skip lesions or local recurrence along the extremity. In such cases, no conservative intervention with removal of all apparent injuries would ensure adequate margins because of the micro-dissemination in evolution.

Minor (and now questionable) criteria for amputation are:
1. Extra-compartmental sarcomas (hand, foot, wrist, ankle, elbow, knee). Formerly, these sites represented an absolute indication for ablative surgery because in theory it was considered impossible to achieve wide surgical margins in these location having no natural anatomical barriers. Currently, a more aggressive surgical approach, with en bloc resection of all structures (from the skin surface, deep to the bone surface, through the muscular-tendon plane) and reconstruction at the same time of the most important functional structures. This requires that several, previously described, reconstructive techniques are used and combined in a "tailor-made" eclectic combination to achieve an effective limb salvage without jeopardize oncological results.
2. Sarcomas with massive involvement of several compartments. Ablative surgery should be recommended when neo-adjuvant local treatments for tumour control and shrinkage (pre-operative radio and/or chemo-therapy, extracorporeal perfusion with necrotizing agents with or without hyperthermia) have failed. Often, these treatments provide a total or partial mass reduction allowing conservative surgery in 80–90 % of cases.
3. Patients in whom biopsy massively contaminated or infected the compartment. The risks of improperly performed biopsy have been well demonstrated in a multi-centre study of Mankin et al. [25]: 18 % of diagnostic errors, 19 % of complications after treatment of the tumour, 10 % of poor results and 3 % of amputations, which could have been avoided. To avoid such risks, we recommend needle biopsy (under ultrasound or CT guidance) or intra-operative biopsy.

Surgical Radicalization

One dilemma is the strategy to adopt in patients after a marginal or intralesional excision performed improperly for diagnostic purposes in absence of a detectable local recurrence. Currently, there is a unanimous agreement to recommend a surgical radical excision associated with radiotherapy [16, 23, 29, 48]. Radicalization consists of a wide removal of skin and muscle all around the site of the original tumour together with the scar tissue and the area of post-operative haematoma. If there is not documentation of the original tumour extension, we invite the patient to design it on the skin. The extension of post-operative haematoma is better appreciated in MRI study. The radicalization should be accomplished within 3 months of the initial surgery. Persistence of macro- or microscopic tumour areas is detected in 35–59 % of the cases. Despite the radicalization, the risk of local recurrence is higher (1.5–3 times higher) in patients with neoplastic nodules in the operative scar. Patients subject to radicalization do not, however, appear to have a final prognosis (survival at 5 years) worse that the patients operated correctly from outset [19, 38].

Basic Concepts of Radiotherapy

Importance

Radiation therapy alone (60 Gy or more) does achieve local control only in 33 % of patients and at the cost of significant morbidity [41].

In the United States, there is a tendency to perform adjuvant radiotherapy regardless of tumour grading and obtained surgical margin [39]. In Europe, particularly in Scandinavia, it is reserved to all sarcoma of intermediate or high malignancy and in low grades only if surgery is inadequate [19, 34].

Radiation therapy, even if it has no effect on the prognosis, has proved to be an excellent adjuvant treatment which ensures a better local control after resection. Pisters et al. [30], in a randomized, prospective study showed that local control at 5 years was best if treated by surgery and radiation therapy (82 %) compared to patients treated with surgery alone (69 %) patients. Gustafson [19] has demonstrated the effectiveness of radiotherapy to improve local control after marginal resection (decrease of local recurrence from 60 to 30 %). Stotter et al. [37] confirmed this beneficial effect not only after surgery with inadequate margins (decrease from 56 to 34 %) but also in surgery with adequate margins (decrease from 29 to 11 %) also. Radiotherapy can sterilize the tumour cells present in the peri-tumour pseudocapsule and potential tumour microfoci (skip lesions) on the outskirts of the tumour. Evidence-based recommendations for local therapy were given by Pisters et al. [31, 32].

Radiation Therapy Techniques

Radiation therapy can be done pre-, peri- or post-operatively.

Pre-operative Radiotherapy

Generally 5,000–5,400 cGy are delivered on the target original volume (180–200 cGy/day in 28–30 sessions). This treatment is generally associated with an overdose on critical areas, administered under three different modalities:
1. by conventional post-operative radiotherapy (1,000–1,600 cGy), indicated when present multiple and separate tumour areas at high risk;
2. brachytherapy peri- post-operative (1,500 cGy 45–50 h), which is preferred for selectively irradiating major and deep neurovascular structures;
3. by intra-operative radiotherapy (1,250–1,750 cGy in a single shot) in cases where it is not possible to perform an interstitial brachytherapy because of difficulties of positioning and maintenance of the catheter position. Some authors [13] prefer the pre-operative radiotherapy for the following reasons:
    (a) It is currently possible to determine by MRI before the operation the exact extension of the neoplasm (no need as in the

past to place markers clip to show tumour volume);
(b) The radiation is more effective if the tissues are well vascularized (haematoma and surgery could alter the peritumoural oxygenation, thus diminish the effect of ionizing radiation);
(c) It is possible to restrict the target volume (5 cm around the tumour edges are considered sufficient) and thus reduce the number of joints in the field of radiation.
(d) It reduces the risk and consequence of intra-operative contamination (because of the necrotic effect on tumoral cells and formation of a thicker pseudocapsule).

However, there are two disadvantages regarding this technique: the first is to leave the tumour in place for a long time especially in cases where the irradiation is not effective; the second is the exposure to a higher rate of post-surgical local complications (from 14 to 43 %) [5, 13]. Local control is obtained from 78 to 95 % of cases and according to Bujko et al. [5], the best results are obtained on the lower limbs, in elderly patients, and in association with interstitial brachytherapy.

Post-operative Radiotherapy

It can be done in three different ways: external only, brachytherapy alone or combined (brachytherapy followed by external irradiation) [4, 28].

The post-operative external beam radiotherapy. This is the conventional method, indicated to treat large areas at tumor risk. The total doses used are of the order of 60–70 Gy, with fractions of 180–200 cGy. They are distributed in space in a concentric way: approximately 46 Gy in 23 fractions on the initial target, 56 Gy in 28 fractions on the intermediate target volume, 60–66 Gy in 30–33 fractions on the final target volume. The initial target volume should include all the anatomical compartment or, when it is too wide, the tumour bed with longitudinal margins of 5–10 cm from the poles of the tumour. The vicinity of anatomical barriers, such as the bony structures and fascial septa influence the margins of irradiation, which in any event shall not be less than 2 cm.

The intermediate target volume consists of the tumour bed plus a peripheral area of 4 cm. The final target volume represents the major risk area (i.e. the tumour bed with a margin of about 2 cm). In the limbs avoid the irradiation of the full circumference of the extremity to avoid distal lymphoedema (at least one-third of the circumference should be spared). Avoid if possible the irradiation of the circumference of the long bones when they are included in the volume to treat, to avoid fracture. The spinal dose should not exceed 40 Gy/4 weeks and that of the small intestine or colon 50 Gy/5 weeks. Local control varies from 78 to 92 %. Local complications range from 6 to 16 %. Cheng et al. [6] showed that there is no difference between radiotherapy pre-and post-operative as well in terms of survival without symptoms (56 vs. 67 %) and local control (83 vs. 91 %). However pre-operative radiotherapy also produces a higher rate of complications (31 vs. 8 %). Regardless of the mode of administration, pre- or post-operative, the current trend is more and more versus hyperfractionated doses (in two or three daily sessions): this technique may reduce the negative effects on healthy tissues or increase the total doses and therefore local control (obtained in 92–95 % of the cases).

Post-operative Radiotherapy can also be practised with *interstitial brachytherapy*, either exclusively (4,000/4,500 cGy in 90–110 h), or combining it (1,500 cGy 45–50 h) to conventional external radiotherapy. Interstitial brachytherapy is a simple, fast, effective, non-expensive and it is particularly suitable in the following situations:

1. When the dissection is close to important neurovascular structures. In this case, catheters can be placed directly in contact with these structures to deliver high doses while maintaining their anatomical and functional integrity.
2. When performing a major resection of superficial tissues (longitudinal amputation) and the loss of substance is rebuilt by free flap. In this case, only the deep bed must be irradiated while the (reconstructed) superficial planes must be, as far as possible, spared to maintain their viability.

3. In the treatment of child tumours located next to the meta-epiphyses of the long bones, to limit the damage to the growth cartilage.
4. In adults with peri-articular location. With external beams, most of the joint receives a high dose of radiation (with possible evolution of sub-chondral necrosis, chondromalacia, articular fibrosis). With brachytherapy, radiation is concentrated only in the more peripheral areas at major risk. Brachytherapy alone (full doses concentrated in a small area) allows excellent local control at the level of the central tumour area at major risk (local recurrence *in-situ*: 4 %); However, it is less secure in more peripheral areas (local recurrences outside the field 30 %) [20]. The risk of local recurrence at the level of the margins of the treatment field is due to the rapid fall of the dose on the periphery. High doses resulted in very frequent local complications at the level of the wound (35 %) particularly (22 %) if the radioactive material is applied early, and less frequently (14 %) if it is deferred to a week from intervention. Combined therapy (brachytherapy + EBRT) allows more balanced treatment both of the core and peripheral areas and allows an increase of the doses without significant increase in the risk of complications. Even if Alekhteyar et al. [2] reported overall comparable results for both methods (brachytherapy alone *versus* brachytherapy combined with external radiation therapy), the author recommends the latter when surgical margins are contaminated. Our experience has shown that the combination (brachytherapy + post-operative radiotherapy) produces a sharply reduced percentage of local recurrences (2.5 versus 12.5 % with radiotherapy conventional pre- and post-operative and 23 % with surgery alone). This effect has been noted not only in patients whose margins were inadequate, but also in patients treated with wide resection (3 % local recurrence against 16 %). The functional outcome was satisfactory in almost all of the patients (90 %), although with more aggressive combination treatment, the percentage of local complications was increased (from 13 to 26 %) and the percentage of complications requiring surgery (from 66 to 85 %) [4].

Intra-operative Radiation Therapy

Intra-operative Radiation Therapy is based on the application of a direct beam of electrons on the surgical field immediately after removing the tumour with a total dose of 10–20 Gy. This dose is complemented by a secondary external radiotherapy (35–40 Gy). In pelvic or retroperitoneal tumours the intestine can be lifted far away from the field of irradiation during the intra-operative treatment, which allows higher doses. This technique is recommended in cases where it is not possible to use the interstitial brachytherapy because of difficulties of placement of catheters or retroperitoneal tumours [46]. In a randomized study by the *National Cancer Institute*, this method, compared to the conventional external radiotherapy, reduced the rate of local recurrence (from 80 to 40 %) and enteritis (from 50 to 13 %), but was subject to a high rate of post-irradiation neuropathies (60 % compared to 5 % with the conventional technique).

Current Strategy

Pre-and post-operative radiation therapy showed comparable efficiency. However the higher rate of surgical complications after pre-operative radiotherapy justify our current trend to perform immediate excision of the neoplasm associated with interstitial brachytherapy, supplemented by external radiation in 3 weeks.

This order is reversed (pre-operative radiotherapy followed by excision and intra-operative brachytherapy) in selected cases:
1. to reduce the volume of highly radiosensitive tumours (Rhabdomyosarcoma, Mesenchimal Chondrosarcoma, Liposarcoma Mixoide, Ewing, etc.). In these cases, the role of pre-operative radiotherapy must be compared to the new loco-regional techniques (neo-adjuvant chemotherapy, hyperthermia, extracorporeal perfusion chemotherapy, etc.).

2. When a motor unit transplant is planned in order to have an effect of muscular cover, but also recovery of contractile capacity. It is important to not irradiate the free motor unit preventing its re-innervation and avoiding fibrosis of the transplanted muscle. Interstitial brachytherapy can also administered as a post-operative burst which is important to sterilize the deep area at major risk. Like others, we found that free flaps can be used concomitantly with brachytherapy without major risk of failure of the micro-anastomosis. It is however useful, in such cases, to place the micro-anastomosis out of the field of radiation.

Loco-regional Treatments

Several combination of local regional treatment have been proposed to reduce the tumour mass.

Neo-adjuvant Chemotherapy ± Radiation Therapy

The rationale for neo-adjuvant chemotherapy is: that it may help to shrink the tumour, it treats immediately the micrometastasis, and may give prognostic information regarding chemo-response of the tumour. However the response is often limited and unpredictable: in these patients the delay of surgery may be worrisome. Pisters received a complete response in only 8 patients out of 89 treated with multi-drug neo-adjuvant treatment (dacarbazine, doxorubicin, cyclophosphamide).

Some authors have proposed using doxorubicin in monochemotherapy associated with radiotherapy. In advanced cases, Badellino et al. [3] observed a response that allowed conservative surgery in 40 % of patients. In the standard case [12], this technique has allowed the conservation of the limb in 90 % of cases, with a low rate of local recurrence (<10 %) but with a high rate of wound complications. There were no differences between the results (percentages of necrosis, conservative surgery, local recurrence and complications) of intravenous or intra-arterial administration of doxorubicin. Induced necrosis seems to be a prognostic factor. A scheme based on three pre-operative cycles of MAID (mesna, doxorubicin and ifosfamide and decarbazine) combined with 44 Gy, showed a 3 years survival of 75 % and only 5.7 % of local recurrence in wide resections. However, in case of tumour response, combining pre-operative chemo- and radiotherapy it is impossible to establish the individual contribution.

Loco-regional Isolated Perfusion with Recombinant Tumour Necrosis Factor (rTNFα)

Experimentally, the effective antitumoural activity (selective destruction of tumour vessels) of the rTNF has been demonstrated. However, the maximum doses are approximately ten times lower than those which have been experimentally effective in animals. For this reason, the treatment must be performed by infusion isolating the limb. There is a synergic effect between the rTNFα and the melphalan [11, 26, 44], doxorubicin [10], interferon [11, 44] and hyperthermia [10, 11, 26, 44]. The hyperthermic infusion of rTNFα interferon γ and melphalan resulted in 35 % complete and 50–60 % partial response, allowing a conservative surgery in many patients candidates for amputation (85–90 % of cases) with a modest risk of local recurrence (13 %) [11, 17, 26, 44]. Similarly, with the rTNFα and doxorubicin hyperthermic perfusion, 60 % of patients showed a very good reduction (by 75 %) and 28 % a good enough reduction in tumour mass, which made possible a conservative intervention in 75 % of cases [10]. The resulting necrosis can be evaluated satisfactorily with FDG-PET conducted before and after treatment [44]. This technique is not devoid of risks associated with cardiovascular or respiratory toxicity and kidney failure (due to an increase in the secondary myoglobin in rhabdomyolysis) which, although reversible, limits the application. Currently, the method is reserved for sarcoma of soft tissues locally advanced in an attempt to avoid amputation or very scattered sarcomas, trying to stop the local progression even temporarily.

Adjuvant Chemotherapy

The literature has 11 controlled studies on adjuvant treatment of sarcoma of soft tissues, including 6 based on the use of the monochimotherapie (doxorubicin) and 5 of a multi-drug therapy with doxorubicin. Only five of these studies (Rizzoli, NCI, EORTC, Foundation Bergonia) showed a significant difference in terms of survival without evidence of disease between chemotherapy and control group. In addition, in two of these studies (EORTC, NCI), this difference was more related to a decrease in local recurrence than metastasis. Only two (Rizzoli, Foundation Bergonia) studies have shown a correlation between chemotherapy and overall survival. However, these studies have been criticized because of the small number of patients and the terms of randomization. For this reason, there is still a doubt on the effectiveness of adjuvant chemotherapy. Tierney et al. [42] conducted a metanalysis of the cases reported in the literature (1,546 patients) and found in the chemotherapy group a reduction of the life risk of 41 % at 5 years (equivalent to about 12 % of absolute improvement in survival). In a randomized study of a multi-drug therapy (epirubicin, high dose ifosfamide) in patients at high risk, the difference in terms of the favourable outcome for the chemotherapy group has been so significant that the randomization was interrupted: however these results were not confirmed at the long term [15].

Conclusion

Surgery is still the gold standard in treatment of soft tissue sarcoma. Radiotherapy is useful as adjuvant or neo-adjuvant treatment in selected cases. Neo-adjuvant or adjuvant chemotherapy has demonstrated controversial and/or unpredictable results. The surgery should be aggressive trying to remove the tumour with adequately wide margins. Often the aggressive oncological approach is feasible only if complex and eclectic reconstructions are available. Due to its rarity and its complex and multidisciplinary treatment patients with this pathology should be referred to a superspecialist centre.

References

1. Abbatucci JS, Mandard AM, Bouliee N, Vernhes JC, Lozier JC (1990) End results in 130 cases of soft tissue sarcomas of the limbs and trunk walls treated by a systematic radio-surgical association. Multivariate analysis of prognostic factors. Chir Organi Mov 75(1):146–149
2. Alekhteyar KM, Leung DM, Brennan MF, Harrison LB (1996) The effect of combined external bean radiotherapy and brachytherapy on local control and wound complications in patients with positive microscopic margin. Int J Radiat Oncol Biol Phys 36(2):321–324
3. Badelino F, Canavese G, Palumbo R, Vecchio C, Catturich A, Grimaldi A, Raffo P, Villani G, Di Somma C, Gipponi M, Tomei D, Rosato F, Toma S (1997) Surgery after concomitant radio-chemio therapy treatment in advanced soft tissue sarcomas (STS); feasibility and activity of a multimodality limb sparing protocol. In: International Society of limb salvage, IXth symposium. New York
4. Beltrami G, Rüdiger HA, Mela MM et al (2008) Limb salvage surgery in combination with brachytherapy and external beam radiation for high-grade soft tissue sarcomas. Eur J Surg Oncol 34:811–816
5. Bujko K, Suit MD, Springfield DS, Convery K (1993) Wound healing after preoperative radiation for sarcomas of tissue. Surg Gynecol Obstet 176:124
6. Cheng EY, Dusenbery KE, Winters MR, Thompson RC (1996) Soft tissue sarcomas: preoperative versus postoperative radiotherapy. J Surg Oncol 61(2):90–99
7. Choong PFM, Pritchard DJ, Rock MG, Sim FH, Frassica FJ (1995) Survival after pulmonary metastatectomy in soft tissue sarcoma: prognostic factors in 214 patients. Acta Orthop Scand 66(6):561–568
8. Choong PFM, Gstafson P, Rydholm A (1995) Size and timing of local recurrence predicts metastases in soft tissue sarcoma. Growth rate index retrospectively analyzed in 134 cases. Acta Orthop Scand 66(2):147–152
9. Choong PFM, Gustafson P, Willelm M (1995) Prognosis following locally recurrent soft tissue sarcoma. A staging system based on primary and recurrent tumor characteristics. Int J Cancer 60:33–37
10. Di Filippo F, Lise M, Rossi CR, Vaglini M, Azzarelli A, Anzà M, Santinami M, Cavaliere F, Giannarelli D, Schiratti M, Vecchiato A, Psailor A, Quagliolo V, Cavaliere R (1997) Hyperthemic autoblastic perfusion with a TNF and dexorubicina for the treatment of soft tissue limb sarcoma in candidates for amputation: results of I study. Proc Am Soc Clin Oncol 16:501–1800
11. Eggermont AM, Schraffordt Koeps M, Lienard D, Kroon BB, Van Geel AM, Hoekstra MJ, Lejeune FJ (1994) Isolated limb perfusion with high dose tumor necrosis factor alpha in combination with interferon – gamma and melphalan for non resectable extremity soft tissue sarcomas: a multicenter trial. J Clin Oncol 14(10):2653–2665

12. Eilber FR, Eckandt JJ, Rosen G, Fu YS, Seeger LL, Selch MT (1993) Neoadjuvant chemotherapy and radiotherapy in the multidisciplinary management of soft tissue sarcomas of the extremity. Surg Oncol Clin North Am 2(4):611–620
13. Eilber FR, Eckandt JJ, Rosen G, Selch M, Fu YS (1995) Preoperative therapy for soft tissue sarcoma. Hematol Oncol Clin North Am 9(4):418–423
14. Engellau J, Bendahl P-O, Persson A et al (2005) Improved prognostication in soft tissue sarcoma: independent information from vascular invasion, necrosis, growth pattern, and immunostaining using whole-tumour sections and tissue microarrays. Hum Pathol 36:994–1002
15. Frustaci S, Gherlinzoni F, De Paoli A, Pignatti G, Zmerly M, Azzarelli A, Comandone A, Buonadonna A, Olmi P, Ippolito V, Barbieri E, Apice G, Zakotmic B, Bacci G, Picci P (1997) Preliminary results o fan adjuvant randomized trial on high risk extremity soft tissue sarcomas. Proc Am Soc Clin Oncol 16:468–1785
16. Goodland JR, Fletcher CD, Smith MA (1996) Surgical resection of primary soft tissue – sarcoma- incidence of residual tumor in 95 patients needing re – excision after local resection. J Bone Join Surg Br 78(4):658–661
17. Grunhagen DJ, de Wilt JHW, Graveland WJ et al (2006) Outcome and prognostic factor analysis of 217 consecutive isolated limb perfusions with tumour necrosis factor-alpha and melphalan for limb-threatening soft tissue sarcoma. Cancer 106:1776–1784
18. Gustafson P, Akerman M, Alvegard TA et al (2003) Prognostic information in soft tissue sarcoma using tumour size, vascular invasion and microscopic tumour necrosis – the SIN-system. Eur J Cancer 39:1568–1576
19. Gustafson P (1994) Soft tissue sarcoma, epidemiology and prognosis in 508 patients. Acta Orthop Scand 65(Suppl 259):2–31
20. Habrand JL, Gerbaulet A, Pejonic MH (1991) Twenty years experience of interstitial iridium brachytherapy in the management of soft tissue sarcomas. Int J Radiat Oncol Biol Phys 20:405–411
21. Kawaguehi N, Matumoto S, Manabe J (1995) New method of evaluating the surgical margin and safety margin for muscolo-skeletal sarcoma, analysed on the basis of 457 surgical cases. J Cancer Res Clin Oncol 121:555–563
22. Lack E, Steinberg SM, White DE, Kimsellon T, Glatstein E, Chang AE, Rosenberg SA (1989) Extremity soft tissue sarcomas: analysis of prognostic variables in 300 cases and evaluation of tumor necrosis as a factor in stratifying higher-grade sarcomas. J Surg Oncol 41:263–273
23. Lawis JJ, Leung D, Woodruff JM, Breunan MF (1997) Extremity soft tissue sarcoma: are two operations better than one? In: International Society of Limb Salvage. IXth international symposium. New York
24. Mandard AM, Petiot JF, Marnay J, Mandard JC, Hassle J, De Ranieri E, Dupin P, Merlin P, De Ranieri J, Tangery A, Boulier M, Abbatucci JS (1989) Prognostic factors in soft tissue sarcomas. Cancer 63:1437–1451
25. Mankin HJ, Mankin CJ, Simon MA (1996) The hazards of the biopsy revisited. J Bone Joint Surg Am 78(5):656–663
26. Meller I, Gutman M, Schlush L, Abu Abid E, Kolender Y, Merimsky O, Imber M, Isakov J, Klausner JM (1997) Hyperthermic isolated limb perfusion with high dose necrosis factor alpha and melphalan as a limb preserving modality in patients with extensive soft tissue sarcomas. In: International Society of Limb Salvage, transaction IXth symposium, New York
27. Mintzer DM, King JJ, Alavi A et al (2007) Utility of PET scan in predicting chemotherapeutic response in soft tissue sarcoma patients. ASCO annual meeting proceedings part I. J Clin Oncol 25(18S, June 20 supplement):10021
28. Muhic A, Hovgaard D, Petersen MM et al (2008) Local control and survival in patients with soft tissue sarcomas treated with limb sparing surgery in combination with interstitial brachytherapy and external radiation. Radiother Oncol 88:382–387
29. Noria S, Davis A, Kandel R, Levesque J, O'Sullivan B, Wunder J, Bell R (1996) Residual disease following unplanned excision of soft tissue sarcoma of an extremity. J Bone Joint Surg Am 78(5):650–655
30. Pisters PW, Harrison LB, Leung DII, Woodruff JM, Casper ES, Brennan MF (1996) Long term results of a prospective randomized trial of adjuvant brachytherapy in soft tissue sarcoma. J Clin Oncol 14(3):859–868
31. Pisters PWT, O'Sullivan B, Maki RG (2007) Evidence based recommendations for local therapy for soft tissue sarcomas. J Clin Oncol 25:1003–1008
32. Pisters PWT, Patel SR, Varma DGK, Evans HL, Respondek PM, Chen MP, Nguyen HTB, Feig BW, Hunt K, Pollack A, Zagons G, Pollock RE, Benjamin RS (1997) Pathologic complete response following preoperative multimodality therapy for stage IIIB extremity soft tissue sarcoma. Proc Am Soc Clin Oncol 16:499–1795
33. Rydholm A (1997) Prognostic factor in soft tissue sarcoma. Acta Orthop Scand 68(Suppl 273):148–155
34. Rydholm A (1997) Surgery without radiotherapy in soft tissue sarcoma. Acta Orthop Scand 273(68):117–119
35. Schwarzbach MH, Hormann Y, Hinz U et al (2005) Results of limb-sparing surgery with vascular replacement for soft tissue sarcoma in the lower extremity. J Vasc Surg 42:88–97
36. Sim FII, Frassica FJ, Frassica DA (1994) Soft tissue tumors, diagnosis evaluation and management. J Am Acad Orthop Surg 2(4):202–211
37. Stotter AT, A'Hern RP, Fischer C, Mott AF, Fallowfield ME, Westbury G (1990) The influence of local recurrence of extremity soft tissue sarcoma on metastasis and survival. Cancer 65:1119–1129
38. Sugiura H, Takahashi M, Katagiri H et al (2002) Additional wide resection of malignant soft tissue tumours. Clin Orthop 394:201–210

39. Suit HD (1989) The George Edelstym memorial lecture. Radiation in the management of malignant soft issue tumors. Clin Oncol 1:5–10
40. Szendroi M, Zoltan S, Kinga K, Zsuzsa P (2010) Diagnosis and treatment of soft tissue sarcoma. In: Bentley G (ed) European instructional course lectures. 11th EFORT Congress, Madrid, pp 37–49
41. Tepper JE, Smit HD (1985) Radiation therapy alone for sarcoma of soft tissue. Cancer 56:475–479
42. Tierney JF, Mosseri V, Stewart LA, Souhami RL, Parmar MK (1995) Adjuvant chemotherapy for soft tissue sarcoma; review and meta-analysis of the published result of randomized clinical trials. Br J Cancer 72(2):469–475
43. Van Geel AN, Egermont MM, Hanssens PEJ et al (2003) Factors influencing prognosis after initial inadequate excision (IIE) for soft tissue sarcoma. Sarcoma 7:159–165
44. Van Giunkel RJ, Hoekstra MJ, Pruim J, Nieweg OE, Molenaar WM, Paans AM, Willemsen AT, Vallburg W, Koops IIS (1996) FDG RET too evaluate response to hyperthermic isolated limb perfusion for locally advanced soft-tissue sarcoma. J Nucl Med 37(6): 984–990
45. Vraa S, Keller J, Nielsen OS et al (2001) Soft tissue sarcoma of the thigh. Surgical margin influences local recurrence but not survival in 152 patients. Acta Orthop Scand 72:72–77
46. Willet CG, Suit MD, Tepper JE (1991) Intraoperative electron beam radiation therapy for retroperitoneal soft tissue sarcoma. Cancer 68:278–283
47. Zagara GK, Ballo MT, Pisters PW et al (2003) Surgical margins and reresection in the management of patients with soft tissue sarcoma using conservative surgery and radiation therapy. Cancer 97: 2544–2553
48. Zormig C, Peiper M, Schroder S (1995) Reexcision of soft tissue sarcoma after inadequate initial operation. Br J Surg 82(2):278–279

Part III

Trauma

Biologics in Open Fractures

Christian Kleber and Norbert P. Haas

Introduction

The successful management of open fractures continues to represent a surgical and reconstructive challenge due to high rate of infection (<50 %), poor soft tissue coverage, impaired fracture healing, non-union and secondary amputation [1]. Although open fractures are severe but rare injuries, the potential risk for detrimental consequences and serious handicaps, which in turn, cause major socio-economic costs, is high [2, 3]. The two main problems in management of open fractures are infections and impaired fracture healing. Historically the treatment and major clinical problems in open fractures changed from infectious to reconstructive and bone healing complications. Cornerstones of open fracture treatment have been the invention of simple sterility measures like hand disinfection (Semmelweis 1818–1865), skin disinfection by iodine solutions (Grossich 1849–1926), wearing of rubber gloves (Friedrich 1864–1916), sterilization of operation instruments (Schimmelbusch 1860–1895) and the invention of antibiotic agents (discovery of Penicillin by Fleming et al. and first clinical use by Florey and Chain et al. which won the Nobel prize 1945). Due to the improved methods of limb reconstruction the rate of secondary amputations after open fractures has decreased and reconstruction protocols for non-unions and bone segmental defects have improved over the last decade. The paradigm change, that not bone but soft tissue coverage, responsible for vascularity, microcirculation and immune response are crucial for complete recovery, improved the outcome of open fractures in the last decades. Nevertheless, limb salvage in contrast to primary amputation is still associated with an increased rate of complications and sometimes large numbers of necessary surgeries [4]. Osteomyelitis and osteitis are still the major factor for non-union and re-hospitalization after open fractures. Prognostically relevant are the amount of initial bone loss, fracture type, grade of soft tissue injury and defect, deficiency of bone vascularity, type of microbiological contamination, compartment syndrome, concomitant vascular injury or peripheral vascular occlusive disease, co-morbidities (diabetes, adiposity), connective tissue diseases, iatrogenic factors (NSAID therapy, corticosteroid use), smoking and social background [5]. Owing to scientific progress new biologics, from debridement devices to coated implants and recombinant growth factors are available to positively influence the clinical course of open fractures and assist the surgeon in order to fully rehabilitate patients. In the following chapters we provide an overview of diagnosis, actual treatment concepts and available biologics in the treatment of open fractures.

C. Kleber (✉) • N.P. Haas
Center for Musculoskeletal Surgery,
Charité – Universitätsmedizin Berlin,
Augustenburger Platz 1, 13353 Berlin, Germany
e-mail: christian.kleber@charite.de;
norbert.haas@charite.de

Diagnosis of Impaired Fracture Healing and Infectious Complications

The initiation and observation of the early bone healing process (reactive/reparative phase) without calcification is difficult to diagnose and observe on conventional X-ray or CT-scan. New techniques like ultrasound and MRI are useful to assess the granulation tissue, callus formation and lamellar bone deposition. A test for early diagnosis of deranged or impaired fracture healing is not available. Recent studies try to understand the regulatory mechanisms (cytokines, adoptive immune system, biomechanics) of the bone healing process in order to predict impaired fracture healing and develop new targets to accelerate bone healing.

The early diagnosis of infectious complications or impaired fracture healing is difficult. Beside clinical examination with rubor, calor, dolor and pus, several clinical tests assist in confirming infectious complications. Despite a high sensitivity all tests have a low specificity:

Blood tests (CRP, WBC)	80–90 % sensitivity	60 % specificity
3-phase scintigraphy	100 % sensitivity	25 % specificity
MRI	100 % sensitivity	60 % specificity

In contrast sequestra and intra-/extramedullary fat globules on MRI are a specific signs of osteomyelitis [6, 7]. The combination of microbiological wound swabs, tissue tests and histological investigations, normally acquired while during interventions are the most reliable, but invasive diagnostics. But correct procedure to prove the presence of pathogens is crucial. Specimens must be obtained under strict sterile conditions. Bearing and transportation of the specimens must be organized. Large probe volumes and numbers, no superficial swabs and short transportation time can increase the detection rate. The specimens should be taken before administration of antibiotic agents or an antibiotic window (>24 h) should be obtained. New highly specific bacterial PCR tests may assist in proving low-grade infections and biofilm pathogens in the future.

Management of Open Fractures and Clinical Guidelines

In the following two sections we outline the current clinical practice and use of biologics in open fractures. The major goals in treatment of open fractures are to prevent infectious complications, assure fracture healing and restore function (Fig. 1).

The "Gold standard" for prevention of infection after open fractures is the combination of radical surgical debridement with initially calculated antibiotic therapy. Due to changes in the microbiological spectrum, today we see more Gram-negative infections in open fractures than 20 years ago, and therefore a combined antibiotic therapy should be administered (section "Systemic Antibiotic Therapy"). Not only the incidence of infectious complications after open fractures depends on the soft tissue injury severity and grade of open fracture (classifications of Tscherne/Oestern and Gustilo/Anderson), but also the initial surgical treatment [8–14]:

1. Debridement, primary wound closure and definitive osteosynthesis (grade I/II open fractures Tscherne/Oestern and Gustilo/Anderson)
2. Staged therapy algorithm (grade II–IV open fracture Tscherne/Oestern, grade II–IIIc Gustilo/Anderson) with debridement, primary shortening, temporary fracture stabilization (external fixator), re-vascularization, temporary wound closure, programmed debridement and soft tissue conditioning, plastic surgery and definitive osteosynthesis
3. In the subsequent phase of typical complications (septic/aseptic non-union) radical debridement, removal of osteosynthesis implants, segmental resection, antibiotic-loaded bone cement (PMMA) spacer implantation, reconstruction of bone segmental defects with bone substitutes and growth factors are needed (section "Bone Segmental Defects, Impaired Fracture and Bone Healing").

Debridement

Debridement is one of the cornerstones of limb salvage, wound and fracture healing in open fractures.

An open fracture is a traumatology emergency. The first surgical debridement should be performed within 6 h after trauma. Notably, the radical surgical debridement in specialized centres has had a stronger impact on the outcome compared to the time-point of initial surgery. Serially-performed debridement every 48 h until negative microbiological culture results produced decreased infection and complication rates. Additive tools like high pulsatile lavage (Jet-lavage) and the hydrosurgical scalpel are reported controversially. Some publications report reduced infection rates, others fear additional soft tissue injury due to hydrostatic pressure and dissemination of pathogens in deep, primary not contaminated and infected, compartments. Intramedullary reaming, with a cortical window for decompression and decreased risk of septic complications, is used in septic non-unions with an affected bone canal. The new RIA (Reamer-Irrigator-Aspirator) is an elegant way to debride intramedullary long-bone osteomyelitis because of simultaneous suction while reaming [15]. The classical intra-operative methylene blue application is useful to label fistulae for radical excision.

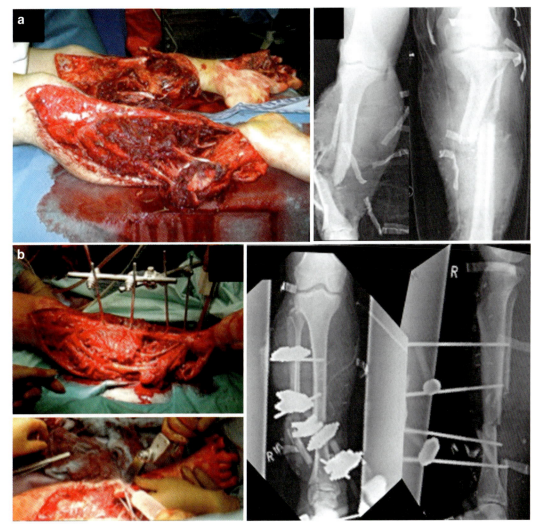

Fig. 1 (**a**) Male 23 year old cyclist overrun by train: subtotal amputation both legs – open amputation left leg – replantation, primary shortening, external fixator (**b**) secondary amputation toes – free flap – skin graft – nailing and plating – fracture healing 1 year after trauma (**c**)

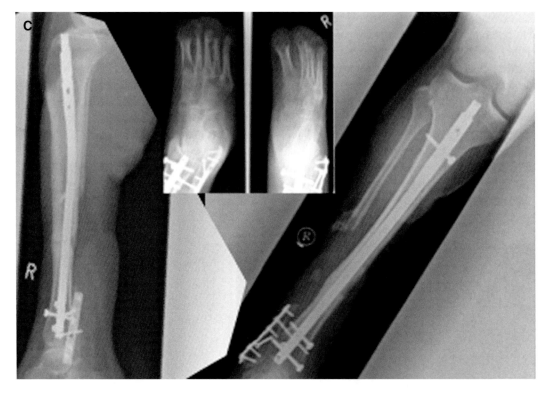

Fig. 1 (continued)

Wound Closure

The time point for wound closure and successful soft tissue management are crucial to prevent secondary complications after open fractures. In contrast, ambitious wound closure can provoke secondary necrosis. Open wound management with sterile gauze has the disadvantage of moist milieu and danger of secondary infections, especially with hospital pathogens. Therefore, we think an individual concept of wound closure should be performed:

In type I/II open fractures we should strive for primary wound closure, which according to the literature, is associated with lower infection rates.

In type III–IV open fractures primary wound closure is normally not possible. Temporary soft tissue coverage can be achieved by artificial skin (Epigard) or negative pressure wound therapy (NPWT). NPWT can reduce the infection rate by up to 20 % [16, 17]. NPWT in type II–IV open fractures (negative pressure-50–150 mmHg) can reduce the defect size and soft tissue oedema. Furthermore, NPWT protects the wound from secondary contamination and hospital acquired infections. Definitive wound closure should be achieved within 1 week for type III–IV open fractures.

Chronic wounds are a domain of modern wound management with occlusive wound dressings, enzymatic wound cleaning, secretory absorption and facilitation of granulation tissue formation. Silver-coated gauze has positive effects on wound healing and protection from secondary infections. Silver is an antimicrobial agent which has been used for nearly 20 years. Nanocrystalline silver dressing has been developed to prevent wound adhesions, control bacterial growth up to 7 days and improve healing of burn wounds. Furthermore, silver-coated sponges may reduce Gram-positive infections.

Infection-Associated Complications in Open Fractures

Systemic Antibiotic Therapy

The early use of systemic antibiotic therapy together with debridement is the cornerstone of successful open fracture management and prevention of secondary complications. It can significantly reduce the soft tissue infection rate up to 60 % in open fractures [18, 19]. The calculated antibiotic therapy should start as soon as possible after trauma, but at least within 3 h after injury [20]. According to the severity of soft tissue injury, contamination, environment of the injury and grade of open fracture, the antibiotic therapy should be chosen:

In type I/II open fractures short-term antibiotics for Gram-positive pathogens (Cephalosporin or Clindamycin) is advised.

Type III–IV open fractures need additional Gram-negative antibiotic therapy (aminoglycoside, fluoroquinolones) due to high incidence of Gram-negative pathogens. Therefore, calculated antibiotic therapy until positive culture results and afterwards adaption according to microbiogramme should be performed. According to the EAST report antibiotic therapy should be stopped 24 h after soft tissue coverage in type I/II and 72 h after wound closure in type III open fractures.

For the duration of antibiotic therapy in chronic infections and osteomyelitis no hard evidence exists [21]. But the principle of antibiotic therapy are:

Hit early and hard (high dose)
Use combination antibiotics
Favour bactericide antibiotics
Use antibiotics with good bone and biofilm penetration:
Excellent: Fluoroquinolones, clindamycin, rifampicin, fusidic acid, metronidazole
Fair: Betalactam antibiotics, gylcopeptides, fosfomycin and sulfonamids
Poor: Aminoglycosides

Some antibiotic agents have negative impact on bone healing and should be avoided (e.g. fluoroquinolones). Additionally to systemic antibiotic therapy another form of systemic antimicrobial therapy, the hyperbaric oxygen therapy (HBOT), can be used. HBOT uses oxygen in supra-atmospheric pressure to treat bacterial infections. Positive effects of HBOT have been described for necrotizing fasciitis, osteomyelitis, skin grafts, flaps and other forms of traumatic ischaemia [22].

Local Antibiotic Therapy

Local antibiotic deliverance, e.g. sponge, fleece, PMMA cement/chains/spacers, has the advantage of high antibiotic concentration at the infection focus and less systemic complications [23]. Most of the antibiotic carrier systems (sponge) are biodegradable and must not be removed. Soaking of antibiotic-loaded sponges before implantations precisely decrease the antibiotic concentration in the sponge and should not be performed [24]. PMMA bone cement loaded with antibiotics (tobramycin, gentamycin, vancomycin) was able to reduce the infection rate after open fractures due to 10–30-fold higher local concentrations compared to systemic application [25]. But the release of antibiotics is temporary. In some studies, 3–4 weeks after implantation, bacteria and biofilm colonized the PMMA spacer. Early infection of implants, in some cases, have been successfully been treated by debridement and local antibiotic agents without removal of the implant.

To summarize, positive effects for the treatment of open fractures are known but in general due to lack of randomized trials the reduction of infection and osteomyelitis rate in open fractures is arguable.

Bone Segmental Defects, Impaired Fracture and Bone Healing

Beside infectious complication the delayed- or non-union of open fractures is the second major clinical task in open fracture treatment.

Septic vs. aseptic and atrophic versus hypertrophic non-unions are known. According to the individual pattern of impaired fracture healing, specific treatment should be performed. The bases for fracture healing are adequate cellular environment, vascularization, sufficient growth factors, bone matrix, soft tissue coverage and mechanical stability. In delayed or non-union one of these factors is abnormal. The effectiveness of treatment depends on the detailed analysis of the impaired bone healing in order to reveal the responsible factor. Mostly, the reason for aseptic delayed or non-union is wrong osteosynthesis with no biomechanical stability leading to secondary pseudarthrosis. Hypertrophic aseptic non-unions are treated with intra-or extramedullary osteosynthesis. Atrophic non-union is more difficult to treat, because of a poor biological environment. In cases of infection-associated pseudarthrosis a staged therapy algorithm with radical debridement, segmental bone resection, temporary external stabilization and secondary reconstruction of the bone defect is recommended. Shortening of the leg is a possibility but limited by vascular kinking. Another classical method to reconstruct large bone segmental defects is bone segmental transport by Ilizarov or external fixator. The disadvantages are pin-track infections, discomfort and the long time period needed for bone segmental transport (1 mm per day). A staged approach to reconstruct large diaphyseal bone segmental defects (<25 cm) was described by Masquelet [26]. After initial resection of pathological bone, an antibiotic-loaded PMMA cement spacer is inserted into the bone defect in order to induce a pseudosynovial membrane. In a second operation the membrane around the cement spacer is preserved, the cement spacer removed and the membrane filled with bone graft. The pseudomembrane protects the spongy graft from resorption and favours it's vascularity and corticalisation.

The optimal bone substitute to reconstruct non-unions or bone segmental defects is controversial. It´s properties should be osteoconductive, osteo-inductive and biodegradable to be replaced by autologous bone [27]. Osteoconductive means a three-dimensional structure, which has biomechanical properties and serves as a scaffold for new bone ingrowth. A synonym is osteo-integration. Osteo-inductive means the promotion of differentiation of osteoprogenitor cells into osteoblasts and the acceleration of new bone formation. BMP is the most famous osteo-inductive growth factor (section "Bone Morphogenetic Proteins (BMPs)"). Osteogenesis means the ingrowth of cells and guided tissue and bone regeneration for optimal healing [28]. Recently, industrial partners offer an array of products with big regional worldwide differences.

Autologous Bone Grafts

Autologous bone grafts are taken from the patient him/herself and transferred to another anatomical body region. Autologous bone graft from iliac crest, rib, skull, mandible, fibula are limited in supply, but are the only bone substitutes which are osteo-conductive, inductive and osteogenic. Autografts, especially from the iliac crest, have a high co-morbidity rate (24 % pain, 65 % haematoma) [29, 30]. Although, harvesting bone from iliac crest is time-consuming and expensive, it is still the gold standard for bone substitutes in a bone defects up to 3 cm in size [31]. In autologous grafting, de-fatting of the bone chips (Jet-lavage) is important to improve the integration rate. In the future antibiotic or growth factor-loaded autologous grafts might be available. Another elegant way to harvest bone is the reamer-irrigator-aspirator (RIA). Developed to reduce fat embolism and thermal necrosis after reaming of long-bone fractures, due to reduction of intramedullary pressure, RIA can harvest autologous bone from long bones together with mesenchymal stem cells [32]. Additionally, reaming itself has been shown to improve bone healing in tibial shaft fractures in some studies [31]. Large bone defects (>3 cm) need primary mechanical stability and perfusion. Vascularized grafts (fibula), autologous/allogenic grafts (strut grafts), custom- made implant or bone segmental transport by Ilizarov fixator, are possible solutions.

Allogenic Bone Grafts

Allografts are bone or bone substitutes from another human, transferred to the patient. Allografts are used in up to 35 % of all bone transplantations [33]. Mostly, cadaveric bone or donor bone from hip arthroplasty is obtained and stored in a bone bank. To avoid the transmission of e.g. HIV, hepatitis and prions, the allografts are processed which weakens the osto-inductive properties of the graft and maybe the mechanical stability. The limited osteoconductive capacity leads to failure of ingrowth of the transplant in 15–20 % [34]. In general, three different types of allografts (fresh or fresh-frozen bone, freeze-dried bone grafts (FDBA), demineralized freeze-dried bone grafts (DFDBA)) in different application forms (cancellous, corticocancellous, structural cortical graft) are available. Irradiation of bone grafts reduces the incorporation rate from 80 to 100 % in non-irradiated grafts to 40 % irradiated grafts [34]. De-mineralized freeze-dried bone grafts lose their biomechanical stability after processing. Allogenic strut grafts (fibula) are used more seldom, especially in large bone segmental defects (>3 cm). Analogous to autologous grafts the future perspectives are antibiotic, chemotherapeutic or growth factor-loaded bone grafts. Allogenic, compared to autologous bone grafts, are not limited in size/amount but carry risks of transfection and have lower osteoinduction properties.

Xenogenic Bone Grafts

Xenogenic bone graft is derived from animals, mostly bovine or coral in origin. Due to transfection issues the xenogenic bone substitutes, analogous to allografts are processed to eradicate viruses, prions or bacteria. Therefore, xenogenic grafts have no osteo-inductive and comparable osteoconductive properties to allogenic bone grafts.

Synthetic Bone Grafts

Industry produces synthetic bone grafts created from calcium phosphate, calcium-sulphate, bioactive glass, polymers and composites. Some products are loaded with antibiotics or growth factors. Compared to synthetic bone grafts 10–20 years ago, the modern grafts are osteoconductive and biodegradable for 6–18 months whilst not weakening osteosynthesis or grafting. Some studies report similar mechanical properties to bone. Today, synthetic bone grafts are used in joint reconstruction surgery (proximal tibial fractures) with comparable biomechanical and socioeconomic properties to autologous and allogenic grafts.

Platelet-Rich Therapies (PLT)

Platelet-rich therapies are autologous blood products with enriched concentration of platelets due to a bedside centrifugation process (platelet-rich plasma by gravitational platelet separation) [35]. Furthermore, the processed platelet concentrate can be in-vitro activated by e.g. thrombin adjunct. After intra-operative preparation PLT is directly located to the critical fracture site. PLT promotes bone healing via release of various growth factors (PDGF, TGF-β) [36]. A recent Cochrane database analysis revealed only two trials with insufficient evidence to recommend routine use of PLT in non-union [35]. Actually, no controlled study is available investigating the application of PLT in delayed- or non-union after open fractures.

Bone Morphogenetic Proteins (BMPs)

BMP's are members of the TGF-β family. As growth factors with osteoconductive and osteoinductive effects, BMP's induce bone and cartilage formation and play a key role in osteoblast differentiation, accelerating bone regeneration and fracture healing. The clinical use and approval by the American FDA underscores the effectiveness of BMP in problematic bone healing situations.

Mostly BMPs are used in atrophic delayed or non-unions [37]. Commercially available are BMP-2 and -7. The application of recombinant BMP-2/7 in clinical studies showed enhanced fracture healing in scaphoid, fibula, distal tibial fractures and spine fusions. Due to short half-life the drug delivery, actually a bovine collagen sponge or biodegradable polyurethane scaffold, is a scientific task [38, 39]. Also the combination of BMPs with new implants and autologous graft was shown to be a safe procedure with good results [40]. With further scientific research new growth factors like PDGF are potential targets for clinical use in the future.

Coated Implants

Osteosynthetic implants with the capability of local, controlled drug release pose a feasible and logical way to solve the local and specific problems of infectious or impaired bone healing complications after open fractures. Some titanium implants, especially tibial nails, are covered with biodegradable polylactide and gentamycin. Early promising results from clinical trials are published [1, 41]. In the future this technology might give us the opportunity to treat complications after open fracture with coated implants or even prevent secondary complications. Until then much scientific and investigational work has to be done.

Pulsed Electromagnetic Field (PEMF) and Low Intensity Pulsed Ultrasound (LIPUS)

The indications for PEMP and ultrasound are aseptic, atrophic delayed or non-unions. Exposure of bone cells to pulsed electromagnetic field induces intra-cellular signalling cascades associated with anabolic bone formation (PTH, insulin, IGF-2, LDL, calcitonin receptors) similar to mechanical load [42–44]. Osteoblasts are simulated by PEMF and secret BMP-2/-4 and TGF-beta [45, 46]. The success rate in healing non-union was dependent on the daily timespan used. In 36 % of non-unions treated with less than 3 h a day with PEMF, bone healing was observed, compared to 80 % when the device was used for more than 3 h a day [47]. Furthermore, PEMF is an effective tool in aseptic non-unions after paediatric osteotomies and adult tibial fractures [48, 49]. Beside PEMF also low intensity pulsed ultrasound healing gave rates up to 86 % [50, 51].

Summary Table of Biologics in Open Fractures

Graft	Osteoconductive	Osteoinductive	Osteogenesis	Stability
Autologous	+	+	+	+
Allogenic	+	(+)		+
Xenogenic	+			
Synthetic	+			
RIA	+	+	+	
BMP-2/7		++		
PDGF		+		
PLT		+		
MSC			+	
BMA			+	

RIA reamer-irrigator-aspirator, *BMP* bone morphogenetic protein, *PDGF* platelet-derived growth factor, *PLT* platelet-enriched therapy, *MSC* mesenchymal stem cells, *BMA* bone marrow aspirate

References

1. Schmidmaier G, Lucke M, Wildemann B, Haas NP, Raschke M (2006) Prophylaxis and treatment of implant-related infections by antibiotic-coated implants: a review. Injury 37(Suppl 2):S105–S112
2. Court-Brown CM, Rimmer S, Prakash U, McQueen MM (1998) The epidemiology of open long bone fractures. Injury 29:529–534
3. Schwabe P, Haas NP, Schaser KD (2010) Fractures of the extremities with severe open soft tissue damage. Initial management and reconstructive treatment strategies. Unfallchirurg 113:647–670; quiz 671–672
4. Bosse MJ, MacKenzie EJ, Kellam JF, Burgess AR, Webb LX, Swiontkowski MF, Sanders RW, Jones AL, McAndrew MP, Patterson BM, McCarthy ML, Travison TG, Castillo RC (2002) An analysis of outcomes of reconstruction or amputation after leg-threatening injuries. N Engl J Med 347:1924–1931
5. Taitsman LA, Lynch JR, Agel J, Barei DP, Nork SE (2009) Risk factors for femoral nonunion after femoral shaft fracture. J Trauma 67:1389–1392
6. Davies AM, Grimer R (2005) The penumbra sign in subacute osteomyelitis. Eur Radiol 15:1268–1270
7. Davies AM, Hughes DE, Grimer RJ (2005) Intramedullary and extramedullary fat globules on magnetic resonance imaging as a diagnostic sign for osteomyelitis. Eur Radiol 15:2194–2199
8. Gustilo RB, Merkow RL, Templeman D (1990) The management of open fractures. J Bone Joint Surg Am 72:299–304
9. Court-Brown CM, Wheelwright EF, Christie J, McQueen MM (1990) External fixation for type III open tibial fractures. J Bone Joint Surg Br 72:801–804
10. Gustilo RB, Anderson JT (1976) Prevention of infection in the treatment of one thousand and twenty-five open fractures of long bones: retrospective and prospective analyses. J Bone Joint Surg Am 58:453–458
11. Gustilo RB, Mendoza RM, Williams DN (1984) Problems in the management of type III (severe) open fractures: a new classification of type III open fractures. J Trauma 24:742–746
12. Lenarz CJ, Watson JT, Moed BR, Israel H, Mullen JD, Macdonald JB (2010) Timing of wound closure in open fractures based on cultures obtained after debridement. J Bone Joint Surg Am 92:1921–1926
13. Seligson D, Ostermann PA, Henry SL, Wolley T (1994) The management of open fractures associated with arterial injury requiring vascular repair. J Trauma 37:938–940
14. Sirkin M, Sanders R, DiPasquale T, Herscovici D Jr (2004) A staged protocol for soft tissue management in the treatment of complex pilon fractures. J Orthop Trauma 18:S32–S38
15. Kanakaris NK, Morell D, Gudipati S, Britten S, Giannoudis PV (2011) Reaming irrigator aspirator system: early experience of its multipurpose use. Injury 42(Suppl 4):S28–S34
16. Webb LX, Pape HC (2008) Current thought regarding the mechanism of action of negative pressure wound therapy with reticulated open cell foam. J Orthop Trauma 22:S135–S137
17. Stannard JP, Volgas DA, Stewart R, McGwin G Jr, Alonso JE (2009) Negative pressure wound therapy after severe open fractures: a prospective randomized study. J Orthop Trauma 23:552–557
18. Gosselin RA, Roberts I, Gillespie WJ (2004) Antibiotics for preventing infection in open limb fractures. Cochrane Database Syst Rev:CD003764
19. Gosselin A, Hare L (2004) Effect of sedimentary cadmium on the behavior of a burrowing mayfly (Ephemeroptera, Hexagenia limbata). Environ Toxicol Chem 23:383–387
20. Patzakis MJ, Wilkins J (1989) Factors influencing infection rate in open fracture wounds. Clin Orthop Relat Res 243:36–40
21. Darley ES, MacGowan AP (2004) Antibiotic treatment of gram-positive bone and joint infections. J Antimicrob Chemother 53:928–935
22. Kawashima M, Tamura H, Nagayoshi I, Takao K, Yoshida K, Yamaguchi T (2004) Hyperbaric oxygen therapy in orthopedic conditions. Undersea Hyperb Med 31:155–162
23. Knaepler H (2012) Local application of gentamicin-containing collagen implant in the prophylaxis and treatment of surgical site infection in orthopaedic surgery. Int J Surg 10(Suppl 1):S15–S20
24. Lovering AM, Sunderland J (2012) Impact of soaking gentamicin-containing collagen implants on potential antimicrobial efficacy. Int J Surg 10(Suppl 1):S2–S4
25. Ostermann PA, Henry SL, Seligson D (1993) Value of adjuvant local antibiotic administration in therapy of open fractures. A comparative analysis of 704 consecutive cases. Langenbecks Arch Chir 378:32–36
26. Masquelet AC, Fitoussi F, Begue T, Muller GP (2000) Reconstruction of the long bones by the induced membrane and spongy autograft. Ann Chir Plast Esthet 45:346–353
27. Giannoudis PV, Dinopoulos H, Tsiridis E (2005) Bone substitutes: an update. Injury 36(Suppl 3):S20–S27
28. Retzepi M, Donos N (2010) Guided bone regeneration: biological principle and therapeutic applications. Clin Oral Implants Res 21:567–576
29. Skaggs DL, Samuelson MA, Hale JM, Kay RM, Tolo VT (2000) Complications of posterior iliac crest bone grafting in spine surgery in children. Spine 25:2400–2402
30. Niedhart C, Pingsmann A, Jurgens C, Marr A, Blatt R, Niethard FU (2003) Complications after harvesting of autologous bone from the ventral and dorsal iliac crest – a prospective, controlled study. Z Orthop Ihre Grenzgeb 141:481–486
31. Schmidmaier G, Herrmann S, Green J, Weber T, Scharfenberger A, Haas NP, Wildemann B (2006) Quantitative assessment of growth factors in reaming aspirate, iliac crest, and platelet preparation. Bone 39:1156–1163

32. Bacher A, Mayer N, Klimscha W, Oismuller C, Steltzer H, Hammerle A (1997) Effects of pentoxifylline on hemodynamics and oxygenation in septic and nonseptic patients. Crit Care Med 25:795–800
33. Berven S, Tay BK, Kleinstueck FS, Bradford DS (2001) Clinical applications of bone graft substitutes in spine surgery: consideration of mineralized and demineralized preparations and growth factor supplementation. Eur Spine J 10(Suppl 2):S169–S177
34. Blokhuis TJ, Lindner T (2008) Allograft and bone morphogenetic proteins: an overview. Injury 39(Suppl 2):S33–S36
35. Griffin XL, Wallace D, Parsons N, Costa ML (2012) Platelet rich therapies for long bone healing in adults. Cochrane Database Syst Rev 7:CD009496
36. Kasten P, Vogel J, Geiger F, Niemeyer P, Luginbuhl R, Szalay K (2008) The effect of platelet-rich plasma on healing in critical-size long-bone defects. Biomaterials 29:3983–3992
37. Schmidmaier G, Schwabe P, Wildemann B, Haas NP (2007) Use of bone morphogenetic proteins for treatment of non-unions and future perspectives. Injury 38(Suppl 4):S35–S41
38. Lissenberg-Thunnissen SN, de Gorter DJ, Sier CF, Schipper IB (2011) Use and efficacy of bone morphogenetic proteins in fracture healing. Int Orthop 35: 1271–1280
39. Brown KV, Li B, Guda T, Perrien DS, Guelcher SA, Wenke JC (2011) Improving bone formation in a rat femur segmental defect by controlling bone morphogenetic protein-2 release. Tissue Eng Part A 17:1735–1746
40. Kanakaris NK, Lasanianos N, Calori GM, Verdonk R, Blokhuis TJ, Cherubino P, De Biase P, Giannoudis PV (2009) Application of bone morphogenetic proteins to femoral non-unions: a 4-year multicentre experience. Injury 40(Suppl 3):S54–S61
41. Fuchs T, Stange R, Schmidmaier G, Raschke MJ (2011) The use of gentamicin-coated nails in the tibia: preliminary results of a prospective study. Arch Orthop Trauma Surg 131:1419–1425
42. Schnoke M, Midura RJ (2007) Pulsed electromagnetic fields rapidly modulate intracellular signaling events in osteoblastic cells: comparison to parathyroid hormone and insulin. J Orthop Res 25: 933–940
43. Victoria G, Petrisor B, Drew B, Dick D (2009) Bone stimulation for fracture healing: what's all the fuss? Indian J Orthop 43:117–120
44. Ciombor DM, Aaron RK (2005) The role of electrical stimulation in bone repair. Foot Ankle Clin 10: 579–593, vii
45. Hannouche D, Petite H, Sedel L (2001) Current trends in the enhancement of fracture healing. J Bone Joint Surg Br 83:157–164
46. Kuzyk PR, Schemitsch EH (2009) The science of electrical stimulation therapy for fracture healing. Indian J Orthop 43:127–131
47. Midura RJ, Ibiwoye MO, Powell KA, Sakai Y, Doehring T, Grabiner MD, Patterson TE, Zborowski M, Wolfman A (2005) Pulsed electromagnetic field treatments enhance the healing of fibular osteotomies. J Orthop Res 23:1035–1046
48. Boyette MY, Herrera-Soto JA (2012) Treatment of delayed and nonunited fractures and osteotomies with pulsed electromagnetic field in children and adolescents. Orthopedics 35:e1051–e1055
49. Assiotis A, Sachinis NP, Chalidis BE (2012) Pulsed electromagnetic fields for the treatment of tibial delayed unions and nonunions. A prospective clinical study and review of the literature. J Orthop Surg Res 7:24
50. Nolte PA, van der Krans A, Patka P, Janssen IM, Ryaby JP, Albers GH (2001) Low-intensity pulsed ultrasound in the treatment of nonunions. J Trauma 51:693–702; discussion 702–703
51. Rutten S, Nolte PA, Guit GL, Bouman DE, Albers GH (2007) Use of low-intensity pulsed ultrasound for posttraumatic nonunions of the tibia: a review of patients treated in the Netherlands. J Trauma 62: 902–908

Classification and Algorithm of Treatment of Proximal Humerus Fractures

Herbert Resch and C. Hirzinger

Pathophysiological Considerations and Pre-operative Planning

Knowledge about the relations between the various bony fragments is extremely important not only for the blood supply of the humeral head, but also to benefit from the so-called ligamentotaxis-effect. Consequently, it is important to study the "pattern" of the fracture. It is characterised by the position of the head fragment in relation to the shaft in two planes. Four main fracture patterns can be differentiated involving 93 % of all fractures with a fracture in the surgical neck area:

Each fracture pattern consists of either two, three or four displaced or non- displaced fragments. Fracture pattern + number of fragments = Fracture type.

Varus Avulsion Type

Varus avulsion type (Fig. 1): Most of these fractures are two or three fragment fractures. This type is characterised by complete separation of shaft and head fragments. This is why such fractures are very unstable fractures. Since the head fragment is in varus position, it has to be reduced by a hook. Once the shaft and the head fragment are in alignment, the two K-wires which have been inserted at the beginning ("waiting position"), are drilled to the subchondral bone. In case of a displaced greater tuberosity this fragment has to be reduced also by a hook and fixed by two or three screws.

Varus Impaction Type

Varus impaction type (Fig. 2): The shaft fragment is impacted at the medial part of the head fragment, which is in varus position. In the coronal plane there is no interfragmentary distance on the lateral side whereas head and shaft show anterior angulation in the sagittal plane. These fractures still have some residual stability. Most of these fractures are two-part fractures. Reduction is achieved only by a manual manoeuvre. The K-wires, which are in "waiting position", are introduced at the right moment as soon as reduction is achieved.

Valgus Lateral Impaction Type

Valgus lateral impaction type (Fig. 3): The head fragment is impacted into the metaphysis without major angulation in the sagittal plane. One or both tuberosities are fractured. Reduction is performed by an elevator which is inserted percutaneously through the intertubercular fracture gap. The greater tuberosity is reduced by the

H. Resch (✉) • C. Hirzinger
Department of Traumatology and Sports Injuries,
Paracelsus Medical University Salzburg,
Landeskrankenhaus – Universitätsklinikum Salzburg,
Müllner Hauptstrasse 48, Salzburg 5020, Austria
e-mail: h.resch@salk.at

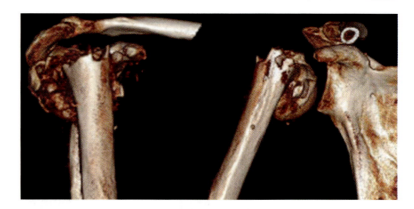

Fig. 1 Varus avulsion-2 fragment fracture: head in varus position, head and shaft separated

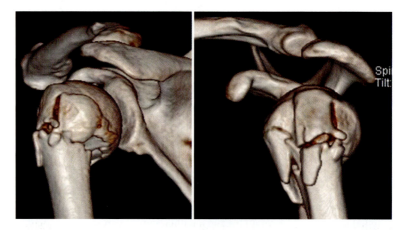

Fig. 2 Varus impaction 2-fragment fracture: head in varus position, shaft impacted, no lateral distance

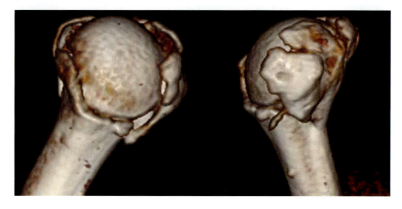

Fig. 3 Valgus lateral impaction

periosteum, which is still intact. After the head fragment has been raised, it is tightened by the rotator cuff (RC). Finally, it is fixed with two or three screws. In cases where the lesser tuberosity is displaced, medially, reduction is performed with the arm placed in an abduction position. The fragment is pulled laterally by a hooked instrument and fixed by one or two screws.

Valgus Posterolateral Impaction Type

Valgus posterolateral impaction type (Fig. 4): This type is characterised by lateral impaction of the head fragment with additional anterior angulation between shaft and head fragment. The head fragment faces laterally and posteriorly. Reduction is similar to the above- mentioned type. This time

Fig. 4 Valgus posterolateral impaction 3-fragment fracture: high fracture level, hinge displaced, lesser tuberosity not fractured

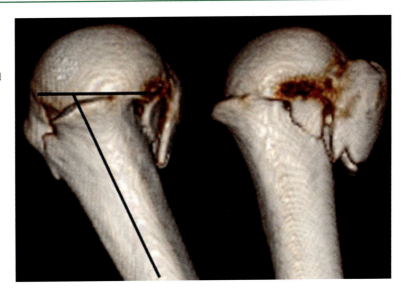

however, the elevator has to be placed not centrally under the head fragment, but in the posterior half.

Treatment Algorithm

Irrespective of the preferred techniques, the following guidelines can be recommended:

Varus Fractures

1. Varus Impaction Fractures: Varus Impaction 2- and 3-fragment fractures are excellent for reconstructive surgery; even in osteoporotic bone conditions, as residual stability still exists (humerusblock, plating, nailing)
2. Varus Disruption Fractures:
   - Varus Avulsion 2 fragment fractures: reconstructive surgery is indicated (humerusblock, plating, nailing)
   - Varus Avulsion 3 fragment fractures: in cases with less severe displacement (no rotational instability of the head), reconstructive surgery is recommended (humerusblock, plating)

   In other cases with severe displacement, reconstructive surgery is indicated in younger patients (humerusblock, plating,). In older patients with osteoporotic bone conditions, prosthetic replacement (reverse shoulder arthroplasty) is recommended.

Valgus Fractures

- Valgus Impaction Fractures: Valgus Lateral Impaction 3- and 4-fragment fractures (<20° sagittal angulation) without horizontal displacement are good indications for reconstructive surgery (humerusblock, plating). The same treatment recommendations can be given for Valgus Posterolateral Impaction fractures (>20° sagittal angulation).
- Valgus Impaction 4-fragment fractures with horizontal displacement in elder patients with osteoporotic bone quality are good indications for reverse prosthetic replacement (reverse shoulder arthroplasty).

Head Split Fractures

Head Split fractures (found in 2.5 %) are the most difficult fractures in terms of reduction and fixation. Despite this, the preferred treatment for younger patients should be reconstructive surgery, whereas in older patients, prosthetic replacement should be the treatment of choice.

Generally speaking, for very old patients (>80 years) suffering from complex fractures, reverse arthroplasty rather than anatomical hemi-arthroplasty should be considered as a treatment option.

Reduction and Fixation of Proximal Humerus Fractures in Our Department [1–3]

The technique is based on percutaneous reduction and fixation. As a pre-requisite, the knowledge of fracture pattern and number of fragments is mandatory. 3D-CT reconstruction is extremely helpful for the understanding of the fracture pattern.

Philosophy of Treatment

The goal of treatment is the change of a severely displaced fracture into a minimally-displaced fracture by manual and percutaneous manoeuvre and fixation of the fragments by minimally-invasive osteosynthesis. Comparably to the conservative treatment, the arm is immobilised in a sling for 3 weeks.

Instruments

Reduction is achieved by manual manoeuvres and by percutaneously-introduced instruments such as simple elevators or hooks. Fixation of the fragments is performed with the so-called Humerusblock (De Puy Synthes). This fixation device contains two K-wires (2.5 mm diameter), which are locked by two scrub screws in the fixation block. The K-wires provide rotational as well as axial stability by a so-called three-point fixation:
1. in the fixation block
2. in the lateral shaft cortex
3. in the subchondral bone.

Before reduction, the Humerusblock is fixed to the shaft and two K-wires are inserted through the cortex of the shaft up to the fracture level, where they remain in a "waiting position".

Indications and Contra-Indications

Good Indications
1. Varus Impacted Fractures
2. Varus Disrupted 2-fragment Fractures and Varus Disruption 3-Fragment Fractures without severe internal rotation deformity (severe displacement of the greater tuberosity)
3. Valgus Lateral Impacted 3- and 4-Fragment Fractures

Less Good Indications
1. Varus Disrupted 3-Fragment Fractures with severe internal rotational deformity
2. Head split fractures
3. Dislocation Fractures

Results

Out of 621 cases operated on between 1999 and 2008, 559 (90 %) of all cases) were treated by percutaneous techniques. Of the remaining 62 cases (10 %), 31 (5 %) had an open reduction internal fixation (ORIF) and the other 31 (5 %) had a hemi-arthroplasty (HAP).

Forty-eight percent of all cases were 70 years or older. Out of 169 patients older than 70 years, 89 were followed up in 2008. Forty-one had a two-part, 32 a three-part and 16 a four-part fracture. According to the Constant score, the average outcome was 81 % in two-part fractures compared to the uninjured side, 85 % in three-part and 69 % in four-part fractures. In 19 fractures (out of 162) unacceptable re-displacement occurred in the early phase and required surgical re-intervention with the same procedure in nine cases and with arthroplasty in ten patients. The results show that of all patients who had a different treatment from minimally-invasive surgery (MIS) from the very beginning (13 patients), 80 % (162 minus 32) of all patients over the age of 70 years could be treated satisfactorily with this technique [4].

Conclusion

The aim of this technique is to change a severely-displaced fracture into a minimally-displaced fracture performed by percutaneous measurements. The post-operative treatment is comparable to conservative treatment with the arm in a sling for 3 weeks. The percutaneous reduction is based on knowledge about the condition of the soft tissue around the fracture. Therefore, the study of the fracture pattern in two planes with 3D-CT scans based on the above mentioned pathophysiological considerations, is a pre-requisite before starting with the surgery. With this technique at least 80 % of all fractures can be treated satisfactorily. Since open techniques with angle stable plates or even HAP have not fulfilled the expectations in osteoporotic bone conditions, this technique is an attractive option.

References

1. Resch H, Povacz P, Fröhlich H, Wambacher M (1997) Percutaneous fixation of three- and four- fractures of the proximal humerus. J Bone Joint Surg Br 79–13: 295–300
2. Resch H, Aschauer E, Povacz P, Ritter E (2000) Closed reduction and fixation of articular fractures of the humeral head. Tech Shoulder Elbow Surg 3:154–162
3. Resch H, Hübner C, Schwaiger R (2001) Minimally invasive reduction and osteosynthesis of articular fractures of the humeral head. Injury 32(1):S-A25–S-A32
4. Bogner R, Huebner C, Matis N, Auffarth A, Lederer S, Resch H (2008) Minimally invasive treatment of three and four part fractures of the proximal humerus in elderly patients. J Bone Joint Surg Br 90:1602–1607

Management of Proximal Tibial Fractures

Christos Garnavos

Introduction

The proximal tibia has been defined as the part of the tibia that extends from the knee joint distally for 1.5 times the medial to lateral joint width [53] (Fig. 1). Fractures that occur in this area are grossly heterogeneous and their prognosis depends on several factors. The most important are:
(a) intra-articular involvement and severity (such as the degree of articular step-off and the extent and separation of condylar fracture lines),
(b) the degree of fracture comminution and extension,
(c) the condition of the soft-tissue envelope,
(d) osteoporosis and
(e) patient's age and co-morbidities [82].

While all these factors should be considered whenever surgeons are dealing with fractures of the proximal tibia, fractures of the tibial plateau are an entity on their own and their management is completely differentiated from meta-diaphyseal fractures that do not extend into the knee joint. Therefore, the current review will be separated in two main parts, the current treatment options for extra-articular proximal tibial fractures followed by the current management of tibial plateau fractures. However, the injury of the soft tissues that surround the proximal tibia is a problem common to both extra- and intra-articular fractures and should be considered seriously prior to fracture treatment.

C. Garnavos, MD, PhD
Department of Orthopaedic,
Evangelismos General Hospital,
45-47 Ipsilandou St, 10676 Athens, Greece
e-mail: cgarn@otenet.gr

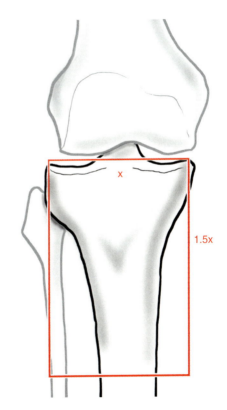

Fig. 1 Drawing that defines the Proximal Tibia (Lindvall et al. [53])

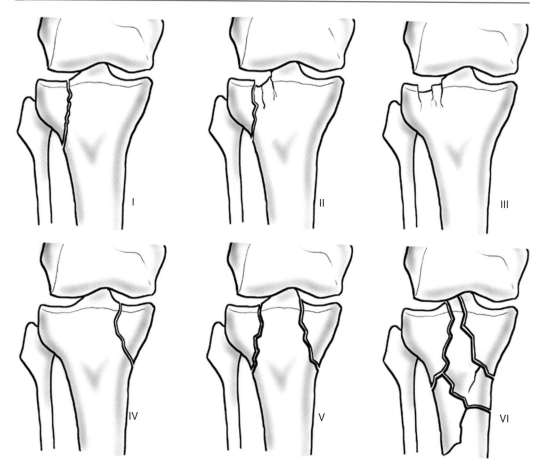

Fig. 2 Schatzker classification of intra-articular (tibial plateau) fractures. The fractures are classified from grades (I–VI) according to the severity and complexity of the bony injury

Epidemiology

Intra-articular proximal tibial fractures account approximately for 1 % of all fractures in the general population and about 8 % of fractures in the elderly and affect males more commonly than females [60]. The causes are road traffic accidents in 52 % of cases, falls in 17 % of cases and sporting or recreational activities in 5 % of cases [16, 60]. The lateral plateau alone is affected from 55 to 70 % of tibial plateau fractures, 10–25 % involve only the medial plateau and 10–30 % are bi-condylar fractures [60]. Approximately, 90 % of all tibial plateau fractures have some sort of soft tissue injury and 1–3 % are open fractures [21]. Extra-articular proximal tibial fractures are estimated to be 5–10 % of all tibial fractures [51].

Classification

Intra-articular proximal tibial fractures are mostly classified with the classifications introduced by Schatzker et al. [72] (Fig. 2) and AO/OTA compendium [58, 72] that also classifies extra-articular proximal tibial fractures (Fig. 3). Extra-articular fractures can be also classified with a simpler classification that we introduced recently (Garnavos classification) and can be used in every-day clinical practice, supplementing the more complicated AO/OTA classification [29].

As already mentioned, the severity of soft tissue injury plays an important role in treatment planning and management and both the Gustilo-Anderson and Tscherne-Gotzen classifications that refer to the soft tissue injury of open or closed fractures respectively, should be considered accordingly [37, 78].

Management of Proximal Tibial Fractures

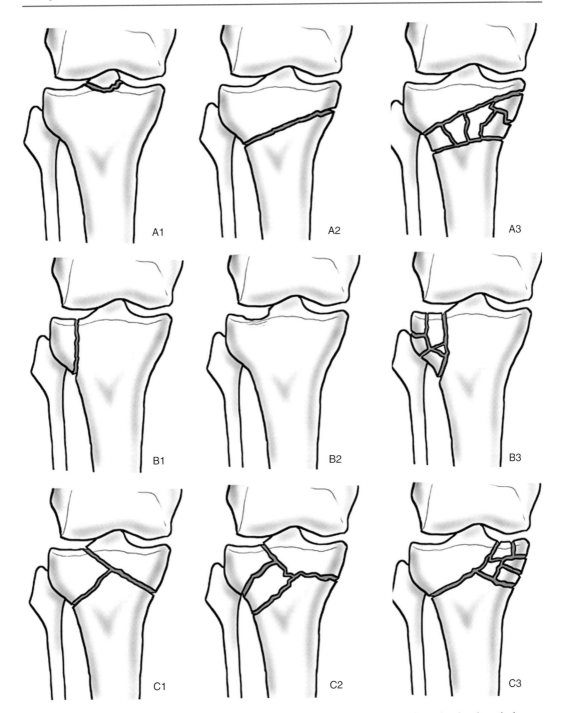

Fig. 3 AO/OTA classification of proximal tibial fractures. (A1–A3) contains fractures that do not involve the articular surfaces of the condyles, (B1–B3) contains unicondylar fractures while (C1–C3) contains more complex bi-condylar fractures

Soft Tissue Injury

Regardless of the pattern of a proximal tibia fracture, the soft tissues around the knee joint can be injured with variable severity (Fig. 4). Open fractures should be managed immediately with clinical assessment of the neurovascular status of the leg and foot, antibiotic administration, adequate irrigation, debridement, provisional reduction and immobilisation of the fracture and coverage of

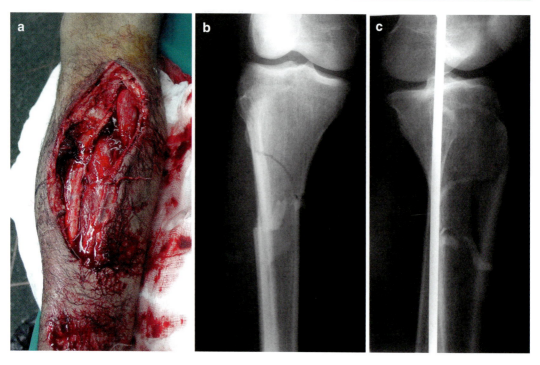

Fig. 4 Open fracture of the proximal tibia. (**a**) Clinical presentation. (**b**) Antero-posterior x-ray. (**c**) Lateral x-ray

exposed bone with healthy soft tissues, utilizing simple or more complex plastic surgical procedures, as soon as possible. Closed fractures may be more challenging to manage, regarding the soft tissue injury, as severe crushing of the soft tissues may not be obvious at the beginning and therefore, careful observation of patients with closed fractures of the proximal tibia is mandatory. Development of excessive oedema and fracture blisters may require intervention, starting with covering with sterile non-adhesive dressings and regular monitoring of the compartments' pressure. Elevation of the leg should follow and definitive surgical fracture fixation should be delayed until improvement of the soft tissue condition.

It has been reported that the incidence of meniscal and ligamentous injuries is high in fractures of the tibial plateau, even in cases that could be treated non-operatively [1, 18, 28, 74].

However, the necessity for diagnosing and treating these injuries in the acute phase, synchronously with the proximal tibial fracture is still controversial with some authors recommending early repair while others advocate an "active neglect" policy initially and repair at a later timing if necessary [5, 12, 58, 59, 80].

It is my opinion that deferring treatment of a significant meniscal or ligamentous injury is not wrong as, within a background of a severe bony injury, one prolongs the operating (and tourniquet?) time and adds to surgical trauma in order to repair non-crucial soft tissue trauma. Most ligamentous or meniscal injuries that accompany fractures of the proximal tibia can be managed satisfactorily with some delay and it is not infrequent that less severe injuries will not require any intervention in the future.

Conservative Management of Proximal Tibial Fractures

Undisplaced or minimally-displaced fractures of the proximal tibia can be managed conservatively with the use of a well moulded long-leg cast, which is applied upon subsidence of the oedema, with the knee in about 10° of flexion and is maintained for 3–4 weeks [70].

At this time the long cast can be replaced with a hinged brace and the patient can start mobilizing the knee joint, under supervision. Initiation of weight-bearing depends on fracture configuration, patient's body mass and co-operation but, generally, touch weight-bearing can be allowed at 4–6 weeks and full weight-bearing at 8–12 weeks from the accident [70].

Because of the short proximal fragment and high incidence of comminution and/or significant intra-articular involvement, angular deformities and/or displacement occur frequently. In addition, the soft tissue envelope that surrounds the proximal tibia is tight and both closed and open fractures impose serious danger for the neurovascular structures that cross the specific anatomical area. For all these reasons, most proximal tibial fractures are not amenable to conservative management. Surgical treatment restores anatomy and allows early mobilization of the knee joint and weight-bearing of the limb.

Operative Management of Proximal Tibial Fractures

All available surgical techniques of osteosynthesis have been used in the management of intra- and extra-articular proximal tibial fractures. While it seems that there is a consensus towards either percutaneous screw fixation or unilateral plating for simpler intra-articular fractures (AO/OTA: 41-B1, 41-B2, 41-B3 or Schatzker types I, II, III and IV), there is a lot of controversy regarding the management of more complex bicondylar (AO/OTA: 41-C1, 41-C2, 41-C3 or Schatzker types V and VI) or proximal extra-articular fractures (AO/OTA: 41-A2, 41-A3, 42-C3). In any case, pre-operative planning must be meticulous, as the surgeon must plan not only the approach and fixation technique but also how to assess the articular reduction if the fracture involves the articular surface. Depending on the surgeon's preference and experience but also on available resources, the assessment of the articular reduction can be accomplished by three different ways;

1. direct visualization (through an arthrotomy),
2. fluoroscopy or
3. arthroscopy.

Simple Intra-Articular Fractures

AO/OTA type 41-B1 or Schatzker type I fractures can be treated with percutaneous screws 1/2 or 1/3 thread, that can apply compression to the split fracture [20, 45, 47]. If the lateral plateau fragment appears displaced, reduction to its anatomical position can be achieved with closed manoeuvres or a bone reduction forceps. Lately, I have treated a series of such fractures with the use of one or two compression bolts that offer great compression and stability to the fracture site and thus allow immediate mobilisation of the knee joint and initiation of partial weight-bearing at 2–3 weeks post-operatively (Fig. 5). By 4–6 weeks from surgery all patients regained full range of motion, commenced full weight-bearing and returned to usual activities. In no case there was any loss of reduction or any other complication and the patients did not report any irritation or problem from the head of the compression bolt.

Intra-Articular Fractures of Intermediate Severity

AO/OTA types 41-B2 and 41-B3 or Schatzker type II, III and IV fractures require more attention, as there is either lateral articular fragmentation or depression (AO/OTA types 41-B2 and 41-B3, Schatzker type II, III) or medial articular fragmentation (Schatzker type IV). The most common technique for the fixation of these fractures is buttress plating [50, 71].

Split-depressed fractures of the lateral tibial plateau (Schatzker type II) can be approached via a limited antero-lateral incision. The fractured lateral tibial condyle can be displaced laterally at the fracture site and the depressed articular surface can be reduced to its proper position under direct vision. The elevated cartilage should be supported with a suitable filler. While autologous bone is unanimously considered as

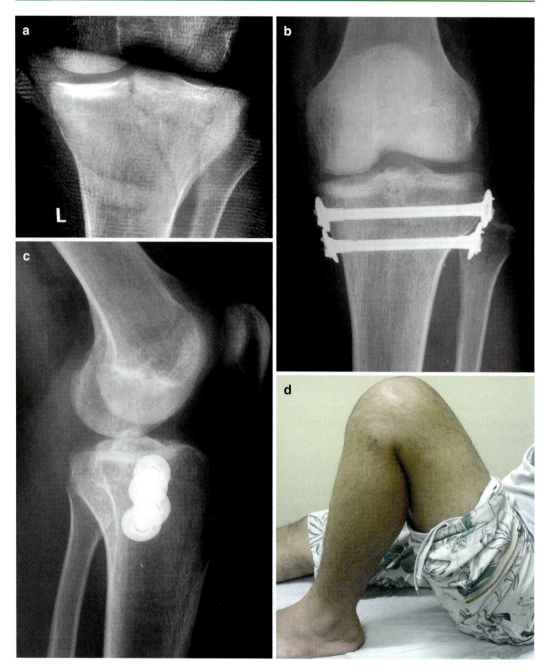

Fig. 5 Management of a Schatzker type I fracture with compression bolts: (**a**) Pre-operative antero-posterior x-ray; (**b, c**) antero-posterior and lateral x-ray at 6 weeks with the patient being fully weight bearing; (**d, e**) knee joint motion was fully restored at 4 weeks post-operatively

Fig. 5 (continued)

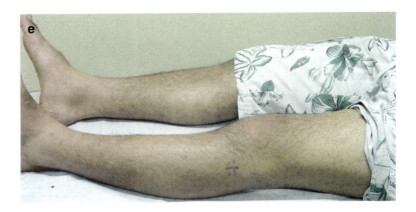

the best grafting material, it requires an additional (graft harvesting) procedure, that could create problems from the donor site. Therefore, alternative grafting options have been proposed, such as allografts, methylmethacrylate, and bone substitutes [17, 26, 33].

Over the last decade I have been using freeze-dried cancellous allograft as filler. This allograft is incorporating within the surrounding metaphyseal bone after a short period of time (8–12 weeks) and has proven strong enough to support sufficiently the restored joint surface (Fig. 6). Furthermore, there have not been any complications that could relate to its use [52].

Following the restoration of the articular surface and grafting, the lateral condyle is reduced and the construct is supported and fixed with a lateral buttress plate. My personal preference for this type of fracture is a traditional non-locking plate with 6.5 mm cancellous screws for the metaphyseal region and 4.5 mm cortical screws for the more distal meta-diaphyseal area. However, recently there is a trend towards locking plates with 3.5 mm "rafting" screws, a more costly option.

Schatzker type III fractures that present with a depressed lateral tibial plateau without separation of the condyle should be treated in a similar manner. The impacted articular surface can be reduced and supported with the selected filler through a fenestration 2–3 cm below the articular surface. The reconstructed area can then be supported with a buttress plate and screws as described above [50, 71] (Fig. 7).

Isolated medial plateau fractures (Schatzker type IV) are usually inferiorly displaced but not impacted. These fractures can be managed with open reduction of the medial fragment through a postero-medial approach and fixation with a simple 3.5 mm buttress plate. Unfortunately, there are not substantive studies dealing with this particular fracture type and we can only find scarce cases in between other types of tibial plateau fractures in relevant studies. However, it is reported that medial plateau fractures have a tendency to displace post-operatively and their prognosis is not as good as Schatzker II and III types [7, 13, 42].

Complex or Bi-Condylar Fractures of the Tibial Plateau

AO/OTA 41C1, 41C2, 41C3 types or Schatzker types V and VI fractures constitute the most difficult group of fractures that involve the tibial plateau, as one or both tibial condyles are usually displaced and/or depressed. Not infrequently, significant soft tissue injury (severe skin contusion, meniscal and ligament tears, neurovascular problems) co-exist. Immediate management should involve elevation and immobilization while skeletal traction, usually through the os calcis, could be used as temporary immobilization and reduction method. Immediate spanning external fixation is used frequently nowadays, whenever feasible, depending on the patient's physical

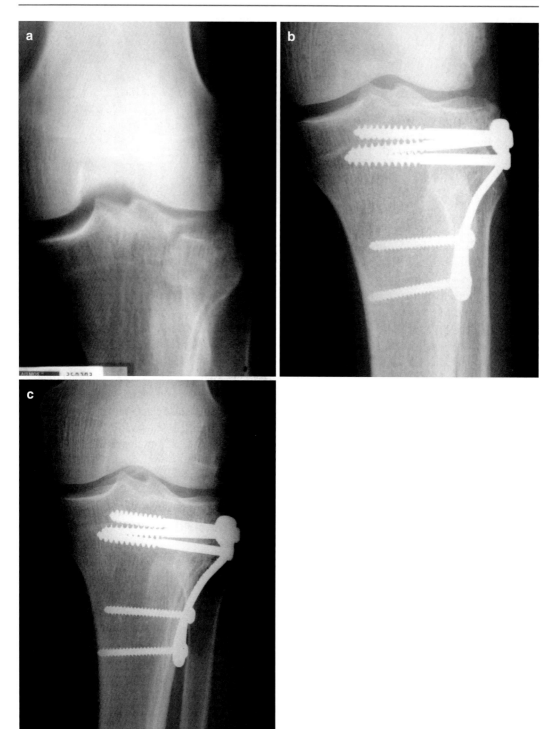

Fig. 6 (**a**) Tomogram of a Schatzker type II split-depressed fracture. (**b**) Immediate post-operative x-ray showing the result of open reduction and internal fixation with traditional plating. The metaphyseal cavity was filled with freeze-dried allograft. (**c**) Six weeks later the allograft is almost fully incorporated

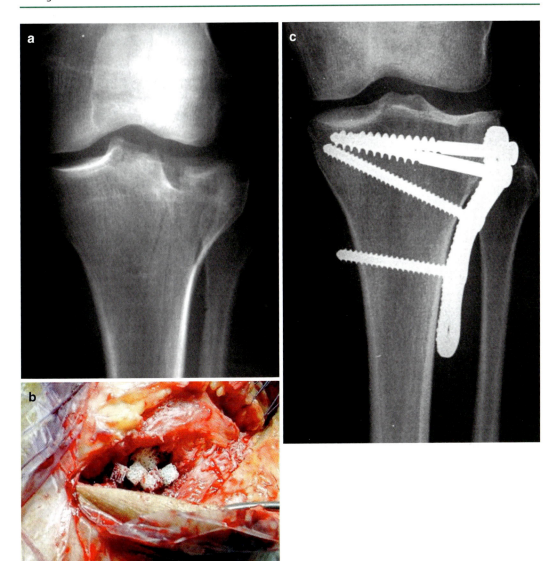

Fig. 7 (**a**) Antero-posterior x-ray of a Schatzker type III depressed fracture. (**b**) Intra-operative picture showing the insertion of freeze-dried allograft within the cavity that was created after the elevation of the impacted articular surface. (**c**) Ten weeks later the allograft is incorporated and the fracture is healed

status and theatre availability. With reduction of the oedema and satisfactory condition of the skin, that usually takes 5–10 days, definitive surgical treatment should be carried out. Plating and external fixation have been traditionally used for the management of complex fractures of the tibial plateau. However, recently, intramedullary nailing, combined with compression bolts, has also been tried with promising results.

Plating Osteosynthesis

The traditional open reduction and internal fixation (ORIF) procedure is still popular although it requires wide exposure of the proximal tibia. However, the extensive iatrogenic injury to the soft tissues compromises their integrity, reduces the blood supply to the fractured bone, does not preserve fracture haematoma and increases the risks of complications, such as knee joint stiffness, infection and non-union. In addition, initial studies regarding plating of proximal tibia fractures revealed that one plate may not provide adequate stability, especially in bi-condylar proximal tibial fractures or extra-articular fractures with a very short proximal fragment. Therefore, dual plating or a composite fixation consisting of lateral plating and a medial external fixator has been proposed for improved stability (Fig. 8). Although these techniques improve the biomechanical properties of the fixation construct, they do not address the problem of the extensive iatrogenic trauma and soft tissue dissection [9, 34, 46].

The introduction and popularization of locking plates over the last decade that can be inserted with minimally-invasive technique (Minimally Invasive Plate Osteosynthesis [MIPO]) changed the concept of plating fixation for complex proximal tibial fractures (Fig. 9). According to the initial reports the percutaneous technique reduced the problems of open plating that predominantly originated from the wide exposure of the proximal tibia while the new plate-screw locking facility seemed to enhance the biomechanical properties of the fixation, especially in osteoporotic bone [8, 15, 48, 69, 73, 75].

Shortly after the introduction of the new plating technique important issues were raised:
- When does the plate/bone distance influence stability?
- All screws locked or combination locked/non-locked screws can suffice?
- Bi-cortical or uni-cortical screws?
- One Locking Plate or Two Conventional Plates for bi-condylar fractures?
- Do poly-axial plates improve outcomes?

Although absolute contact of the locking plate with the bone is not required for a successful fixation, it has been shown that when the plate is positioned at a distance >2 mm from the bone, the stability of the construct is significantly reduced [2].

The issue of all-locked versus hybrid locked/non-locked screw configurations seems sorted out, since a relatively recent biomechanical study confirmed the strong clinical suspicion that the two options were not statistically different with regard to the stability of fixation [25].

While it seems that, in the management of complex fractures of the tibial plateau, bi-cortical screw placement provides a biomechanically superior construct than uni-cortical screw placement, [19] there has been disagreement about the choice of one locking plate or two conventional plates for bi-condylar fractures. Earlier studies supported that there does not seem to be a significant difference in the strength and outcomes of the fixation, [22, 35, 61] while more recent studies reported more stability and less incidence of post-operative mal-alignment and symptomatic hardware irritation with conventional dual plate fixation [41, 43, 66].

Limited evidence from the use of poly-axial plates indicates that these plates perform well with a high rate of fracture union and no evidence of varus collapse [38, 62].

Scepticism followed the initial enthusiasm for the use of the new locking plates with the MIPO technique, as complication rates rose to unexpected figures. So, hardware failure has been reported up to18%, poor fracture reduction was seen up to 23 %, implant removal was necessary up to 30 %, irritation from hardware occurred up to12%, deep infection up to 18 % and superficial infection up to 10 % [36, 43, 67, 76]. Despite these reports, locking plates are considered a significant advancement in the management of complex proximal tibial fractures; [55]. They offer enhanced angular stability while having a low profile and therefore are particularly suitable for osteoporotic fractures. The MIPO technique results in less periosteal stripping and soft tissue preservation. However, alongside the previously reported complications, one should consider also that insertion of a locking plate still requires a lateral approach to the proximal tibia, something that could hamper a future knee arthroplasty procedure [81] while these plates are sometimes difficult to remove. Finally, the parameter of cost-effectiveness in the use of locking plates has yet to be defined.

External Fixation

In the management of complex fractures of the tibial plateau external fixators can be used as temporary knee-bridging devices (Fig. 10) or

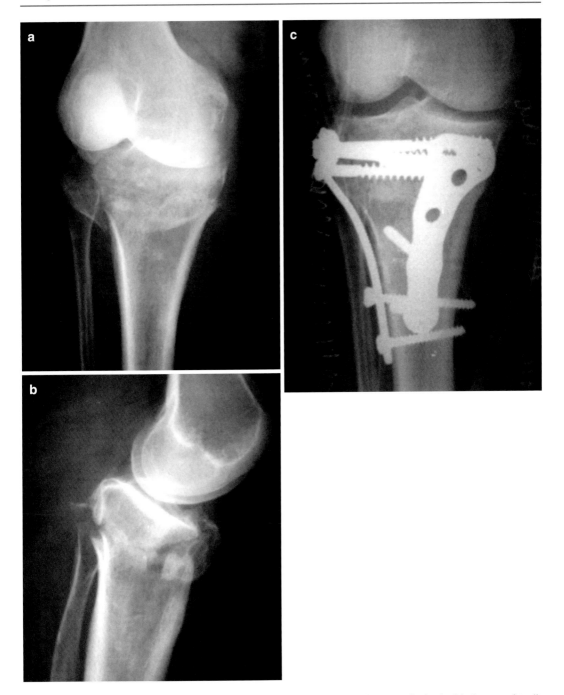

Fig. 8 Comminuted and displaced Schatzker type V bicondylar fracture. (**a**) Antero-posterior x-ray. (**b**) Lateral x-ray. (**c**) Post-operative antero-posterior x-ray showing the good result that was obtained with the use of traditional dual plating

as definitive treatment in the form of Ilizarov-type circular frames or hybrid constructs. Knee-bridging fixators are invaluable devices for the initial management of severe intra-articular fractures of the knee joint but should not be used as definitive treatment, as their prolonged use is likely to create irreversible stiffness of the knee [6, 23, 65, 79].

Since the 1980's and 1990's, ring fixators that allow knee motion have been used successfully in

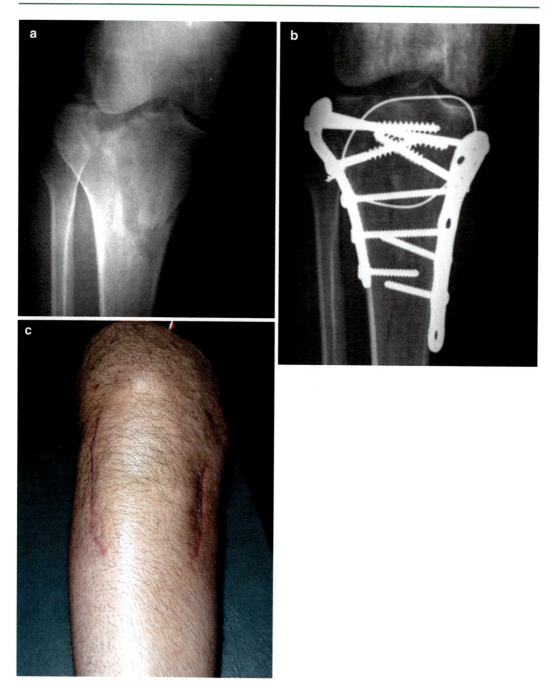

Fig. 9 (**a**) Antero-posterior pre-operative x-ray of a Schatzker type VI complex fracture of the tibial plateau, (**b**) Post-operative antero-posterior x-ray showing restoration and fixation with the double plating technique, (**c**) post-operative clinical picture showing the two incisions, (**d**) Less severe cases like this Schatzker type II fracture can be managed with MIPO technique (**e, f**)

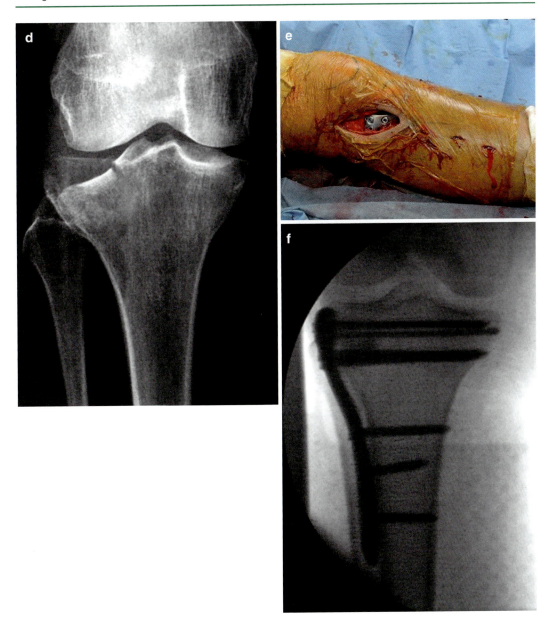

Fig. 9 (continued)

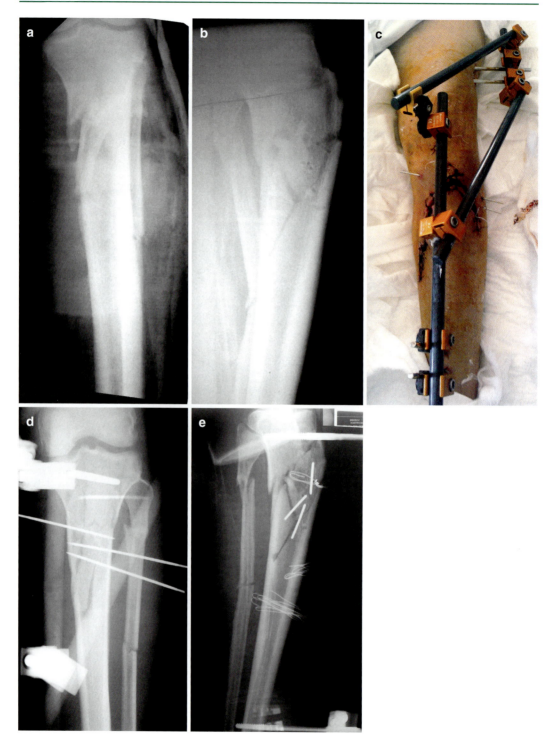

Fig. 10 Knee bridging external fixation in an intra-articular Gustilo-Anderson IIIb open fracture of the proximal tibia. (**a**, **b**) initial antero-posterior and lateral x-rays, (**c**) temporary immobilization with a knee-bridging external fixator, (**d**, **e**) antero-posterior and lateral x-rays after wound debridement and temporary external fixation

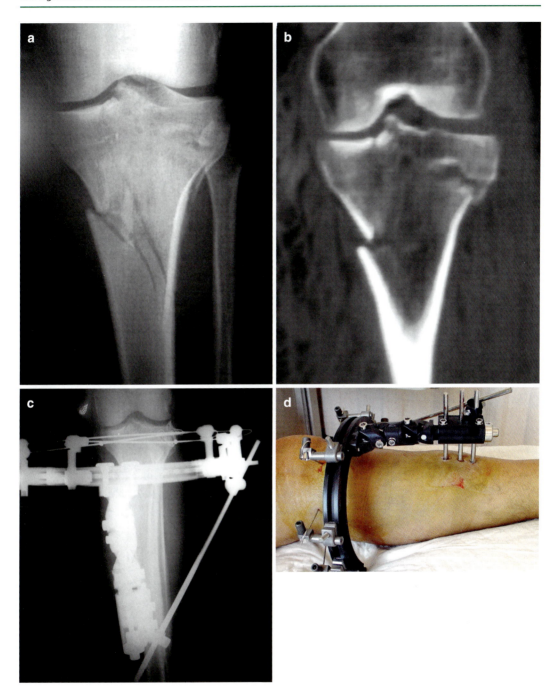

Fig. 11 Definitive management of a Schatzker type VI fracture with hybrid external fixation. (**a**) Initial antero-posterior x-ray, (**b**) CT-image depicting the fracture extension towards the knee joint, (**c, d**) Antero-posterior x-ray and clinical appearance 3.5 months post-injury

the definitive treatment of bicondylar fractures of the tibial plateau [3, 4, 32, 57, 83] (Fig. 11).

The significant advantage of the technique has been the less invasive means of reducing and stabilizing the tibial plateau fracture while gaining good overall limb alignment. Additionally, external fixation has a significantly reduced rate of wound necrosis, compared with the traditional plating technique, it allows early knee motion and weight-bearing whilst it can be removed

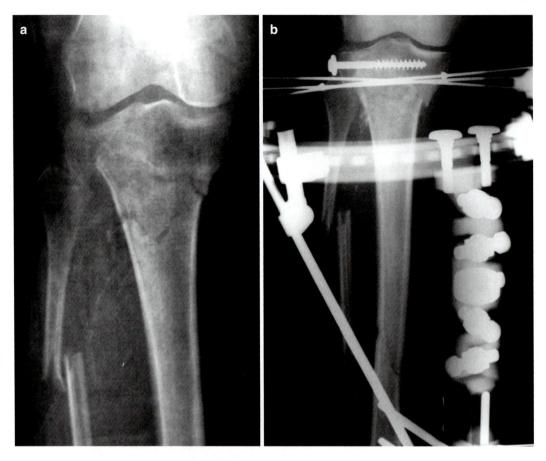

Fig. 12 (**a**) Antero-posterior x-ray showing a Schatzker type VI fracture treated with (**b**) the combination of external with limited internal osteosynthesis

easily in the clinic without anaesthesia [12]. More recent reports recommend the combination of external with limited internal osteosynthesis for more anatomical and stable fixation of the intra-articular element of the fracture [6, 14, 44, 77] (Fig. 12).

Complications that can occur with the use of external fixation in the treatment of bi-condylar tibial plateau fractures include pin-tract infection, inadequate reduction or loss of reduction of the articular surface, joint stiffness and septic arthritis [4, 64] (Fig. 13).

Open Reduction and Internal Fixation or External Fixation for Bi-Condylar Fractures of the Tibial Plateau?

Bearing in mind that the minimally-invasive locking plating technique was not included in the study, a multicentre, prospective, randomized

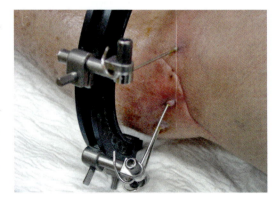

Fig. 13 Pin-track infection is of the most frequent complications of the external fixation

clinical trial showed that traditional dual plating and external fixation techniques provide satisfactory reduction. However, external fixation resulted in a shorter hospital stay, marginally faster return of function and similar clinical outcomes. In addition, the number and severity of complications was higher with open reduction and internal fixation [12].

A more recent attempt for a systematic review of the literature regarding the treatment selection for bi-condylar tibial plateau fractures concluded that hybrid external fixation, theoretically, respects more the soft tissues but the benefit over internal fixation was found modest at best and did not demonstrate improved outcomes. It was also stated that newer fixed angle screw and plate systems are increasingly in use but comparative studies that could determine their role in this complex group of fractures are missing at present [56].

Intramedullary Nailing and Compression Bolts

Since 2005 I have been using intramedullary nailing and compression bolts for the management of bi-condylar fractures of the tibial plateau without significant depression of the articular surface [31]. The technique is minimally-invasive and includes percutaneous reduction and fixation of the intra-articular fracture with a compression bolt positioned with a medio-lateral direction 0.5–1 cm below the articular surface. Intramedullary nailing of the meta-diaphyseal part of the fracture follows, as if the fracture was extra-articular (Fig. 14). The idea was generated by the drawbacks of both conventional and MIPO plating techniques, such as the compromise of soft-tissue integrity, fracture mal-alignment and high infection rate. Another drawback with plating in the event of delaying union of the diaphyseal part of an extended/segmental fracture is that there is no option for dynamisation and finally, removal of a locking plate and screws can be troublesome. Especially in osteoporotic fractures, lateral and/or medial incisions, bulky metalwork and its removal alongside with substantial infection rate can compromise the option of a knee arthroplasty procedure in the future [81]. The technique of external fixation has its own problems, as previously described. More particularly, in osteoporotic patients, loss of reduction or fracture mal-union cannot be considered infrequent problems. Patients at a certain age do not tolerate bulky external fixation devices that can interfere adversely with the mobilisation process of their knee and the rehabilitation programme, whilst the option of a knee arthroplasty in the future could be compromised by infection that can happen in the pin tracks close to the knee joint.

The nail/compression bolt technique offers a number of advantages. It is minimally-invasive and the main incision, that facilitates nail insertion, is short and close to the mid-line, whilst stab incisions are used for the insertion of the compression bolt(s) and locking screws. Therefore, the operation can be performed soon after the accident as it does not interfere significantly with the soft tissues at the metaphyseal area, where many patients develop blisters and abrasions. In addition, scarring should not be a problem in case of a knee arthroplasty operation in the future [81]. Intramedullary implants, being load-sharing devices, distribute axial forces evenly and allow early mobilisation and weight-bearing, an important necessity for elderly patients in particular. Infection rate is much lower after nailing if compared with plating. In the event of an open fracture, intramedullary nailing could facilitate the soft-tissue care better than a plate or a circular frame. Finally, removal of intramedullary nails and compression bolts is usually a straightforward procedure.

Conclusively, the advantages of the nailing/bolt technique are:
1. Minimally-invasive procedure that can be performed as soon as possible after the accident (even with sub-optimal soft-tissue condition)
2. optimal option for extended or segmental fractures and "floating" knee injuries
3. stable fixation that allows rapid mobilisation of both the patient and the knee joint
4. reduced morbidity and complications, such as infection, irritation from the metalwork and re-operation rate; and
5. 'compatibility' of subsequent operations, such as knee arthroplasty (by keeping the knee joint fully mobile, mid-line and straight main incision and easily removable metalwork).

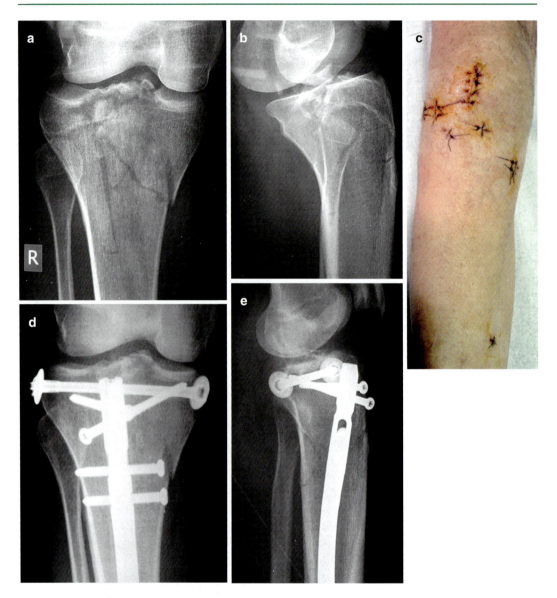

Fig. 14 Bi-condylar (Schatzker type VI) fracture of the proximal tibia treated with intramedullary nailing and a compression bolt. (**a, b**) Initial antero-posterior and lateral x-rays. (**c–e**) Clinical and radiological appearance 2 weeks post surgery. Note the direction of the compression bolt (postero-medial to antero-lateral) that reduces and supports the postero-medial fragment

Over the last 2–3 years we have exploited the potentials of the nailing-bolt technique for the treatment of complex fractures of the tibial plateau in younger patients with more complicated fracture patterns with excellent results (Fig. 15). We have also organized a biomechanical study that compared in vitro the mechanical properties of traditional dual plating, the laterally positioned locking plate and the nail-bolt construct with the results being favourable for the last technique (Lasanianos NG, Garnavos C, Magnisalis E, Kourkoulis S, Babis GC, 2013, A comparative biomechanical study for complex tibial plateau fractures. Nailing and compression bolts versus modern and traditional plating, (accepted for publication in INJURY).

Extra-Articular Proximal Tibial Fractures

Both plating osteosynthesis and external fixation have been popular methods in the management of extra-articular proximal tibial fractures. However, until recently, the effectiveness of these techniques could not be easily assessed, as extra-articular fractures of the proximal tibia, were usually studied as a group with intra-articular proximal tibial, distal tibial or distal femoral fractures[8, 10, 15, 24, 38, 65, 69]. However, over the last few years, a lot of attention has been drawn to the management of proximal extra-articular tibial fractures, as modern minimally- invasive, locking plate osteosynthesis is being challenged by intramedullary nailing, that has been significantly improved. In the classical study by Lang et al. (1995) [51] the authors considered that proximal third tibial fractures should not be nailed, because "these fractures do not appear to respond favourably to intramedullary nailing". However, in the last 10–15 years many things changed. Major problems such as mal-reduction and/or displacement of proximal

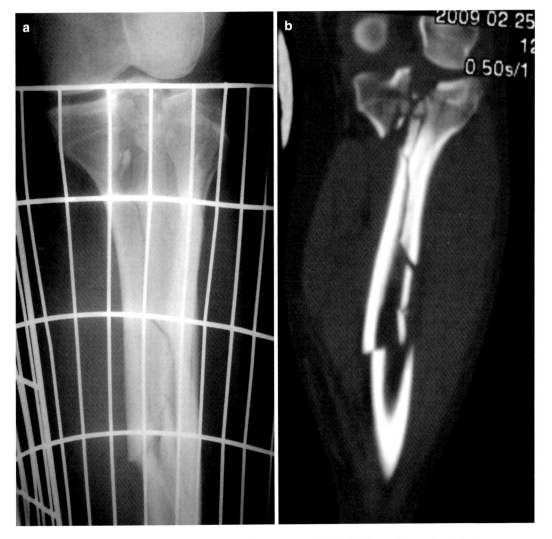

Fig. 15 An extended Schatzker type VI fracture in a 31 year old male patient. (**a**, **b**) Pre-operative antero-posterior x-ray and CT scan. (**c**) Immediate post-operative AP x-ray. (**d–g**) Radiographic and clinical appearance 3 months post-operatively

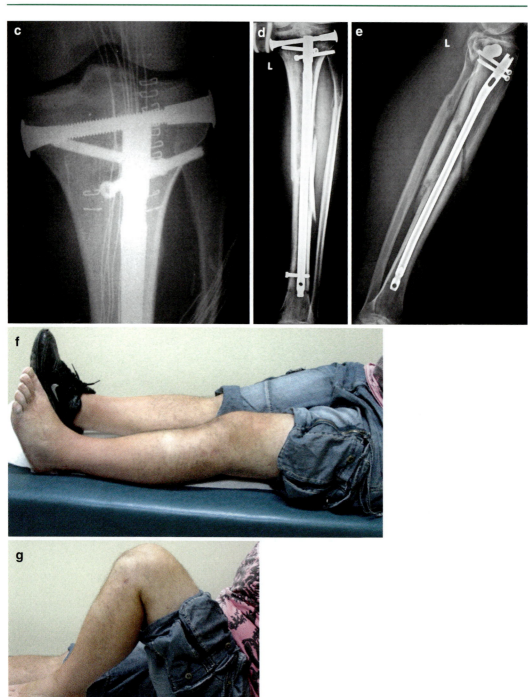

Fig. 15 (continued)

tibial fractures post-nailing were dealt with by new nail designs and improvements/alterations of the surgical technique. Therefore, the proximal bend of the tibial nails (Herzog bend) was positioned more proximally in order to be contained within the short proximal fragment and thus resist its anterior translation. Proposals regarding modifications of the surgical technique include the provisional use of a distractor/external fixator or the supplementary provisional or permanent use of a plate [39, 54, 55, 63, 86]. A popular aid towards fracture reduction and strengthening of the fixation, whilst comprising with the closed technique of intramedullary nailing, has been the introduction of free antero-posterior and/or medio-lateral guidance screws ("blocking" screws) [39, 40, 49, 54, 55, 63, 68]. Another important issue regarding intramedullary nailing of proximal tibia fractures is the location of the entry portal of the nail in the coronal plane. Most researchers support the lateral location always [11, 27, 39, 40, 55, 63] while there have been reports that argue either in favour of the medial insertion or where exactly on the lateral side should the entry portal be located [84, 85]. It has been our observation that in the management of extra-articular proximal tibial fractures with intramedullary nailing, the location of the entry portal on the coronal plane should be parapatellar, lateral or medial, depending on the side where the fracture approximates mostly to the articular surface of the proximal tibia on the antero-posterior (AP) x-ray [30] (Figs. 16 and 17).

Regarding the patient positioning, I favour the free hanging of the leg with the knee in maximum flexion during surgery that facilitates the insertion of the nail as proximal as possible within the sort proximal fragment. However, this position increases the anterior angulation of the fracture due to the action of the patellar tendon on the proximal fragment and furthermore, does not allow adequate antero-posterior visualisation with the image intensifier after the insertion of the nail, as the handle of the nail impinges on the patella and the extension of the knee joint becomes cumbersome. The recently proposed retro-patellar approach that facilitates undisturbed AP and lateral visualization during the whole procedure with the knee in a semi-extended position could be the solution to the problem (Fig. 18). This approach also facilitates better control of fracture reduction and alignment of the leg. Nevertheless, the technique requires special tools for nail insertion and tissue protection whilst there may be the need for manufacturing fracture specific intramedullary nails.

Conclusions

The definition "proximal tibial fractures" refers to a group of grossly heterogeneous injuries regarding the severity of soft tissue and bony injury, treatment requirements and clinical outcomes. These fractures involve the knee joint and their management requires detailed imaging studies and meticulous pre-operative planning, excellent theatre facilities and advanced surgical expertise. Existence of more than one treatment option for each subgroup of these fractures indicates that none guarantees excellent results and a minimal complication rate. Furthermore, new surgical techniques and implants appear constantly, making the evaluation process an ongoing and difficult task. Despite the changes that require constant education and training, our efforts to obtain sort and long term optimal outcomes for our patients can only be obtained if the most appropriate treatment method is be applied to each case individually after careful justification and planning, bearing in mind our resources, limitations and capabilities.

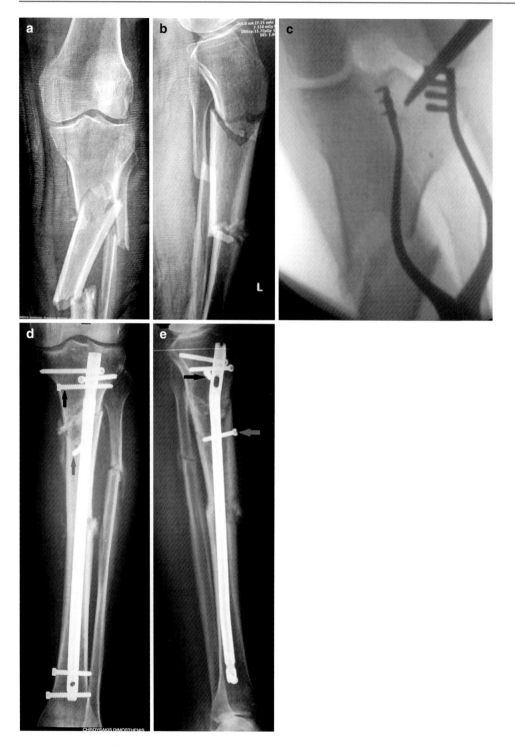

Fig. 16 Extra-articular fracture of the proximal tibia (part of segmental fracture). (**a, b**) Initial antero-posterior and lateral x-rays. (**c**) Intra-operative picture depicting the site of the lateral parapatellar location of the entry point of the nail, as the fracture approximates the knee joint mostly from the lateral cortex. (**d, e**) Antero-posterior and lateral x-rays at 2.5 months post-operatively showing the good alignment of the tibia. The medio-lateral blocking screw (*black arrow*) prohibited the anterior angulation of the proximal fracture while the nail trajectory did not allow its varus/valgus deviation. The second antero-posterior blocking screw (*grey arrow*) contributed towards the reduction of the middle free segment

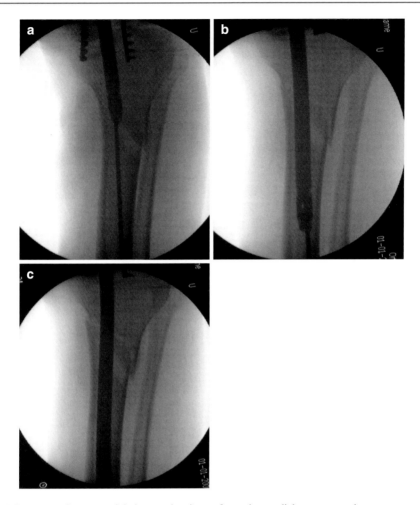

Fig. 17 (**a–c**) Intra-operative sequential pictures showing the impact of nail trajectory to avoidance of varus deformity. The fracture approximates the knee joint mostly from the medial cortex on the antero-posterior x-ray, therefore the entry point of the nail was located medially

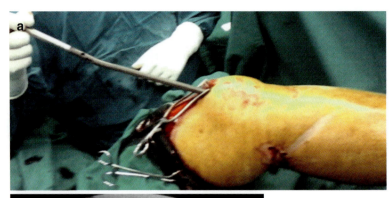
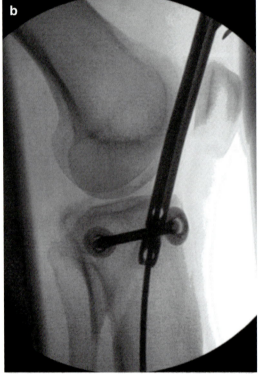

Fig. 18 (a, b) Clinical and radiological pictures showing the nailing of a proximal tibia fracture via the retro-patellar approach

Acknowledgements The author would like to thank Dr. Konstantinos Dudulakis for his contribution with the drawings in the text.

References

1. Abdel-Hamid MZ, Chang CH, Chan YS, Lo YP, Huang JW, Hsu KY, Wang CJ (2006) Arthroscopic evaluation of soft tissue injuries in tibial plateau fractures: retrospective analysis of 98 cases. Arthroscopy 22(6):669–675
2. Ahmad M, Nanda R, Bajwa AS, Candal-Couto J, Green S, Hui AC (2007) Biomechanical testing of the locking compression plate: when does the distance between bone and implant significantly reduce construct stability? Injury 38(3):358–364. doi:10.1016/j.injury.2006.08.058, S0020-1383(06)00546-8 [pii]
3. Ali AM, Yang L, Hashmi M, Saleh M (2001) Bicondylar tibial plateau fractures managed with the Sheffield hybrid fixator. Biomechanical study and operative technique. Injury 32(Suppl 4):SD86–SD91. doi:S0020138301001656 [pii]
4. Babis GC, Evangelopoulos DS, Kontovazenitis P, Nikolopoulos K, Soucacos PN (2011) High energy tibial plateau fractures treated with hybrid external

fixation. J Orthop Surg Res 6:35. doi:10.1186/1749-799X-6-35, 1749-799X-6-35 [pii]
5. Bennett WF, Browner B (1994) Tibial plateau fractures: a study of associated soft tissue injuries. J Orthop Trauma 8(3):183–188
6. Berkson EM, Virkus WW (2006) High-energy tibial plateau fractures. J Am Acad Orthop Surg 14(1): 20–31. doi:14/1/20 [pii]
7. Bhattacharyya T, McCarty LP 3rd, Harris MB, Morrison SM, Wixted JJ, Vrahas MS, Smith RM (2005) The posterior shearing tibial plateau fracture: treatment and results via a posterior approach. J Orthop Trauma 19(5):305–310
8. Boldin C, Fankhauser F, Hofer HP, Szyszkowitz R (2006) Three-year results of proximal tibia fractures treated with the LISS. Clin Orthop Relat Res 445: 222–229. doi:10.1097/01.blo.0000203467.58431.a0
9. Bolhofner BR (1995) Indirect reduction and composite fixation of extraarticular proximal tibial fractures. Clin Orthop Relat Res 315:75–83
10. Buckley R, Mohanty K, Malish D (2011) Lower limb malrotation following MIPO technique of distal femoral and proximal tibial fractures. Injury 42(2): 194–199. doi:10.1016/j.injury.2010.08.024, S0020-1383(10)00636-4 [pii]
11. Buehler KC, Green J, Woll TS, Duwelius PJ (1997) A technique for intramedullary nailing of proximal third tibia fractures. J Orthop Trauma 11(3):218–223
12. Canadian Orthopaedic Trauma Society (2006) Open reduction and internal fixation compared with circular fixator application for bicondylar tibial plateau fractures. Results of a multicenter, prospective, randomized clinical trial. J Bone Joint Surg Am 88(12):2613–2623. doi:10.2106/JBJS.E.01416, 88/12/2613 [pii]
13. Carlson DA (2005) Posterior bicondylar tibial plateau fractures. J Orthop Trauma 19(2):73–78. doi:00005131-200502000-00001 [pii]
14. Catagni MA, Ottaviani G, Maggioni M (2007) Treatment strategies for complex fractures of the tibial plateau with external circular fixation and limited internal fixation. J Trauma 63(5):1043–1053. doi:10.1097/TA.0b013e3181238d88, 00005373-200711000-00013 [pii]
15. Cole PA, Zlowodzki M, Kregor PJ (2004) Treatment of proximal tibia fractures using the less invasive stabilization system: surgical experience and early clinical results in 77 fractures. J Orthop Trauma 18(8):528–535. doi:00005131-200409000-00008 [pii]
16. Court-Brown CM, Caesar B (2006) Epidemiology of adult fractures: a review. Injury 37(8):691–697. doi:10.1016/j.injury.2006.04.130, S0020-1383(06)00323-8 [pii]
17. De Long WG Jr, Einhorn TA, Koval K, McKee M, Smith W, Sanders R, Watson T (2007) Bone grafts and bone graft substitutes in orthopaedic trauma surgery. A critical analysis. J Bone Joint Surg Am 89(3): 649–658. doi:10.2106/JBJS.F.00465, 89/3/649 [pii]
18. Delamarter RB, Hohl M, Hopp E Jr (1990) Ligament injuries associated with tibial plateau fractures. Clin Orthop Relat Res 250:226–233
19. Dougherty PJ, Kim DG, Meisterling S, Wybo C, Yeni Y (2008) Biomechanical comparison of bicortical versus unicortical screw placement of proximal tibia locking plates: a cadaveric model. J Orthop Trauma 22(6):399–403. doi:10.1097/BOT.0b013e318178417e, 00005131-200807000-00005 [pii]
20. Duwelius PJ, Rangitsch MR, Colville MR, Woll TS (1997) Treatment of tibial plateau fractures by limited internal fixation. Clin Orthop Relat Res 339:47–57
21. Egol KA, Koval KJ, Zuckerman JD (eds) (2010) Handbook of fractures. Lippincott Williams & Wilkins, Philadelphia
22. Egol KA, Su E, Tejwani NC, Sims SH, Kummer FJ, Koval KJ (2004) Treatment of complex tibial plateau fractures using the less invasive stabilization system plate: clinical experience and a laboratory comparison with double plating. J Trauma 57(2):340–346. doi:00005373-200408000-00022 [pii]
23. Egol KA, Tejwani NC, Capla EL, Wolinsky PL, Koval KJ (2005) Staged management of high-energy proximal tibia fractures (OTA types 41): the results of a prospective, standardized protocol. J Orthop Trauma 19(7):448–455; discussion 456, doi:00005131-200508000-00003 [pii]
24. Ehlinger M, Adam P, Bonnomet F (2010) Minimally invasive locking screw plate fixation of non-articular proximal and distal tibia fractures. Orthop Traumatol Surg Res 96(7):800–809. doi:10.1016/j.otsr.2010.03.025, [pii] S1877-0568(10)00147-7
25. Estes C, Rhee P, Shrader MW, Csavina K, Jacofsky MC, Jacofsky DJ (2008) Biomechanical strength of the Peri-Loc proximal tibial plate: a comparison of all-locked versus hybrid locked/nonlocked screw configurations. J Orthop Trauma 22(5):312–316. doi:10.1097/BOT.0b013e31817279b8, 00005131-200805000-00005 [pii]
26. Finkemeier CG (2002) Bone-grafting and bone-graft substitutes. J Bone Joint Surg Am 84-A(3):454–464
27. Freedman EL, Johnson EE (1995) Radiographic analysis of tibial fracture malalignment following intramedullary nailing. Clin Orthop Relat Res 315:25–33
28. Gardner MJ, Yacoubian S, Geller D, Suk M, Mintz D, Potter H, Helfet DL, Lorich DG (2005) The incidence of soft tissue injury in operative tibial plateau fractures: a magnetic resonance imaging analysis of 103 patients. J Orthop Trauma 19(2):79–84. doi:00005131-200502000-00002 [pii]
29. Garnavos C, Kanakaris NK, Lasanianos NG, Tzortzi P, West RM (2012) New classification system for long-bone fractures supplementing the AO/OTA classification. Orthopedics 35(5):e709–e719. doi:10.3928/01477447-20120426-26
30. Garnavos C, Lasanianos N (2011) Proximal tibia fractures and intramedullary nailing: the impact of nail trajectory to varus/valgus deformity. Injury

42(12):1499–1505. doi:10.1016/j.injury.2011.05.003, S0020-1383(11)00183-5 [pii]
31. Garnavos C, Lasanianos NG (2011) The management of complex fractures of the proximal tibia with minimal intra-articular impaction in fragility patients using intramedullary nailing and compression bolts. Injury 42(10):1066–1072. doi:10.1016/j.injury.2011.03.024, S0020-1383(11)00119-7 [pii]
32. Gaudinez RF, Mallik AR, Szporn M (1996) Hybrid external fixation of comminuted tibial plateau fractures. Clin Orthop Relat Res 328:203–210
33. Gazdag AR, Lane JM, Glaser D, Forster RA (1995) Alternatives to autogenous bone graft: efficacy and indications. J Am Acad Orthop Surg 3(1):1–8
34. Gerber A, Ganz R (1998) Combined internal and external osteosynthesis a biological approach to the treatment of complex fractures of the proximal tibia. Injury 29(Suppl 3):C22–C28
35. Gosling T, Schandelmaier P, Marti A, Hufner T, Partenheimer A, Krettek C (2004) Less invasive stabilization of complex tibial plateau fractures: a biomechanical evaluation of a unilateral locked screw plate and double plating. J Orthop Trauma 18(8):546–551. doi:00005131-200409000-00011 [pii]
36. Gosling T, Schandelmaier P, Muller M, Hankemeier S, Wagner M, Krettek C (2005) Single lateral locked screw plating of bicondylar tibial plateau fractures. Clin Orthop Relat Res 439:207–214. doi:00003086-200510000-00036 [pii]
37. Gustilo RB, Anderson JT (1976) Prevention of infection in the treatment of one thousand and twenty-five open fractures of long bones: retrospective and prospective analyses. J Bone Joint Surg Am 58(4):453–458
38. Haidukewych G, Sems SA, Huebner D, Horwitz D, Levy B (2007) Results of polyaxial locked-plate fixation of periarticular fractures of the knee. J Bone Joint Surg Am 89(3):614–620. doi:10.2106/JBJS.F.00510, 89/3/614 [pii]
39. Hak DJ (2011) Intramedullary nailing of proximal third tibial fractures: techniques to improve reduction. Orthopedics 34(7):532–535. doi:10.3928/01477447-20110526-19
40. Hiesterman TG, Shafiq BX, Cole PA (2011) Intramedullary nailing of extra-articular proximal tibia fractures. J Am Acad Orthop Surg 19(11):690–700. doi:19/11/690 [pii]
41. Higgins TF, Klatt J, Bachus KN (2007) Biomechanical analysis of bicondylar tibial plateau fixation: how does lateral locking plate fixation compare to dual plate fixation? J Orthop Trauma 21(5):301–306. doi:10.1097/BOT.0b013e3180500359, 00005131-200705000-00003 [pii]
42. Honkonen SE (1995) Degenerative arthritis after tibial plateau fractures. J Orthop Trauma 9(4):273–277
43. Jiang R, Luo CF, Wang MC, Yang TY, Zeng BF (2008) A comparative study of Less Invasive Stabilization System (LISS) fixation and two-incision double plating for the treatment of bicondylar tibial plateau fractures. Knee 15(2):139–143. doi:10.1016/j.knee.2007.12.001, S0968-0160(07)00197-4 [pii]
44. Katsenis D, Dendrinos G, Kouris A, Savas N, Schoinochoritis N, Pogiatzis K (2009) Combination of fine wire fixation and limited internal fixation for high-energy tibial plateau fractures: functional results at minimum 5-year follow-up. J Orthop Trauma 23(7):493–501. doi:10.1097/BOT.0b013e3181a18198, 00005131-200908000-00002 [pii]
45. Keogh P, Kelly C, Cashman WF, McGuinness AJ, O'Rourke SK (1992) Percutaneous screw fixation of tibial plateau fractures. Injury 23(6):387–389
46. Koval KJ, Helfet DL (1995) Tibial plateau fractures: evaluation and treatment. J Am Acad Orthop Surg 3(2):86–94
47. Koval KJ, Sanders R, Borrelli J, Helfet D, DiPasquale T, Mast JW (1992) Indirect reduction and percutaneous screw fixation of displaced tibial plateau fractures. J Orthop Trauma 6(3):340–346
48. Krettek C, Gerich T, Miclau T (2001) A minimally invasive medial approach for proximal tibial fractures. Injury 32(Suppl 1):SA4–SA13
49. Krettek C, Stephan C, Schandelmaier P, Richter M, Pape HC, Miclau T (1999) The use of Poller screws as blocking screws in stabilising tibial fractures treated with small diameter intramedullary nails. J Bone Joint Surg Br 81(6):963–968
50. Lachiewicz PF, Funcik T (1990) Factors influencing the results of open reduction and internal fixation of tibial plateau fractures. Clin Orthop Relat Res 259:210–215
51. Lang GJ, Cohen BE, Bosse MJ, Kellam JF (1995) Proximal third tibial shaft fractures. Should they be nailed? Clin Orthop Relat Res (315):64–74
52. Lasanianos N, Mouzopoulos G, Garnavos C (2008) The use of freeze-dried cancelous allograft in the management of impacted tibial plateau fractures. Injury 39(10):1106–1112. doi:10.1016/j.injury.2008.04.005, S0020-1383(08)00182-4 [pii]
53. Lindvall E, Sanders R, Dipasquale T, Herscovici D, Haidukewych G, Sagi C (2009) Intramedullary nailing versus percutaneous locked plating of extra-articular proximal tibial fractures: comparison of 56 cases. J Orthop Trauma 23(7):485–492. doi:10.1097/BOT.0b013e3181b013d2, 00005131-200908000-00001 [pii]
54. Liporace FA, Stadler CM, Yoon RS (2013) Problems, tricks, and pearls in intramedullary nailing of proximal third tibial fractures. J Orthop Trauma 27(1):56–62. doi:10.1097/BOT.0b013e318250f041
55. Lowe JA, Tejwani N, Yoo B, Wolinsky P (2011) Surgical techniques for complex proximal tibial fractures. J Bone Joint Surg Am 93(16):1548–1559
56. Mahadeva D, Costa ML, Gaffey A (2008) Open reduction and internal fixation versus hybrid fixation for bicondylar/severe tibial plateau fractures: a systematic review of the literature. Arch Orthop Trauma Surg 128(10):1169–1175. doi:10.1007/s00402-007-0520-7
57. Mallik AR, Covall DJ, Whitelaw GP (1992) Internal versus external fixation of bicondylar tibial plateau fractures. Orthop Rev 21(12):1433–1436

58. Marsh JL, Slongo TF, Agel J, Broderick JS, Creevey W, DeCoster TA, Prokuski L, Sirkin MS, Ziran B, Henley B, Audige L (2007) Fracture and dislocation classification compendium - 2007: Orthopaedic Trauma Association classification, database and outcomes committee. J Orthop Trauma 21(10 Suppl):S1–S133. doi:00005131-200711101-00001 [pii]
59. Marsh JL, Smith ST, Do TT (1995) External fixation and limited internal fixation for complex fractures of the tibial plateau. J Bone Joint Surg Am 77(5):661–673
60. Moore TM, Patzakis MJ, Harvey JP (1987) Tibial plateau fractures: definition, demographics, treatment rationale, and long-term results of closed traction management or operative reduction. J Orthop Trauma 1(2):97–119
61. Mueller KL, Karunakar MA, Frankenburg EP, Scott DS (2003) Bicondylar tibial plateau fractures: a biomechanical study. Clin Orthop Relat Res 412:189–195. doi:10.1097/01.blo.0000071754.41516.e9
62. Nikolaou VS, Tan HB, Haidukewych G, Kanakaris N, Giannoudis PV (2011) Proximal tibial fractures: early experience using polyaxial locking-plate technology. Int Orthop 35(8):1215–1221. doi:10.1007/s00264-010-1153-y
63. Nork SE, Barei DP, Schildhauer TA, Agel J, Holt SK, Schrick JL, Sangeorzan BJ (2006) Intramedullary nailing of proximal quarter tibial fractures. J Orthop Trauma 20(8):523–528. doi:10.1097/01.bot.0000244993.60374.d6, 00005131-200609000-00001 [pii]
64. Papagelopoulos PJ, Partsinevelos AA, Themistocleous GS, Mavrogenis AF, Korres DS, Soucacos PN (2006) Complications after tibia plateau fracture surgery. Injury 37(6):475–484. doi:10.1016/j.injury.2005.06.035, S0020-1383(05)00232-9 [pii]
65. Parekh AA, Smith WR, Silva S, Agudelo JF, Williams AE, Hak D, Morgan SJ (2008) Treatment of distal femur and proximal tibia fractures with external fixation followed by planned conversion to internal fixation. J Trauma 64(3):736–739. doi:10.1097/TA.0b013e31804d492b, 00005373-200803000-00023 [pii]
66. Partenheimer A, Gosling T, Muller M, Schirmer C, Kaab M, Matschke S, Ryf C, Renner N, Wiebking U, Krettek C (2007) Management of bicondylar fractures of the tibial plateau with unilateral fixed-angle plate fixation. Unfallchirurg 110(8):675–683. doi:10.1007/s00113-007-1271-1
67. Phisitkul P, McKinley TO, Nepola JV, Marsh JL (2007) Complications of locking plate fixation in complex proximal tibia injuries. J Orthop Trauma 21(2):83–91. doi:10.1097/BOT.0b013e318030df96, 00005131-200702000-00001 [pii]
68. Ricci WM, O'Boyle M, Borrelli J, Bellabarba C, Sanders R (2001) Fractures of the proximal third of the tibial shaft treated with intramedullary nails and blocking screws. J Orthop Trauma 15(4):264–270
69. Ricci WM, Rudzki JR, Borrelli J Jr (2004) Treatment of complex proximal tibia fractures with the less invasive skeletal stabilization system. J Orthop Trauma 18(8):521–527. doi:00005131-200409000-00007 [pii]
70. Sarmiento A, Kinman PB, Latta LL, Eng P (1979) Fracutres of the proximal tibia and tibial condyles: a clinical and laboratory comparative study. Clin Orthop Relat Res 145:136–145
71. Savoie FH, Vander Griend RA, Ward EF, Hughes JL (1987) Tibial plateau fractures. A review of operative treatment using AO technique. Orthopedics 10(5): 745–750
72. Schatzker J, McBroom R, Bruce D (1979) The tibial plateau fracture. The Toronto experience 1968-1975. Clin Orthop Relat Res (138):94–104
73. Schutz M, Kaab MJ, Haas N (2003) Stabilization of proximal tibial fractures with the LIS-System: early clinical experience in Berlin. Injury 34(Suppl 1):A30–A35
74. Shepherd L, Abdollahi K, Lee J, Vangsness CT Jr (2002) The prevalence of soft tissue injuries in nonoperative tibial plateau fractures as determined by magnetic resonance imaging. J Orthop Trauma 16(9): 628–631
75. Stannard JP, Wilson TC, Volgas DA, Alonso JE (2003) Fracture stabilization of proximal tibial fractures with the proximal tibial LISS: early experience in Birmingham, Alabama (USA). Injury 34(Suppl 1):A36–A42
76. Stannard JP, Wilson TC, Volgas DA, Alonso JE (2004) The less invasive stabilization system in the treatment of complex fractures of the tibial plateau: short-term results. J Orthop Trauma 18(8):552–558. doi:00005131-200409000-00012 [pii]
77. Subasi M, Kapukaya A, Arslan H, Ozkul E, Cebesoy O (2007) Outcome of open comminuted tibial plateau fractures treated using an external fixator. J Orthop Sci 12(4):347–353. doi:10.1007/s00776-007-1149-7
78. Tscherne H, Gotzen L (1984) Fractures with soft tissue injuries. Springer, New York
79. Tscherne H, Lobenhoffer P (1993) Tibial plateau fractures. Management and expected results. Clin Orthop Relat Res (292):87–100
80. Vangsness CT Jr, Ghaderi B, Hohl M, Moore TM (1994) Arthroscopy of meniscal injuries with tibial plateau fractures. J Bone Joint Surg Br 76(3): 488–490
81. Vince KG, Abdeen A (2006) Wound problems in total knee arthroplasty. Clin Orthop Relat Res 452:88–90. doi:10.1097/01.blo.0000238821.71271.cc, 00003086-200611000-00017 [pii]
82. Watson JT (1994) High-energy fractures of the tibial plateau. Orthop Clin North Am 25(4):723–752
83. Watson JT, Ripple S, Hoshaw SJ, Fhyrie D (2002) Hybrid external fixation for tibial plateau fractures: clinical and biomechanical correlation. Orthop Clin North Am 33(1):199–209, ix
84. Weninger P, Tschabitscher M, Traxler H, Pfafl V, Hertz H (2010) Influence of medial parapatellar nail insertion on alignment in proximal tibia fractures-special consideration of the fracture level. J Trauma 68(4):975–979. doi:10.1097/TA.0b013e3181a4c1f0

85. Weninger P, Tschabitscher M, Traxler H, Pfafl V, Hertz H (2010) Intramedullary nailing of proximal tibia fractures-an anatomical study comparing three lateral starting points for nail insertion. Injury 41(2):220–225. doi:10.1016/j.injury.2009.10.014, S0020-1383(09)00537-3 [pii]

86. Wysocki RW, Kapotas JS, Virkus WW (2009) Intramedullary nailing of proximal and distal one-third tibial shaft fractures with intraoperative two-pin external fixation. J Trauma 66(4):1135–1139. doi:10.1097/TA.0b013e3181724754, 00005373-200904000-00027 [pii]

Surgical Treatment of Pelvic Ring Injuries

Jan Lindahl

Introduction

Unstable pelvic ring disruptions result from high energy trauma and are often associated with multiple concomitant injuries [12, 37, 41]. Haemorrhage, head injury, pelvic soft tissue trauma (open fractures), and primary system complications are responsible for high mortality rates [4, 33, 51]. If the patient is haemodynamically unstable, the primary goals are to control airways, to establish adequate ventilation, and to maintain circulation. The external fixation frame may have a role in partial stabilization of the pelvic ring, reducing pelvic volume, increasing tamponade, and, thereby, reducing bleeding [2, 3, 9, 16, 56]. Once the patients are stabilized, careful assessment and definitive treatment of the pelvic ring injuries can be done.

In the 1970's, external fixation devices became popular as definitive treatment of unstable pelvic ring injuries [15, 24, 45, 46]. Later it became clear that an external frame applied anteriorly could not restore enough stability to an unstable (Type-C) disruption of the pelvic ring to allow mobilization of the patient without risking re-displacement of the fracture [23, 26, 32, 49, 55]. Therefore methods of open reduction and internal fixation (ORIF) were introduced [13, 22, 29, 36, 48, 54]. More recently, closed reduction and percutaneous screw fixation techniques have been developed [7, 42, 43]. Internal fixation has become the preferred method in the treatment of unstable posterior pelvic ring injuries [22, 29, 37, 50], but the indications for fixation of the anterior pelvic ring injuries have varied [20, 30, 42, 44]. The latest results of type C injuries seem to favour internal fixation of displaced and unstable rami fractures and symphyseal disruptions in conjunction with posterior fixation to achieve better stability of the whole pelvic ring [21, 27, 35].

Classification of Pelvic Ring Injuries

According to the AO/ASIF classification system, the pelvic ring fractures are graded into three types, A, B, and C, in order of increasing severity [48, 49].

Type A injuries are stable including avulsion fractures, fractures of the iliac wing, and transverse fractures of the sacrum below SI-joints.

Type B injuries are rotationally unstable but vertically and posteriorly stable. They may be caused by external rotatory forces ("**open book**" **injuries**) or internal rotatory forces (**lateral compression injuries**).

Type C unstable injuries are complete disruptions of the posterior sacro-iliac complex, involving vertical shear forces. Posterior pelvic ring injuries form the basis of the subgroups; fractures of the ilium C1-1, sacroiliac

J. Lindahl, MD
Pelvis and Lower Extremity Trauma Unit,
Helsinki University Central Hospital,
Topeliuksenkatu 5, Helsinki 00260, Finland
e-mail: jan.lindahl@pp.inet.fi, jan.lindahl@hus.fi

dislocation or fracture dislocation C1-2, and sacral fractures C1-3. The posterior injury may be bilateral. The bilateral posterior lesion may be vertically unstable on one side and stable on the other (type C2) or vertically unstable on both sides (type C3).

Bleeding Pelvis

Major pelvic injuries are associated with a high risk of venous and arterial bleeding. In patients with blunt pelvic trauma exsanguinating extraperitoneal bleeding remains the leading cause of early death during the first 24 h after trauma at hospital. Patients "in extremis" are at the biggest risk to die. This patient group is characterized by absent vital signs or a severe shock with initial systolic blood pressure of <70 mmHg and/or requiring mechanical resuscitation or catecholamines despite >12 blood transfusions within the first 2 h after admission [17].

Emergency treatment includes provisional pelvic ring stabilization combined with haemorrhage control. Mechanical stabilization of the pelvic ring might be acheived by pelvic binder application or by an anterior external frame or a posterior pelvic C-clamp, depending on the local resources available. In patients "in extremis" the damage control surgery concept with direct extraperitoneal pelvic packing is recommended [17, 34, 40], whereas in moderately unstable patients or in patients where persistent haemodynamic instability occurs, despite shock therapy and mechanical stabilization, arterial injury is ruled out by angiography followed by embolization of bleeding pelvic arteries.

Massive Bleeding

The rapid control of massive arterial bleeding associated with pelvic ring injuries remains a challenge for emergency trauma care. Bleeding usually originates from the presacral venous plexus or directly from the bony edges and can be relatively massive [19]. However, being a low-pressure system, venous bleeding eventually stops, particularly when the intra-abdominal pressure exceeds the venous pressure. Arterial bleeding occurs in up to 30 % of haemodynamically unstable patients and can originate from a variety of sources. In our series massive bleeding of the 49 consecutive patients treated with angiographic embolization originated in 86 % of the cases from the internal iliac artery or its main branches, in 4 % of the cases from the external iliac artery or its main branches, and in 10 % of the cases from the main branches of the internal and external iliac arteries. Two-thirds of the patients had more than one bleeding artery and one-third had arterial bleeding from both sides of the pelvic ring. Life-threatening bleeding from pelvic or acetabular fractures in pediatric patients is rare (2.8 %), and does not contribute to the overall mortality [53].

Emergency Treatment

Pelvic fracture bleeding can be temporised with a pelvic binder or an external fixator. An anterior external frame can restore pelvic bony stability in certain (but not all) pelvic fracture types. It tamponades effectively non-arterial bleeding from bone edges and pelvic veins but does not stop arterial bleeding. By reducing the pelvic ring, restoring the pelvic volume, and providing temporary stabilization to the fracture and soft tissue injury, pelvic haemorrhage can be controlled by three mechanisms. Stabilizing the pelvic ring can prevent dislodgement of haemostatic clots. Fracture reduction also re-opposes bleeding osseous surfaces, thus promoting clot formation and decreasing blood loss. Pelvic fracture reduction reduces the pelvic and potential retroperitoneal volume, thus tamponading haemorrhage from most non-arterial sources [3, 9, 11, 16, 56].

The operative ligation of the internal iliac artery is fraught with hazard. Direct visualization of its main branches is difficult. Direct exploration of the retroperitoneal haematoma releases any tamponade and allows small arterioles and veins that had been tamponaded to bleed again. Thus, transcatheter embolization has become the standard method of treating blunt pelvic bleeding. In patients in whom bleeding can be identified

Surgical Treatment of Pelvic Ring Injuries

Fig. 1 Algorithm for treating patients with severe pelvic haemorrhage [10]. *DCS* damage control surgery, *PRBC* packed red blood cells

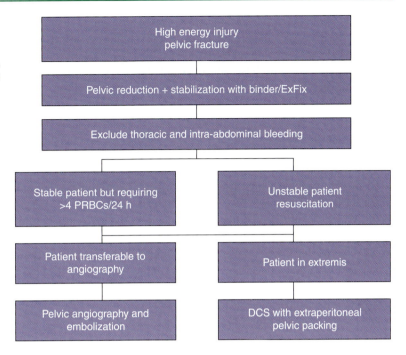

transcatheter embolization definitively treats the bleeding. Because of extensive collateral circulation, the main internal iliac artery can be occluded. If the patient is in extremis due to massive bleeding, pelvic packing is the first option at the early phase [8, 17, 34]. On the other hand, repair of the injury to the external iliac artery should always be attempted, because of a significant risk of limb loss.

Scandinavian algorithm for treating patients with severe pelvic hemorrhage is presented in Fig. 1 [10].

External Fixation of Pelvic Ring Injuries

Anterior External Fixators

Clinical applications of pelvic external fixators comprise the resuscitation phase, initial fracture stabilization, and sometimes also definitive fixation. Blood loss following pelvic fracture can be reduced through early application of an anterior external fixator. It can also prevent undesirable movement at the site of the fracture and reduce pain. Pins can be inserted into the iliac crest percutaneously or through small incisions. Guide-wires (K-wires) applied along the inner and outer aspects of the iliac wing help the insertion of the pins into the bone. The frame that connects the pin groups (two pins on each side) can be assembled very quickly.

In a comparison of the stiffness of current anterior external fixation systems with a human pelvic replica of aluminium with a type C injury, Ponsen et al. [38] found that stability provided by any external fixator was low. Single bar systems were stiffer and performed better than frame configurations. The difference was ascribed to the use of 6 mm pins instead of 5 mm ones (two pins of 6 mm gave 15 % more stiffness than three pins of 5 mm), as well as to the use of stiffer bars instead of more slender rods of the frames. The position of the pins, cranial or ventral, was not of significance.

C-Clamps

The pelvic C-clamp designed by Reinhold Ganz has a sliding bar and is intended to be applied to the posterior aspect of the pelvis opposite the sacro-iliac joints. The pelvic stabilizer has two arms attached and is connected by a central ratchet gear. The specially designed pins attached to the end of this device through additional articulation are intended for insertion either at the back of the pelvis or anteriorly in the dense column of the bone above the acetabulum [1].

Biomechanical studies have shown that the C-clamps are more effective in type C pelvic ring injuries than the standard anterior external fixator to achieve compression at the sacro-iliac joints [1]. On the other hand, the data in a cadaveric study showed that an anterior external fixator and pelvic clamps were equally effective in reducing the pelvic volume and pubic diastasis in "open book" injuries [11]. Most severe complications associated with the application of the C-clamps have been penetration of the fixation pin into the confines of the pelvis and cut-out into the sciatic notch [11]. Surgeon practice on cadavers or with a pelvic model before clinical use will help to ensure safe application of both devices. Special surgical skills are needed if a C-clamp is used in the trauma (emergency) room.

Surgical Treatment of Pelvic Ring Injuries

Open reduction and internal fixation (ORIF) have become the method of choice for stabilization of type C pelvic injuries. All type C injuries, most of type B "open book" injuries, and severely displaced type-B lateral compression injuries are treated surgically. Also some comminuted severely displaced iliac wing fractures (type A) might need surgical treatment (Fig. 2). Biomechanical studies have shown that the best stability in type C pelvic ring fractures can be achieved by internal fixation of the posterior and anterior pelvic ring injuries [25, 49]. Also radiological and functional results have indicated that external fixation alone is of limited value in the definitive treatment of type C injuries [23, 26, 32]. The latest clinical results of type C injuries seem to favour internal fixation of displaced and unstable rami fractures and symphyseal disruptions in conjunction with posterior fixation to achieve better stability of the whole pelvic ring [21, 27, 35].

Internal Fixation of Posterior Pelvic Ring Injuries

Sacral Fractures (C1.3)

The Denis classification system is the most commonly used system for sacral fractures [6]. It divides the fractures into three zones: alar (zone 1), foraminal (zone 2), and central (zone 3). There is a correlation between the fracture course and the rate of neurological deficit: transalar 5 %, transforaminal 28 %, and central 56 % [6]. For stabilization of vertical sacral fractures iliosacral screw fixation is of gold standard. Ilio-iliacal

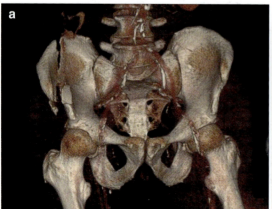 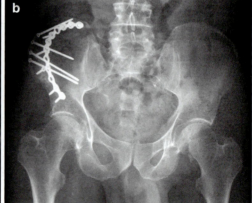

Fig. 2 Open reduction and internal fixation of severely displaced and comminuted iliac wing fracture (A2) with lateral femoral cutaneous nerve injury (**a**). Follow-up X-ray 1 year later (**b**)

Surgical Treatment of Pelvic Ring Injuries

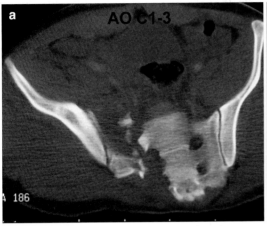
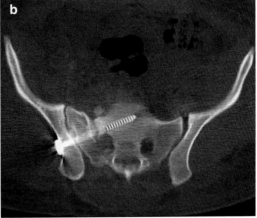

Fig. 3 Severely displaced comminuted transforaminal sacral fracture (C1-3) with lumbosacral plexus injury indicates open reduction and simultaneous cleaning of sacral foramina of small fragments and iliosacral screw fixation. Pre-op (**a**) and post-op CT (**b**) pictures of an 18 years-old male after crush injury

fixation techniques, sacral bars extra-osseously or intra-osseously, ilio-iliacal plate osteosynthesis, and ilio-iliacal internal fixator are alternative methods for sacral fracture fixation. Direct plate osteosynthesis of sacral fractures has also been described.

Displaced sacral fractures with neurological compromise are stabilized with the patient in the prone position with two cannulated partially threaded or fully threaded iliosacral screws across the fracture line into the S1 vertebral body under fluoroscopic guidance [29] (Fig. 3). The posterior longitudinal skin incision is made slightly lateral to the mid-line and clearly medial to the posterior superior iliac crest. The fascia is opened longitudinally without cutting the muscles. The sacral fracture is observed, and the fracture line is cleaned. Decompression of sacral nerve roots is needed in transforaminal sacral fractures when pre-operative CT shows bony fragments in sacral canal. The vertical and anterior-posterior displacement is reduced with forceps. Iliosacral screws are inserted percutaneously through a separate small skin incision lateral to the posterior superior iliac spine to avoid large soft tissue stripping on the lateral aspect of the iliac wing and wound complications.

Minimally-displaced lateral sacral fractures can be treated with closed reduction techniques and percutaneous iliosacral screw fixation either in prone or supine position depending on the fracture pattern of the whole pelvic ring and concomitant injuries (Fig. 4). The screws should be placed at least past the mid-line of the sacrum. Navigation shows promising results compared to fluoroscopy-guided screws, but only a very few trauma centres use this technique routinely.

Sacro-Iliac Dislocation and Fracture-Dislocation (C1.2)

An anterior approach through an incision along the iliac crest offers a good method for reduction and plate fixation of sacro-iliac dislocation and fracture-dislocation [29, 49]. After reduction of the SI-joint with pelvic clamps, anterior plate fixation with two 4.5 mm reconstruction plates or other 4.5 mm 3-hole plates is carried out (Fig. 5). Simultaneous plate fixation of rami fractures and symphysis pubis disruption is possible. Iliosacral screws can be used with the patient in the prone position, but the control of reduction of the SI-joint using posterior approach is difficult with mere finger palpation through the sciatic notch.

Trans-Iliac Fractures (C1.1)

Trans-iliac fractures are fixed with anterior 3.5 mm reconstruction plates or long 3.5 mm cortical screws or both using the iliac window approach.

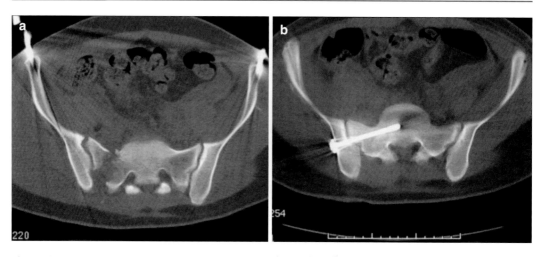

Fig. 4 Minimally-displaced transalar sacral fractures without neurologic deficits (**a**) treated with closed reduction techniques and percutaneous iliosacral screw fixation under fluoroscopic guidance (**b**)

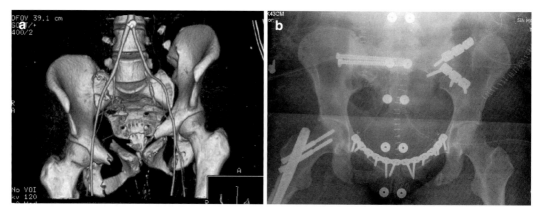

Fig. 5 Bilateral type C3 pelvic ring injury (**a**). The first stage was simultaneous anterior plating of the left SI-joint and bilateral rami fractures through intrapelvic approach and approach along the iliac wing (iliac window). The second stage was open reduction and iliosacral screw fixation of the transforaminal sacral fracture with S1 nerve root injury on the *right* side (**b**)

Internal Fixation of Anterior Pelvic Ring Injuries

"Open Book" Injuries (B1, B3.1)

Biomechanical testing of "open book" injuries by McBroom and Tile [49] showed that external fixators cannot give such stability as does internal fixation. In addition, different external frame configurations did not provide significant advantages. The best stability can be achieved by using two plates over the symphysis [49]. Clinical results have shown that two 3.5 mm reconstruction plates or one 4.5 mm symphyseal plate (4 holes or 6 holes) are safe fixation methods for type B open book injuries with external rotational instability (Fig. 6).

Disruption of the symphysis pubis is exposed through either a vertical or a transverse Pfannenstiel's type skin incision [29]. A vertical incision is chosen when the anterior fixation is combined with laparotomy. Because of cosmetic reasons, a transverse skin incision is otherwise the choice for symphyseal disruption or juxta-symphyseal fractures of the rami. The mid-line between the rectus abdominis muscles is opened, and the prevesical area is exposed. The insertions of the rectus abdominis muscles can be incompletely detached from the pubis on their inner

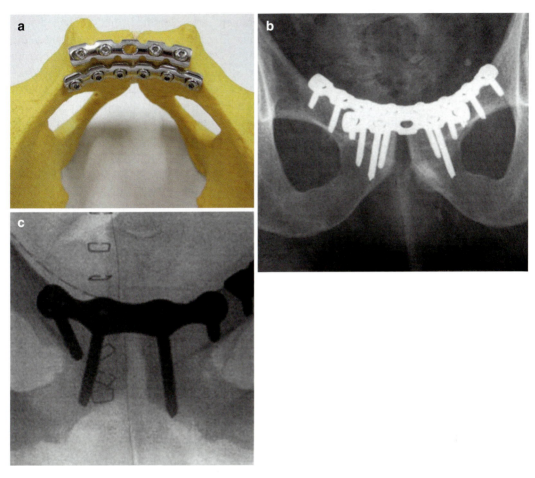

Fig. 6 Disruption of the symphysis pubis is reduced and fixed with two 3.5 mm reconstruction plates (**a**, **b**) or one 4.5 mm symphyseal plate (**c**)

aspects, whereas their lateral and outer parts of attachments are left intact. The symphyseal plates are placed under the rectus sheaths.

Type B Lateral Compression Injuries (B2, B3.2)

In type B lateral compression injury the hemipelvis is usually driven into inward and upward rotation causing slight shortening of the lower limb. The posterior sacro-iliac complex is commonly impacted, and there is no vertical instability. Lindahl et al. [26] evaluated 62 patients with a displaced lateral compression injury treated with an external fixator and found that poor radiological results correlated with poor functional results. More than 10 mm of vertical displacement and shortening at the site of the fracture in the rami were poor prognostic signs [26]. Minimally-displaced lateral compression injuries can be treated conservatively.

Intrapelvic Approach

Displaced lateral fractures of the pubic rami (in type B and C injuries) are approached through an intrapelvic approach [20, 27]. This anterior extraperitoneal approach, which is used in acetabular fracture surgery as well, is also called Stoppa approach [5]. It gives direct visualization of the superior rami, the anterior column, the quadrilateral surface, and the posterior border of the posterior column of the acetabulum (Fig. 7). Intrapelvic approach is a less invasive approach without muscle detachment. An additional approach along the iliac crest (iliac window) makes simultaneous

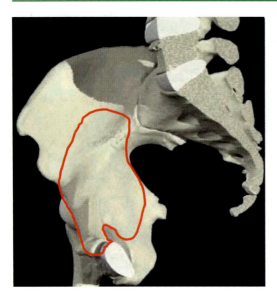

Fig. 7 Through intrapelvic approach the superior ramus, the anterior column and the quadrilateral surface of the acetabulum (area within *red line*) can be visualized

reduction and internal fixation of displaced transiliac fractures and SI-joint dislocation and fracture-dislocation possible. An additional iliac window gives also good access for reduction and fixation of the anterior column fracture component affecting the iliac wing without dissecting the external iliac vessels, the femoral nerve, and the iliopsoas muscle.

The lateral rami fractures are exposed through the low mid-line approach by extending the dissection laterally as described by Hirvensalo et al. [20], and Lindahl and Hirvensalo [27]. The dissection laterally below the rectus muscle is continued subperiosteally along the superior ramus. The corona mortis vessels on the inner aspect of the lateral superior ramus are ligated whenever they are present. The iliopectineal fascia is detached along the linea terminalis to facilitate exposure of the anterior column of the acetabulum. The external iliac vein and artery, the iliopsoas muscle, and the femoral nerve are lifted slightly anteriorly with a retractor and left undisturbed. No dissection or separation of these vulnerable structures is necessary. The underlying obturator nerve and vessels entering the obturator foramen are identified and protected. By remaining close to the pelvic brim and using subperiosteal stripping only, the risk of injuring the external iliac vein and other essential structures can be avoided. If a concomitant acetabular fracture is present, the anterior column and the quadrilateral surface can also be exposed. In bilateral rami fractures both sides are exposed.

After reduction the pubic rami fractures are fixed with a curved reconstruction plate with 3.5-mm screws placed along the pelvic brim (linea terminalis) (Fig. 8). Fixation of lateral fractures of the superior ramus with a long intramedullary 3.5 mm cortical screw is an alternative method especially in cases with good bone quality and a simple fracture without comminution. Bilateral fractures of the rami are fixed either by using two separate plates, one on each side, or with one longer plate over both rami fractures and the symphysis pubis (Fig. 5). In patients with a contaminated open fracture or severe comminution and osteoporosis, fixation of the rami fractures can be done with an anterior external fixator. The fixator is removed after 6–10 weeks. Bladder injury is not considered a contra-indication to simultaneous reconstruction and anterior internal fixation.

Post-operative Care

Mobilization with crutches is started within 1–2 days in type C1 injuries without weight-bearing on the injured side and if allowed by the associated injuries of the lower legs. In type C injuries full weight-bearing is started after 8–12 weeks. The load is increased gradually based on the fracture type and radiographic follow-up. In type C3 injuries the walking exercises with crutches are started after 8–12 weeks based on the type of the posterior pelvic ring injury.

In "open book" injuries mobilization with crutches is started early with weight-bearing within the limits of pain. Partial weight-bearing is allowed after plate fixation of the rami fractures of type B lateral compression injuries and full weight-bearing after 6 weeks.

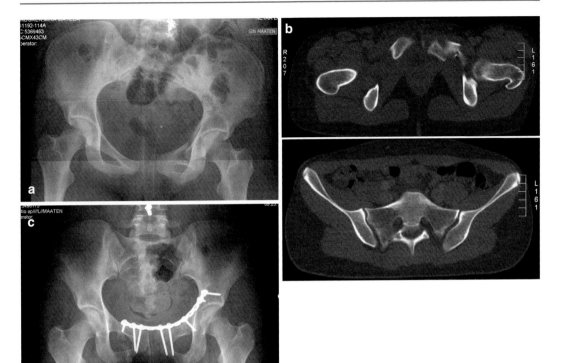

Fig. 8 Disruption of the symphysis pubis and comminuted lateral rami fracture (**a,b**) on the left side (type B injury) were reduced and fixed with one 12 hole 3.5 mm reconstruction plate. Radiological follow-up 5 months post-op showed good fracture healing (**c**)

Outcome of Surgical Treatment

In a systematic review of the literature over the last 30 years (1975–2007), Papakostidis et al. [35] investigated the correlation between the clinical outcome of different types of pelvic ring injuries and the method of treatment. No relevant randomised controlled trials (RCTs) were found. Twenty-seven case series of 818 retrieved reports met their inclusion criteria. They concluded that fixation of all the injured elements of the pelvic ring yields better anatomical results. However, the current literature was insufficient to provide "clear" evidence for choosing the optimal treatment of unstable pelvic ring injuries.

In type C injuries internal fixation of displaced and unstable rami fractures and symphyseal disruptions in conjunction with posterior fixation seems to yield better stability for the whole pelvic ring [25, 27, 49]. Several authors have associated good reduction result with favourable long-term results [26, 27, 31, 39, 50]. Denis et al. [6] and Lindahl and Hirvensalo [27] documented the permanent lumbosacral plexus injury as a strong prognostic factor.

Good reduction together with proper stabilization allows early mobilization, prevents complications, and, thereby, leads to a short hospital stay and an early start of rehabilitation. The clinical results suggest that special attention should be paid to properative planning, reduction of the fracture, decompression of the nerve roots, and stable fixation of all main fracture components.

Open Pelvic Fractures

In open pelvic fractures there is a connection between the skin, perineum, rectum or vagina laceration and the fracture. Evaluation of soft tissues is necessary for both closed and open fractures. The severity of the soft tissue injury thus helps to determine the timing of surgical intervention, the type of fixation, and the prognosis. A high percentage of patients with open pelvic fractures are polytraumatized patients. Their resuscitation should first focus on saving the life and the limb and after that on the long-term normal functional outcome.

Open fractures with severe soft tissue injury (loss of muscle coverage) at the site of the posterior or anterior pelvic injury need immediate surgical treatment: surgical debridement with jet lavage and external fixation for emergency skeletal stabilization in conjunction with other resuscitative efforts. Indications for emergency diverting colostomy are extended perineal soft tissue injuries and severe rectal lacerations.

Definitive reduction and internal fixation of the posterior injury to the pelvic ring can be performed when the patient is stabilized. Severe soft tissue loss might need soft tissue coverage with vascularized rotational or vascularized free tissue (muscle) grafting. It is recommended to be carried out at the same operation by a plastic surgeon. Depending on the severity and location of the soft tissue injury the anterior injury to the pelvic ring might be treated either with an external fixator or with internal fixation. The appropriate treatment of these difficult injuries requires a team of an Orthopaedic trauma surgeon and Plastic surgeons with a 24 h' service.

Initially the patients should be protected with tetanus prophylaxis and intravenous antibiotics (usually a second-generation cephalosporin or clindamycin). In severe Gustilo-Anderson type III fractures, the addition of aminoglycosides for 3–5 days reduces the surviving population of reproducing bacterial cells [1]. In severely contaminated wounds (farm or railroad injuries), triple antibiotic coverage with the addition of metronidasol is recommended.

Concomitant Injuries

Bladder Injuries

The emergency treatment of extraperitoneal bladder ruptures is non-surgical – catheter drainage. Relative surgical indications are bladder neck involvement, bone fragments in the bladder, and bone entrapment of the bladder wall [14, 28]. When the anterior injury to the pelvic ring needs internal fixation, simultaneous reconstruction of the bladder and rami fracture or disruption of the symphysis pubis can be performed within the first few days. Intraperitoneal bladder ruptures are treated surgically due to risk of peritonitis (emergency indication if possible). Bladder injuries have no acute influence on mortality.

Urethral Injuries

Partial posterior urethral tears can be treated non-surgically with catheter drainage (suprapubic or urethral catheter). Primary open re-alignement is not recommended acutely. Secondary re-alignement is associated with fewer incidences of strictures, re-stenosis, incontinence, and impotence [4, 28]. Urethral injuries have no acute influence on mortality; neither are they associated with emergency reconstructive indications.

Morel-Lavallee Soft Tissue Lesion

The Morel-Lavallee lesion is a severe closed degloving soft-tissue injury in which the skin and subcutaneous tissue are separated from the underlying fascia, creating a space filled with blood and necrotic fat.

Closed de-gloving soft tissue injuries can be treated with a minimally-invasive technique; percutaneous drainage, debridement (plastic brush) within 3 days post-injury, and haemovac drain (removed when drainage <30 mL/24 h) [52] or with a more radical surgical technique with an incision over the whole length of the lesion, debridement, extensive irrigation, tending sutures, and wound drainage [47].

The Morel-Lavallee lesion does not effect mortality. The healing rate is high with drainage, debridement, irrigation, and adequate wound management (closed or open unclear), but there is an influence on morbidity.

Organisation of Pelvic Trauma Care

Frequently, Orthopaedic injuries are the determining factor for ultimate disability and quality of life for the injured trauma patient. A designated Orthopaedic trauma system and regionalization are important factors in promoting optimal care and better outcomes. Finland is a relative small country with 5.4 million inhabitants. The public health care system is hierarchical and based on 54 community hospitals (primary hospitals), 16 central hospitals (secondary hospitals), and 5 university hospitals (tertiary hospitals) that have the largest responsibilities [18].

The treatment of unstable pelvic ring fractures is a major challenge even without vascular or neurological compromise, as these fractures are rare injuries and the caseload is small at primary and secondary hospitals. Therefore the definitive treatment of unstable pelvic ring and acetabular fractures has been centralized at five university trauma hospitals in Finland. Only uncomplicated and simple fractures might be treated at some central hospitals. This has improved the level of care and optimized the cost-benefit ratio of the financial input to trauma care by increasing the caseload and re-allocating resources.

References

1. Alonso JE, Jackson L, Burgess AR, Browner BD (1996) The management of complex orthopedic injuries. Surg Clin North Am 76:879–903
2. Bircher MD (1996) Indications and techniques of external fixation of the injured pelvis. Injury 27(Suppl 2):S-B3–S-B19
3. Burgess AR, Eastridge BJ, Young JWR, Ellison TS, Ellison PS Jr, Poka A, Bathon GH, Brumback RJ (1990) Pelvic ring disruptions: effective classification system and treatment protocols. J Trauma 30:848–856
4. Chapple C, Barbagli G, Jordan G, Mundy AR, Rodrigues-Netto N, Pansadoro V, McAninch JW (2004) Consensus on genitourinary trauma. Consensus statement on urethral trauma. BJU Int 93:1195–1202
5. Cole JD, Bolhofner BR (1994) Acetabular fracture fixation via a modified Stoppa limited intrapelvic approach: description of operative technique and preliminary treatment results. Clin Orthop 305:112–123
6. Denis F, Davis S, Comfort T (1988) Sacral fractures: an important problem: retrospective analysis of 236 cases. Clin Orthop Relat Res 227:67–81
7. Ebraheim NA, Rusin JJ, Coombs RJ, Jackson WT, Holiday B (1987) Percutaneous computer tomography-stabilization of pelvic fracture: preliminary report. J Orthop Trauma 1:197–204
8. Ertel W, Keel M, Eid K, Platz A, Trentz O (2001) Control of severe hemorrhage using C-clamp and pelvic packing in multiply injured patients with pelvic ring disruption. J Orthop Trauma 15:468–474
9. Evers BM, Cryer HM, Miller FB (1989) Pelvic fracture hemorrhage. Priorities in management. Arch Surg 124:422–424
10. Gaarder C, Naess PA, Christensen EF, Hakala P, Handolin L, Heier HE, Ivancev K, Johansson P, Leppäniemi A, Lippert F, Lossius HM, Opdahl H, Pillgram-Larsen J, Røise O, Skaga NO, Søreide E, Stensballe J, Tønnessen E, Töttermann A, Örtenwall P, Östlund A (2008) Scandinavian guidelines – "the massively bleeding patient". Scand J Surg 97:15–36
11. Ghanayem AJ, Stover MD, Goldstein JA, Bellon E, Wilber JH (1995) Emergent treatment of pelvic fractures. Comparison of methods for stabilization. Clin Orthop Relat Res 318:75–80
12. Gilliland MD, Ward RE, Barton RM, Miller PW, Duke JH (1982) Factors affecting mortality in pelvic fractures. J Trauma 22:691–693
13. Goldstein A, Phillips T, Sclafani SJA, Scalea T, Duncan A, Goldstein J, Panetta T, Shafton G (1986) Early open reduction and internal fixation of the disrupted pelvic ring. J Trauma 26:325–333
14. Gomez RG, Ceballos L, Coburn M, Corriere JN, Dixon CM, Lobel B, McAninch J (2004) Consensus on genitourinary trauma. Consensus statement on bladder injuries. BJU Int 94:27–33
15. Gunterberg B, Goldie I, Slätis P (1978) Fixation of pelvic fractures and dislocations: an experimental study on the loading of pelvic fractures and sacro-iliac dislocations after external compression fixation. Acta Orthop Scand 49:278–286
16. Gylling SF, Ward RE, Holcroft JW, Bray TJ, Chapman MW (1985) Immediate external fixation of unstable pelvic fractures. Am J Surg 150:721–724
17. Gänsslen A, Hildebrand F, Pohlemann T (2012) Management of hemodynamic unstable patients "in extremis" with pelvic ring fractures. Acta Chir Orthop Traumatol Cech 79(3):193–202
18. Handolin L, Leppäniemi A, Vihtonen K, Lakovaara M, Lindahl J (2006) Finnish trauma audit 2004: current state of trauma management in Finnish hospitals. Injury 37:622–625
19. Henry SM, Tornetta P III, Scalea TM (1997) Damage control for devastating pelvic and extremity injuries. Surg Clin North Am 77:879–895
20. Hirvensalo E, Lindahl J, Böstman O (1993) A new approach to the internal fixation of unstable pelvic fractures. Clin Orthop Relat Res 297:28–32
21. Hirvensalo E, Lindahl J, Kiljunen V (2007) Modified and new approaches for pelvic and acetabular surgery. Injury 38:431–441
22. Kellam JF, McMurtry RY, Paley D, Tile M (1987) The unstable pelvic fracture: operative treatment. Orthop Clin North Am 18:25–41

23. Kellam JF (1989) The role of external fixation in pelvic disruptions. Clin Orthop Relat Res 241:66–82
24. Lansinger O, Karlsson J, Berg U, Måre K (1984) Unstable fractures of the pelvis treated with a trapezoid compression frame. Acta Orthop Scand 55:325–329
25. Leighton RK, Waddell JP, Bray TJ, Chapman MW, Simpson L, Martom RB, Sharkey NA (1991) Biomechanical testing of new and old fixation devices for vertical shear fractures of the pelvis. J Orthop Trauma 5:313–317
26. Lindahl J, Hirvensalo E, Böstman O, Santavirta S (1999) Failure of reduction with an external fixator in the treatment of injuries of the pelvic ring: long-term evaluation of 110 patients. J Bone Joint Surg Br 81B:955–962
27. Lindahl J, Hirvensalo E (2005) Outcome of operatively treated type-C injuries of the pelvic ring. Acta Orthop 76(5):667–678
28. Lynch TH, Martinez-Pineiro L, Plas E, Serafetinides E, Turkeri L, Santucci RA, Hohenfellner M (2005) EAU guidelines on urological trauma. Eur Urol 47:1–15
29. Matta JM, Saucedo T (1989) Internal fixation of pelvic ring fractures. Clin Orthop Relat Res 242:83–97
30. Matta JM (1996) Indications for anterior fixation of pelvic fractures. Clin Orthop Relat Res 329:88–96
31. McLaren AC, Rorabeck CH, Halpenny J (1990) Long-term pain and disability in relation to residual deformity after displaced pelvic ring fractures. Can J Surg 33:492–494
32. Mears DC, Fu F (1980) External fixation in pelvic fractures. Orthop Clin North Am 11:465–479
33. Mucha P, Welch TJ (1988) Hemorrhage in major pelvic fractures. Surg Clin North Am 68:757–773
34. Papakostidis C, Giannoudis PV (2009) Pelvic ring injuries with haemodynamic instability: efficacy of pelvic packing, a systematic review. Injury 40(S4):553–561
35. Papakostidis C, Kanakaris NK, Kontakis G, Giannoudis PV (2009) Pelvic ring disruptions: treatment modalities and analysis of outcomes. Int Orthop 33:329–338
36. Pohlemann T, Bosch U, Gänsslen A, Tscherne H (1994) The Hannover experience in management of pelvic fractures. Clin Orthop Relat Res 305:69–80
37. Pohlemann T, Gänsslen A, Schellwald O, Culemann U, Tscherne H (1996) Outcome after pelvic ring injuries. Injury 27(Suppl 2):S-B31–S-B38
38. Ponsen KJ, van Dijke GAH, Joosse P, Snijders CJ (2003) External fixators for pelvic fractures. Comparison of the stiffness of current systems. Acta Orthop Scand 74:165–171
39. Ragnarsson B, Olerud C, Olerud S (1993) Anterior square-plate fixation of sacroiliacdisruption. 2–8 years follow-up of 23 consecutive cases. Acta Orthop Scand 64:138–142
40. Riska EB, von Bonsdorff H, Hakkinen S, Jaroma H, Kiviluoto O, Paavilainen T (1979) Operative control of massive haemorrhage in comminuted pelvic fractures. Int Orthop 3:141–144
41. Rothenberger DA, Fischer RP, Strate RG, Velasco R, Perry JF Jr (1978) The mortality associated with pelvic fractures. Surgery 84:356–361
42. Routt MLC, Simonian PT, Grujic L (1995) The retrograde medullary superior pubic ramus screw for the treatment of anterior pelvic disruptions: a new technique. J Orthop Trauma 9:35–44
43. Routt MLC, Simonian PT (1996) Closed reduction and percutaneous skeletal fixation of sacral fractures. Clin Orthop Relat Res 329:121–128
44. Routt ML, Simonian PT (1996) Internal fixation of pelvic ring disruptions. Injury 27(Suppl 2): S-B20–S-B30
45. Slätis P, Karaharju E (1975) External fixation of the pelvic girdle with a trapezoid compression frame. Injury 7:53–56
46. Slätis P, Karaharju E (1980) External fixation of unstable pelvic fractures: experiences in 22 patients treated with a trapezoid compression frame. Clin Orthop Relat Res 151:73–80
47. Steiner CL, Trenz O, Labler L (2008) Management of Morel-Lavallee lesion associated with pelvic and/or acetabular fractures. Eur J Trauma Emerg Surg 34:554–560
48. Tile M (1988) Pelvic ring fractures: should they be fixed? J Bone Joint Surg Br 70B:1–12
49. Tile M (1995) Fractures of the pelvis and acetabulum, 2nd edn. Williams & Wilkins, Baltimore
50. Tornetta P III, Matta JM (1996) Outcome of operatively treated unstable posterior pelvic ring disruptions. Clin Orthop Relat Res 329:186–193
51. Tscherne H, Regel G (1996) Care of the polytraumatised patient. J Bone Joint Surg Br 78B: 840–852
52. Tseng S, Tornetta P III (2006) Percutaneous management of Morel-Lavallee lesions. J Bone Joint Surg Am 88:92–96
53. Tuovinen H, Söderlund T, Lindahl J, Laine T, Åström P, Handolin L (2011) Severe pelvic fracture-related bleeding in pediatric patients: does it occur? Eur J Trauma Emerg Surg. doi:10.1007/s00068-011-0140-3 [Published online August]
54. Ward EF, Tomasin J, Vander Griend RA (1987) Open reduction and internal fixation of vertical shear pelvic fractures. J Trauma 27:291–295
55. Wild JJ, Hanson GW, Tullos HS (1982) Unstable fractures of the pelvis treated by external fixation. J Bone Joint Surg Am 64A:1010–1020
56. Wolinsky PR (1997) Assessment and management of pelvic fracture in the hemodynamically unstable patient. Orthop Clin North Am 28:321–329

Part IV
Paediatrics

Anatomical Reconstruction of the Hip with SCFE, Justified by Pathophysiological Findings*

Reinhold Ganz, Kai Ziebarth, Michael Leunig, Theddy Slongo, and Young-Jo Kim

Introduction

It is commonly agreed that prevention of further slipping and iatrogenic necrosis is the major focus in surgical treatment of slipped capital femoral epiphysis (SCFE) [2, 20]. Mild slips do well with pinning in situ [3] and larger slips may need corrective osteotomies when re-modelling will

---

Erwin Morscher Honorary Lecture. EFORT Congress Berlin, May 23–26th., 2012
*Short and rewritten version of manuscript Clin Orthop Relat Res DOI 10.1007/s11999-013-2818-9

R. Ganz, MD (✉)
Faculty of Medicine, University of Bern,
Walchstrasse 10, 3073 Guemligen, Switzerland
e-mail: rd.ganz@bluewin.ch

K. Ziebarth, MD
Orthopaedic Department,
Inselspital, University of Bern,
3010 Bern, Switzerland
e-mail: kai.ziebarth@insel.ch

M. Leunig, MD
Orthopaedic Department, Schulthess Klinik,
Lengghalde 2, 8008 Zurich, Switzerland
e-mail: michael.leunig@kws.ch

T. Slongo, MD
Department of Paediatric Surgery,
Children's Hospital, University of Bern,
3010 Bern, Switzerland
e-mail: theddy.slongo@insel.ch

Y.-J. Kim, MD
Department of Orthopaedic Surgery,
Children's Hospital,
Boston, MA, USA
e-mail: young-jo.kim@childrens.harvard.edu

---

not lead to improved internal rotation [32]. More recently, this concept came under fire with the recognition, that even mild slips lead to early acetabular damage [5, 15, 29] due to impingement of the cam configuration of the anterior head-neck junction [8]. The high incidence of avascular necrosis in clinically unstable slips is thought to be most likely the result of a vascular injury at the time of epiphyseal separation [2, 13, 19, 24, 26]. Although time to surgery in such hips could not be confirmed to be a cause of epipyseal necrosis, there is a general recommendation for emergency treatment, at least to puncture the joint capsule and evacuate a hematoma [18, 22, 32]. Unintended or attempted reduction of a clinically unstable slip is considered to influence the perfusion and increase the risk of epiphyseal necrosis [4]; when complete reduction was achieved the rate of necrosis reached 58 % [30]. Dunn [6] related this to bone apposition at the posterior neck, apparently overstretching the retinacular vessels during the process of reduction.

While standard surgery of SCFE does not include routine arthrotomy, pathophysiological knowledge was mainly based on clinical and radiological findings. New insights were possible with routine arthrotomy, surgical dislocation and execution of an extended retinacular flap for subcapital reduction [7, 9].

We present here the intra-operative findings of 119 hips of 116 patients treated in three institutions (Childrens' Hospital Bern and Boston, Orthopaedic Department Schulthess Clinic

Zurich) between 1996 and 2011. The perceptions may serve as justification for our treatment concept consisting in:
1. Pinning in situ and open or arthroscopic offset restoration for stable slips under 30° [17],
2. surgical dislocation and extended retinacular flap for anatomical epiphyseal reduction after resection of bone apposition at the posterior neck for stable slips over 30° and as an emergency treatment for all slips with clinical signs of an unstable slip [9].

Patients and Methods

Patients' records and radiographs served as the bases for this study. Mean age at surgery was 12 years, 55 % were male patients. Duration of symptoms averaged 16 weeks with a range from 0 to 156 weeks. The average slip angle was 53° (range 15–90°); 35 hips showed a disconnected epiphysis at capsulotomy. In 105 hips subcapital reduction was performed, 14 stable slips with an angle of 30° or less were treated open or arthroscopically with in situ fixation of the epiphysis and anterior osteochondroplasty. Follow-up time was 31 months with a range of 12–108 months. Subcapital reduction was performed in all institutions according to the technique described in details by Leunig et al. [16] (Fig. 1). The retinacular flap is at least twice as long as with the Dunn technique [6] with the advantage of better visual control and less adverse forces on the retinacular flap and the embedded vessels during manipulations for posterior bone resection and reduction of the epiphysis.

Damage to the acetabular cartilage was quantitatively described or recorded using a form sheet (Fig. 2). Disconnection of the epiphysis was visually and manually tested at capsulotomy. Time from injury to surgery in the subgroup of disconnected epiphyses was subdivided into four groups: less than 8 h, 8–24 h, 2–8 days and more than 8 days. Laser-Doppler flowmetry (LDF) was used to record perfusion of the epiphysis at capsulotomy and after anatomical reduction [23]. Drill holes in the epiphysis were used to observe bright red bleeding when LDF was not available [10] and when spontaneous bleeding from epiphyseal bone or from the resection surface of the round ligament could not be observed. Bone apposition at the posterior neck in disconnected epiphyses was radiographically evaluated and compared with statements in the operative notes about bone resection at the posterior neck.

Since clinical stability of SCFE does not necessarily correlate with intra-operative stability [31] we named clinical stability or clinical instability when it refers to the Loder Classification [18] and used the terms stable or disconnected epiphysis when it referred to the intra-operative confirmation of stability or instability.

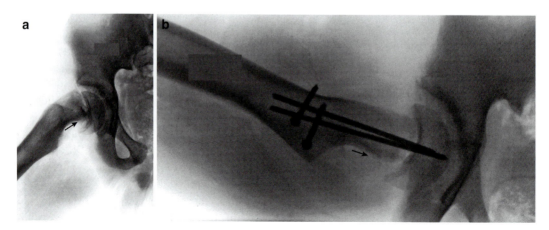

Fig. 1 Disconnected SCFE with sudden pain while running but no other symptoms. (**a**) Lateral view with substantial posterior shift and angulation of the epiphysis. *Arrow* pointing to bone apposition at the posterior neck. (**b**) Postoperative lateral view showing the line of bone resection (*arrow*) and anatomical reduction of the epiphysis

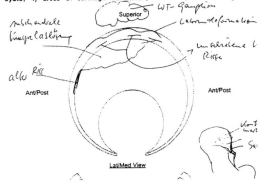

Fig. 2 Section of an original form sheet in use for documentation of intra-operative labrum and cartilage damage as well as for intracapsular treatment aspects

Results

Intracapsular blood was inconsistently observed in the 35 hips with disconnected epiphysis, in only one operative note the haematoma is described as being under pressure; intracapsular blood was also observed in some stable slips and was interpreted as impingement injury to the acetabular rim or synovial villi. All 35 disconnected epiphyses showed rupture of the anterior periosteum, however in only one case did this rupture continue deep into the retinacular tissue threatening vascular injury to the epiphysis. LDF performed immediately after capsulotomy did not reveal signs of epiphyseal perfusion nor did signs of perfusion return after reduction.

In nearly 90 % of all slips damage to the acetabular rim and adjacent cartilage was documented and in nearly 75 % this damage was substantial. There was a tendency, however not significant, for the hips with longer duration of symptoms or higher slip anglesto have more cartilage damage. Damage in disconnected epiphyses was significantly less severe.

Details about the epiphyseal perfusion were recorded in 63 of the 70 stable hips treated with subcapital reduction and in 33 of the 35 hips with disconnected epiphyses at capsulotomy. With a minimum follow-up of one year, so far no epiphyseal necrosis was observed in the group of 70 stable slips. In the subgroup of disconnected epiphyses 23 hips showed epiphyseal perfusion at capsulotomy and after reduction, 3 with increased pulsation of the LDF curve after reduction; in 1 of these hips post reduction perfusion became positive again only after removal of a substantial part of the bone apposition of the posterior neck which first was overlooked (Fig. 3). In six hips there was no epiphyseal perfusion before but clear perfusion after reduction, in one hip with synovitis and difficulties with manual reduction however only after substantial shortening of the neck. Four hips, including the one with an avulsed retinaculum, did not show signs of perfusion at capsulotomy nor after reduction. Three went on to necrosis of the epiphysis and one showed perfusion at revision for metal failure 6 weeks after the first surgery. This hip has a 7 year follow-up with normal structure of the femoral head [28]. When the perfusion profile of the disconnected epiphyses is contrasted with the time to surgery, the six hips with intact perfusion before and after reduction have been operated within the 8 h limit, while epiphyses showing perfusion only after reduction are in the groups with longer intervals. The two epiphyses undergoing necrosis were in the group with longest interval, however in this group were also two hips with perfect perfusion before and after reduction (Table 1).

The final aspect of interest was the bone apposition at the posterior neck in slips with disconnection of the epiphysis. Such bone formation could be observed even in cases in which clinical symptoms before the injury had been denied or had been reported with a duration of 4 weeks or less. 30 of 32 (93%) operative reports contained information about resection of posterior bone apposition. Only in two hips bone apposition could not be detected at the posterior neck and for three hips no information was given. From 20 available pre-operative lateral radiographs with acceptable quality only in 14 could signs of bone apposition on the posterior neck be identified (Fig. 1). For the remaining six however, the operative reports contain information about posterior bone resection.

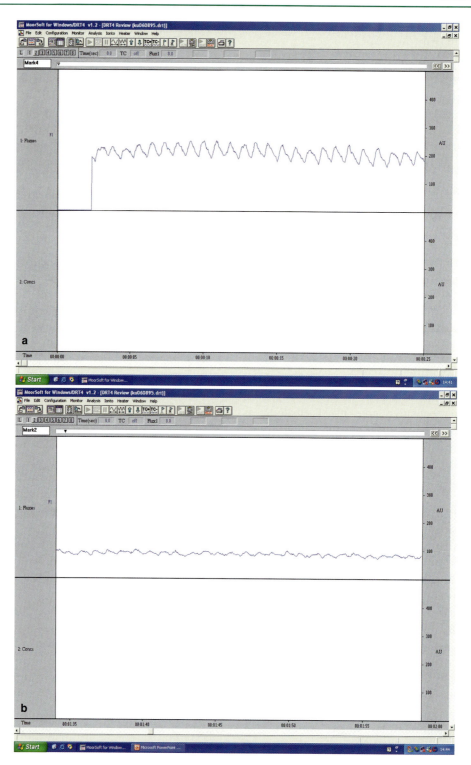

Fig. 3 Laser-Doppler flowmetry (LDF) curves during surgery on a case of SCFE. (**a**) Normal pulsation at capsulotomy. (**b**) Somewhat reduced pulsation after preparation of the extended retinacular flap, probably related to spasm during manipulation. (**c**) Sudden curve drop and loss of pulsation at reduction, due to incomplete resection of bone apposition at the posterior neck (*arrow*). (**d**) Re-established normal pulsation after complete posterior bone resection (*arrow*)

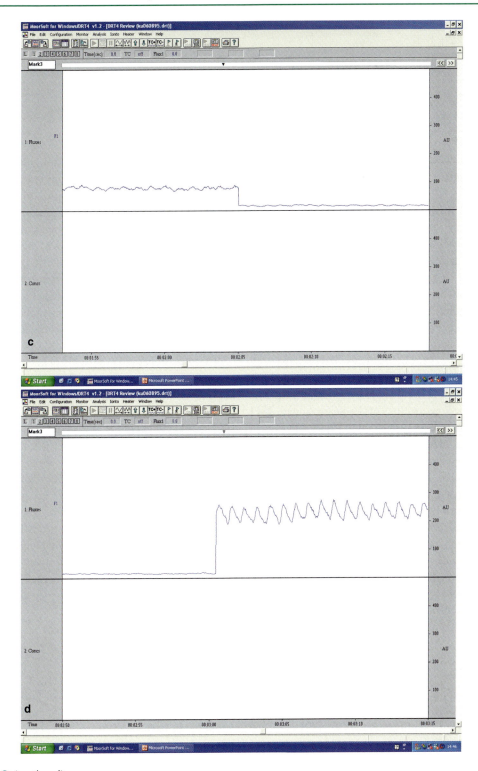

Fig. 3 (continued)

Time to surgery	Insufficient information	<8 h	8–24 h	2–8 days	>8 days
	6		6	4	13	4
Perfusion at capsulotomy	6	6	0	9	2
Perfusion after reduction	6	6	3	3	2
Perfusion at re-operation after 6 weeks				1	
Epiphyseal necrosis				1[a]	2

Table 1 Unstable SCFE (n=27): influence of time interval injury – surgery on epiphyseal perfusion

[a]Case with avulsed retinaculum

Discussion

Pinning in-situ and eventual intertrochanteric correction for malposition of the leg using the smallest possible approach are the cornerstones of a generally accepted treatment strategy for SCFE [2, 20]. More recently, the recognition that even small slips provoke cam-impingement responsible for the frequently observed acetabular cartilage damage gave rise to doubts about this concept [5, 15, 29]. An up-to-the-minute publication [14] on 176 SCFE hips treated with pinning in-situ reported 12 % re-operations, 33 % pain and an activity score of 5 out of 16 points after a follow-up time of 16 years (range 2–43 years). In our study group only four of the stable slips had intra-operatively no acetabular rim or cartilage damage and the majority had substantial damage. We speculate that such damage will further increase when the acetabulum continues to be exposed to the cam morphology of the head-neck junction, a mechanism which was already anticipated with computer simulation [25]. There was a tendency for severe stable slips to have more damage but these hips were also exposed over a longer time. Even small stable slips are very frequently accompanied with substantial cartilage damage and based on anecdotical information we hypothesise that unrestricted, vigorous hip function plays a role. In a concrete case, the pre-operative radiological diagnosis was SCFE with chondrolysis and the intra-operative findings were extended, full thickness abrasion of the acetabular cartilage while the cartilage of the epiphysis was not affected. With the exposed joint it could be demonstrated how the prominent anterior edge of the metaphysis was grinding into the acetabular cavity especially with internal rotation in flexion; it was very similar to perforating implants producing a similar damage mechanism. As mentioned already by Sankar et al. [27] acetabular damage in hips with disconnected epiphysis was clearly less; in our group nearly 30 % disconnected epiphyses showed no signs of acetabular injury. The time of prodromes was half as long compared with the stable slips, though this aspect may not completely explain the low damage rate. As consequence of these findings we continue to regard impingement as an integral part of the SCFE pathology and treat it even in mild slips.

The risk of avascular necrosis is known to be associated with clinically unstable slips, however striking is the large range of reported necroses from 4.7 to 58 % [11, 12, 21, 30]. With such a spread, assignment of the necrosis to the injury of the initial epiphyseal displacement is difficult to understand, although this is a prevailing opinion [1, 13, 19, 24, 26]. Assuming that continuity of the retinaculum can be understood as equal with intact continuity of the retinacular vessels, we have observed only one case with nearly complete rupture of the retinaculum allowing attribution to the postulated mechanism. In fact, this hip did not show signs of perfusion at capsulotomy before or after reduction and went on to complete necrosis.

Another discussed risk factor for necrosis is the time to surgery, however no statistical significance could be established [20]; nevertheless there is some consensus for urgent surgery and some favour the performance of haematoma evacuation as first step [22]. Our approach does not allow us to discuss the value of releasing the intracapsular pressure preceeding the surgery, however in only one of our operative reports a high intracapsular pressure at capsulotomy was noted. In the majority of our cases with disconnected epiphysis the perfusion remained intact even with an interval longer than 1 week. On the other side the two necroses, despite an intact retinaculum, were in the group with longest interval. The few hips in which perfusion was verified only after reduction show that perfusion can be compromised by kinking, overstretching or spasm of the vessels when the epiphysis is mobile, but this impairment can even be reversible [28]. The implication of such observations is that, with a mobile epiphysis, increased time to surgery increases the risk of deleterious impact of intracapsular pressure, retinacular kinking or overstretching. Therefore urgent surgery for slips clinically diagnosed as unstable is ideal, however longer intervals do not necessarily lead to epiphyseal necrosis. If intra-operatively epiphyseal perfusion is not traceable, resection of bone formation at the posterior neck and epiphyseal reduction should still be performed. One of our cases is an excellent example supporting this approach in which perfusion could be documented only at revision surgery which was necessary for implant failure 6 weeks after surgery. The 7-year result shows a perfectly round femoral head without signs of disturbance of perfusion [28].

The final aspect of our interest was bone formation at the posterior neck, indicating chronicity of the slip process. This localised bone apposition is rarely mentioned in the literature [20, 25], although it is present rather regularly in chronic slips and Dunn [6] already has recommended resecting this new bone as part of the epiphyseal reduction. His consideration was that such prominent bone formation may lead to overstretching of the retinaculum when left in place during epiphyseal reduction. For clinically unstable slips Loder recommended a closed reduction not exceeding the slip angle at last radiography in order to respect reduced soft tissue elasticity due to swelling and synovitis [18]. With the same perception others use "gentle reduction" which in fact is a misnomer because stretching of retinacular tissue would depend more on the amount of achieved reduction and less on the way it was achieved. Our findings suggest that posterior bone apposition is not only regular in stable slips but can be found very frequently in slips with disconnected epiphysis including those in which prodromes were explicitly denied and pre-operative lateral radiographies did not show bone formation at the posterior neck; this may have to do with the fact that patient information can be very unprecise and high quality lateral radiographies are frequently not available. On the other hand, our laser Doppler flowmetry results indicate that resection of excessive bone at the posterior neck is an essential factor to protect or re-establish epiphyseal perfusion during epiphyseal reduction.

In summary, our intra-operative data collected from a large group of SCFE treated with open reduction confirms the high incidence of acetabular cartilage damage even in minor slips and support the surgical approach to stop further slipping together with removal of the impingement pathomorphology. In slips with disconnected epiphysis the injury of this separation is rarely responsible for a later necrosis. Time to surgery plays an indirect role for developing a necrosis, on the other hand intact epiphyseal perfusion can be demonstrated with long intervals. Even clinically unstable slips with denied prodromes may have bone formation at the posterior neck. Resection of bone formation at the posterior neck is the most effective element to protect the perfusion of the epiphysis at anatomical reduction.

References

1. Aronsson DD, Loder RT (1996) Treatment of the unstable (acute) slipped capital femoral epiphysis. Clin Orthop Relat Res 322:99–110
2. Aronsson DD, Loder RT, Breur GJ, Weinstein SL (2006) Slipped capital femoral epiphysis: current concepts. J Am Acad Orthop Surg 14:666–679
3. Carney BT, Weinstein SL, Noble J (1991) Long-term follow-up of slipped capital femoral epiphysis. J Bone Joint Surg Am 73:667–674
4. Davidson RS (1996) SCFE: a review of 432 cases, its treatment and complications. Shrine Surgeons Association. Annual meeting, Philadelphia, Sept 1994 in: Lubicky JP Chondrolysis and avascular necrosis: complications of slipped capital femoral epiphysis. J Pediatr Orthop B 5:162–167
5. Dodds MK, McCormack D, Mulhall KJ (2009) Femoroacetabular impingement after slipped capital femoral epiphysis: does slip severity predict clinical symptoms? J Pediatr Orthop 29:535–539
6. Dunn DM (1978) Replacement of the femoral head by open operation in severe adolescent slipping of the

upper femoral epiphysis. J Bone Joint Surg Br 60: 394–403

7. Ganz R, Gill TJ, Gautier E, Ganz K, Krügel N, Berlemann U (2001) Surgical dislocation of the adult hip: a technique with full access to the femoral head and acetabulum without the risk of avascular necrosis. J Bone Joint Surg Br 83:1119–1124

8. Ganz R, Parvizi J, Beck M, Leunig M, Nötzli H, Siebenrock KA (2003) Femoroacetabular impingement: a cause for osteoarthritis of the hip. Clin Orthop Relat Res 417:112–120

9. Ganz R, Huff TW, Leunig M (2009) Extended retinacular soft tissue flap for intraarticular hip surgery: surgical technique, indications, and results of application. Instr Course Lect 58:241–255

10. Gill TJ, Sledge JB, Ekkernkamp A, Ganz R (1998) Intraoperative assessment of femoral head vascularity after femoral neck fracture. J Orthop Trauma 12: 474–478

11. Gordon JE, Abrahams MS, Dobbs MB, Luhmann SJ, Schonecker PL (2002) Early reduction, arthrotomy and cannulated screw fixation in unstable slipped capital femoral epiphysis treatment. J Pediatr Orthop 22:352–358

12. Herman MJ, Dormans JP, Davidson RS, Drummond DS, Gregg JR (1996) Screw fixation of grade III slipped capital femoral epiphysis. Clin Orthop Relat Res 322:77–85

13. Kallio PE, Mah ET, Foster BK, Paterson DC, LeQuesne GW (1995) Slipped capital femoral epiphysis. Incidence and assessment of physeal instability. J Bone Joint Surg Br 77:752–755

14. Larson AN, Sierra RJ, Yu EM, Trousdale RT, Stans AA (2012) Outcomes of slipped capital femoral epiphysis treated with in situ pinning. J Pediatr Orthop 32:125–130

15. Leunig M, Casillas MM, Hamlet M, Hersche O, Nötzli H, Slongo T, Ganz R (2000) Slipped capital femoral epiphysis. Early mechanical damage to the acetabular cartilage by a prominent femoral metaphysis. Acta Orthop Scand 71:370–375

16. Leunig M, Slongo T, Ganz R (2008) Subcapital realignment in slipped capital femoral epiphysis: surgical hip dislocation and trimming of the stable trochanter to protect the perfusion of the epiphysis. Instr Course Lect 57:499–507

17. Leunig M, Horowitz K, Manner H, Ganz R (2010) In situ pinning with arthroscopic osteoplasty for mild SCFE: a preliminary technical report. Clin Orthop Relat Res 468:3160–3167

18. Loder RT (2001) Unstable slipped capital femoral epiphysis. J Pediatr Orthop 21:694–699

19. Loder RT, Richards BS, Shapiro PS, Reznik LR, Aronsson DD (1993) Acute slipped capital femoral epiphysis: the importance of physeal stability. J Bone Joint Surg Am 75:1134–1140

20. Loder RT, Aronsson DD, Weinstein SL, Breur GJ, Ganz R, Leunig M (2008) Slipped capital femoral epiphysis. Instr Course Lect 57:473–498

21. Lubicky JP (1996) Chondrolysis and avascular necrosis: complications of slipped capital femoral epiphysis. J Pediatr Orthop B 5:162–167

22. Mooney JF III, Sanders JO, Browne RH, Anderson DJ, Jofe M, Feldman D, Raney EM (2005) Management of unstable/acute slipped capital femoral epiphysis: results of a survey of the POSNA membership. J Pediatr Orthop 25:162–166

23. Noetzli HP, Siebenrock KA, Hempfing A, Ramseier LE, Ganz R (2002) Perfusion of the femoral heads during surgical dislocation of the hip: monitoring by laser Doppler flowmetry. J Bone Joint Surg Br 84: 300–304

24. Peterson MD, Weiner DS, Green NE, Terry CL (1997) Acute slipped capital femoral epiphysis: the value and safety of urgent manipulative reduction. J Pediatr Orthop 17:648–654

25. Raab GT (1999) The geometry of slipped capital femoral epiphysis: implication for movement, impingement and corrective osteotomy. J Pediatr Orthop 19:419–424

26. Rhoad RC, Davidson RS, Heyman S, Dormans JP, Drummond DS (1999) Pretreatment bone scan in SCFE: a predictor of ischemia and avascular necrosis. J Pediatr Orthop 19:164–168

27. Sankar WN, Partland TG, Millis MB, Kim YJ (2010) The unstable slipped capital femoral epiphysis. Risk factors for osteonecrosis. J Pediatr Orthop 30: 544–548

28. Schöniger R, Kain MSH, Ziebarth K, Ganz R (2010) Epiphyseal reperfusion after subcapital realignment of an unstable SCFE. Hip Int 20:273–279

29. Sink EL, Zaltz I, Heare T, Dayton M (2010) Acetabular cartilage and labral damage observed during surgical hip dislocation for stable slipped capital femoral epiphysis. J Pediatr Orthop 30:26–30

30. Tokmakova KP, Stanton RP, Mason DE (2003) Factors influencing the development of osteonecrosis in patients treated for slipped capital femoral epiphysis. J Bone Joint Surg Am 85: 798–801

31. Ziebarth K, Domayer S, Slongo T, Kim YJ, Ganz R (2012) Clinical stability of slipped capital femoral epiphysis does not correlate with intraoperative stability. Clin Orthop Relat Res 470: 2274–2279

32. Zilkens C, Jäger M, Bittersohl B, Kim YJ, Millis MB, Krauspe R (2010) Slipped capital femoral epiphysis [in German]. Orthopade 39:1009–1021

Part V

Spine

Treatment of the Aging Spine

Max Aebi

Introduction

The aging of the population in the industrialised countries appears to be a non-reversible phenomenon. Increasing life expectancy, due in a great part to the improvement of healthcare, combined with a drastic decrease in birth rate, has led to this situation [40]. The world demographic situation has shifted from a pattern of high birth rates and high mortality rates to one of low birth rates and delayed mortality [23, 40]. In Europe, the proportion of subjects over 65 was 10.8 % in 1950, 14 % in 1970, 19.1 % in 1995 and is projected by some sources at 30.1 % in 2025 and 42.2 % in 2050 [20]. The proportion of subjects over 75 has grown from 2.7 % in 1950 to 5.2 % in 1995 and is projected at 9.1 % in 2025 and 14.6 % in 2050 [20]. However, this trend is not limited to industrialised countries: The developing countries' share of the world's population above 65 is projected to increase from 59 to 71 %. The global consequences of this distortion of the age pyramid on healthcare development, access and costs are huge [29]. For instance approximately 59 % of US residents over 65 are affected by osteoarthritis, which is the main cause of disability. Back and neck pain are amongst the most frequently encountered complaints of all people and the nature of the spine renders those problems highly complex to investigate and to treat.

Furthermore, osteoporotic compression fractures of vertebral bodies is another increasing problem due to aging of the Western population as well as the Japanese and Chinese population, with an increasing number of severely osteoporotic subjects, mostly women. Recent studies have shown that osteoporotic vertebral fractures are associated with an increased risk of mortality and a decreased quality of life. The prevalence in those fractures is around 39 % in subjects over 65 years [Nat. Center for chronic disease prevention] [31].

Degeneration of the spinal structures induces interactive alterations at many levels: bones, discs, facet joints, ligaments. Some of these degenerative lesions can be responsible for compressive damage to the neural elements as in the case of disc herniations or spinal stenosis.

Disc degeneration begins when the balance between synthesis and degradation of the matrix is disrupted; i.e. at the microscopic level, disc degeneration includes a net loss of water as a consequence of a breakdown of proteoglycans in so-called short chains, which are unable to bind water [30, 34]. Furthermore, there is disruption of collagen fibre organisation, specifically in the annulus, and increased levels of proteolytic enzymes. Disc degeneration can be seen in 20 year-old people in about 16 %, whereas this phenomenon is found in 98 % in 70 year-old people and older [8, 9] (Fig. 1).

M. Aebi
McGill University, Montreal (CND),
Orthopädische Klinik Bern, Hirslanden - Salem Spital,
Schänzlistrasse 39, 3000 Bern 25, Switzerland
e-mail: max.aebi@memcenter.unibe.ch

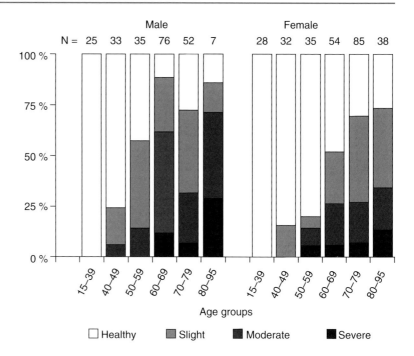

Fig. 1

Women reach the same level of degeneration about 10 years later than men (Fig. 1) [8]. In the aging of the spine there is a predetermined cell viability (endogenous = genetic) and/or decreasing cellular activity in the disc over the years due to exposure of the disc to repetitive mechanical loads [2, 34]. This leads to a loss of extracellular matrix with proteoglycans degrading and decreased capability to bind water. The collagen organisation is dissociated which leads to a loss of the height of the disc. This is always combined with a secondary deterioration of the facet joints, ligaments and muscles. Through this process, the boundaries between the annulus and nucleus are less distinct and the collagen is increasing in the nucleus and replacing the proteoglycans. With that we see concentric fissuring at radial tears which weakens the disc, starting in the third and fourth decade of life. However, there are substantial differences in this whole cascade of events. These changes have clearly biomechanical consequences for the motion segment [2].

The role of vascularisation in the aging spine is most crucial: The nutritional supply of the cells in the disc diminishes because the adjacent vertebral end-plate permeability is decreasing, leading to a blood supply decrease with a secondary tissue breakdown, which starts in the nucleus, and a mechanical impact on the cells (sensitive to mechanical sickness) which leads to a qualitative and quantitative modulation of the matrix proteins [10, 19, 42]. The variation of the proteoglycan content as well as the water content is age-dependent and runs in parallel: more degradation of the proteoglycans, less water content and higher probability of disintegration of the disc (Fig. 2) [18].

The aging of the spine is characterised by two major parallel, however (at least at the beginning), independent processes, which lead to different clinical pictures

1. The reduction of bone mineral density, hence bone mass.
2. The development of degenerative changes of the discoligamentous complex (discs, ligaments, facet joint capsules and facet joints) with consequences of instability, deformity and narrowing of the spinal canal and the exit of the nerve roots (spinal and foraminal stenosis) with secondary neurological problems such as myelopathy, cauda equina and radicular syndromes and disability. Hence, degeneration alone, or in combination with bone mass reduction by osteoporosis and/or metastatic

Fig. 2

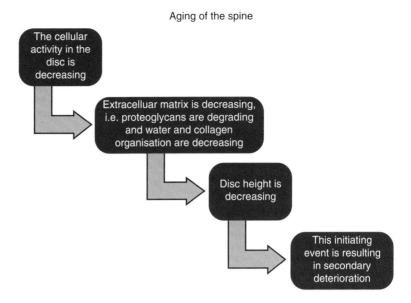

Aging of the spine

tumour involvement, contributes – to a different degree – to the development of a variety of lesions and often to a number of painful and invalidating disorders.

From this short introduction it can be concluded that Orthopaedic surgeons and musculoskeletal specialists as well as dedicated spine specialists are going to face huge problems in treating the numbers of patients affected by diseases which are typical for the aging of the musculoskeletal system.

Typical Disorders of the Aging Spine

Typical disorders of the aging spine are:
- Degenerative disease of the disc(s), **Osteochondrosis** and **disc prolapse**
- **Degenerative disease of the facet joints** with joint incongruences and arthritis, secondary instability and deformity.
- Degenerative **spondylolisthesis** with or without spinal stenosis and instability.
- **Spinal stenosis**, foraminal stenosis due to a narrowing of the spinal canal following hypertrophy of the ligamentum flavum and the joint capsules and the facet joint by itself.
- **Spinal deformities**: scoliosis and/or kyphosis and concomitant secondary instability

- **Osteoporosis** with vertebral compression fractures (VCF) alone or in combination with degenerative defects
- **Pathological fractures** of the vertebrae due to **metastatic** disease
- **Infection** of the spine, spondylodiscitis and spondylitis in the elderly

Disc Degeneration, Osteochondrosis, Disc Herniation

Symptomatic, isolated or multi-level disc degeneration can be seen in the lumbar spine as well as in the cervical spine [13]. The clinically most relevant disc degeneration with subchondral oedema, possible secondary spondylolisthesis and/or translational, rotatory dislocation and consecutive spinal deformity is most frequently seen in the lumbar spine at the level of L3/4 > L2/3 > L4/5 > L1/2. The asymmetrical degeneration may lead to a disc herniation with major or mass dislocation of whole disc fragments (annulus and nucleus parts) leading usually to at least a major neurological complication, such as root compression or cauda compression with significant radicular pain and/or sensomotor deficit.

This pathology can occur in the context of previous surgery in the lower lumbar spine which led to a fusion or at least poorly mobile spinal segment with an overload and stress arising in the adjacent superior or inferior segment with a rapid degeneration of the disc with potential instability, spinal stenosis and possible extrusion of major disc fragments. This can occur as an acute event in almost all those decompressions of the segment and a stabilisation may become necessary [7, 16, 26].

Asymmetrical degeneration of the disc may lead to a further deterioration of adjacent motion segments and may end with a progressive degenerative scoliosis [4], which may need surgical treatment (see below).

Sometimes it is difficult to differentiate the subchondral bony damage from osteoporotic compression fractures. The precise history and clinical examination may lead to a diagnosis as well as STIR sequences of the MRI, CT- Scan and/or bone scintigraphy.

Symptomatic isolated or multi-level disc degeneration can be seen in the lumbar spine as well as in the cervical spine. This disc degeneration with osteochondrosis and sometimes significant subchondral oedema, as expression of inflammation, and occasionally combined with significant disc protrusion, can occur in elderly people primarily without relevant deformity or instability. This degeneration can start in younger age and can be asymptomatic or can be combined with intermittent back pain affecting people sometimes over years and even decades [13].

For some reason, mostly mechanical, disc degeneration can aggravate and become highly symptomatic, specifically when there is a combination with a segmental instability and osteochondritis (Fig. 3). Since these discs are severely degenerated and dehydrated over many years, a herniation consists almost always of a big, combined annulus and fibrotic nucleus sequestrum. The consequence of this disc degeneration may be a secondary deformity, with typical translatory dislocation of vertebrae in a segment or several segments, rotation and scoliosis and/or kyphoscoliosis [4, 13]. It is also possible that disc degeneration and facet joint arthritis can lead to

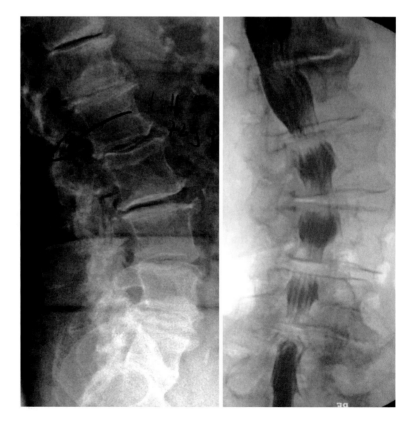

Fig. 3

a degenerative spondylolisthesis [27, 32a, 37]. As long as the disc degeneration is isolated to one or two or three levels without a major deformity, a typical axial "instability" pain occurs, mostly in rotational movements or lifting when upright or when turning in bed during sleep. If conservative treatment with isometric re-inforcement exercises of the abdominal and paravertebral muscles is not successful, surgery may be necessary [32a, b, 36, 38, 41].

There are several surgical options available:
1. minimally invasive, retroperitoneal anterior,
2. posterior as well as
3. far lateral approach surgery as well as combinations. Anterior surgery with stand-alone cages (ALIF), fixed with screws is straight forward in not too adipose patients, and is quite feasible from L3/4, L4/5 and L5/S1, i.e. in the lower lumbar spine. In cases where the patient has had abdominal surgery or is adipose, it is advisable not to do an anterior surgery, but rather a posterior surgery with pedicle fixation and PLIF or TLIF procedure.

In recent years, specifically in elderly people who are frail and where surgery is only an option if everything else does not work, surgery should be limited to a minimum: little blood loss and little surgical trauma and not long anaesthesia time. A far lateral approach (XLIF) may fulfil these requirements [6, 21, 25, 33]. However, to avoid posterior surgery, stand-alone cages need to be used which can be fixed either by an additional plate or with the plate incorporated with the cage (Fig. 4).

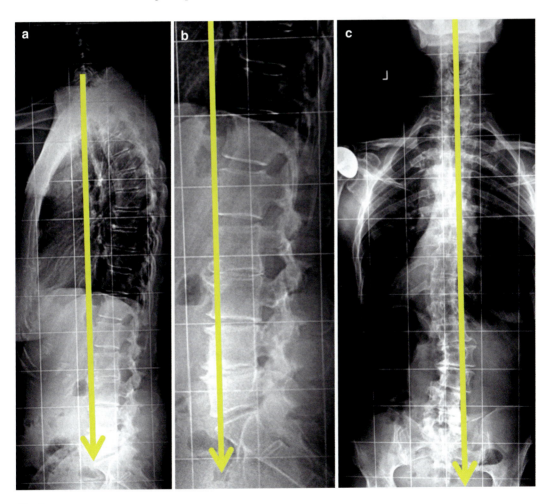

Fig. 4

Fig. 4 (continued)

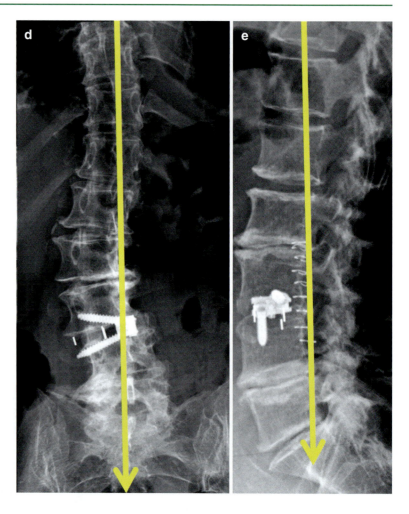

However, ALIF and XLIF surgery is contraindicated in osteoporotic bone, because there is a high probability that the cages will sink into the vertebral bodies [24, 25]. In these cases it is sometimes necessary to do a posterior pedicle screw fixation with cement re-inforcement and even to fill the intervertebral space after removing the disc with cement, i.e. a so-called discoplasty. In some cases where the disc height is significantly reduced and there is significant concomitant facet joint arthritis which participates in the pain generation and if the patient is old with possibly reduced life expectancy and with little demand for physical activity, an interlaminar microsurgical decompression with resection of flavum, capsule and partial arthrectomy, combined with a translaminar facet screw fixation may be sufficient (Fig. 5). This is an atraumatic surgery suitable for very elderly patients with high morbidity and reduced life expectancy and little demand for physical activity, with little blood loss and with one of the major purposes – to control pain – fulfilled by immobilising the facet joints with a screw each.

Spinal Stenosis in the Elderly

Spinal stenosis is a very common condition in the elderly and we have to differentiate between central stenosis, lateral or root canal stenosis, a combination of those two and a combination with or without degenerative spondylolisthesis. There are of course other conditions like the Paget's disease, then degenerative disease, which may cause spinal stenosis with or without neurological

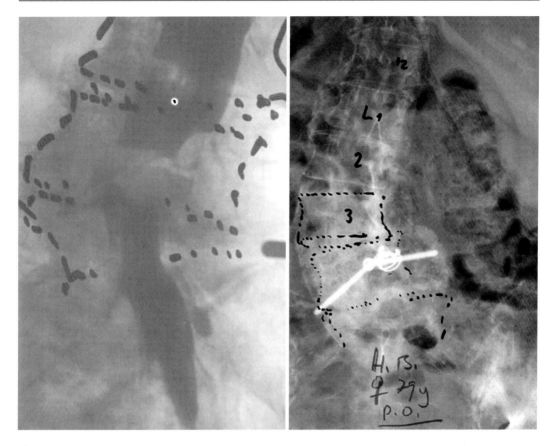

Fig. 5

complications. There is also secondary spinal stenosis due to fracture, mostly osteoporotic fracture, and due to tumour compression of the spinal canal, mostly metastatic disease. Finally, there is iatrogenic stenosis, which can occur as a late result after any spinal surgery at any age. In these cases, spinal stenosis may occur as so-called adjacent segment problem after fusion surgery or be a part of a degenerative deformity (scoliosis and kyphosis) [39].

In most cases, spinal stenosis is due to degenerative changes and/or a pre-existing narrow canal. These changes can lead to symptoms, however, it must be stressed that so-called stenotic images sometimes are present on imaging studies in a number of symptom-free individuals and that the relationship between degenerative lesions, importance of abnormal images and complaints is still unclear. Lumbar stenosis with a claudication symptomatology is also a common reason for decompressive surgery and/or fusion. The investigation of stenotic symptoms should be extremely careful and thorough and should include a choice of technical examinations including vascular investigation. This is of utmost importance, especially if a surgical action is considered, to avoid disappointing results [28].

Surgical management of spinal stenosis can consist of purely decompressive surgery: Here different techniques are available, like classical laminectomy, laminotomy, partial laminectomy, resection of ligamentum flavum and scar tissue, simple foraminal decompression. In recent years it has been suggested in some cases to use a so-called interspinous process distraction. The idea is that with this distraction the foramina are opened and the canal is widened and indirectly decompressed [28, 32b]. The interspinous process distraction also unloads the discs as well as the facet joints. The best patients who are fit

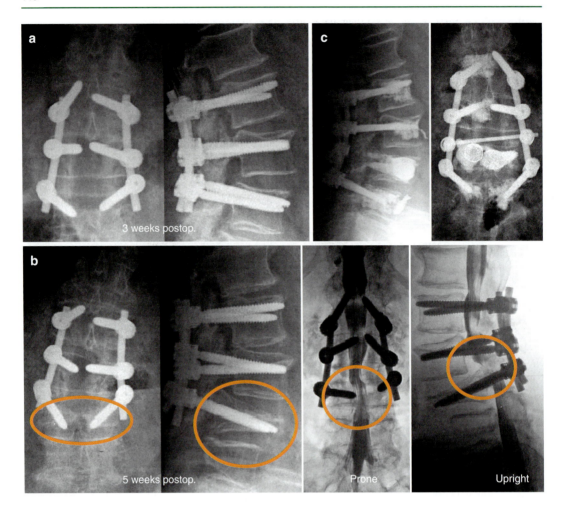

Fig. 6

for this surgery are those with increasing symptoms when doing lumbar extension movements. There is still a quite significant debate whether a decompression needs to be accompanied by instrumentation [28, 32b]. Depending on the osteophyte formations in the anterior column as well as the osteoarthritis of the facet joints and in the absence of any "instability", such as degenerative spondylolisthesis, simple decompression without instrumentation may be sufficient. If there is a need for significant resection of hypertrophic facet joint parts to decompress the dural sac as well as the exiting roots, it may be necessary to stabilise the segment either by simple translaminar/transarticular screw fixation. This is a less rigid fixation than the alternative with pedicle fixation. The risk of the pedicle fixation in spinal stenosis without any deformity and obvious instability is to generate a rigid spine section with a relevant impact on the adjacent segments, including the discs as well as the vertebral bodies [7, 12, 16, 17, 35]. This increases the risk of fatigue fractures in these vertebral bodies and a disruption of the posterior ligament complex as an expression of the aging of ligaments and muscles (Fig. 6).

Obviously, in a severely degenerated cervical spine with spinal stenosis, we may deal with compression of the cord with consecutive myelopathy and/or root compression. The spinal stenosis of the cervical spine often goes together with a deformity usually in kyphosis and sometimes in little scoliotic deformity in the frontal plane. In case there is relevant deformity of the cervical spine combined with a narrow spinal canal, diagnostic traction may be applied to explore how far the deformity can be reduced and the cervical spine can be re-aligned. In cases where this is possible, surgery may be done under traction in the reduced position. In this case there is no manipulation to achieve reduction necessary during the surgery but only the decompressive, and if necessary, the stabilisation part.

Again, also in the cervical spine, there are different ways to address the spinal stenosis. It can be done by an anterior surgery, either by multilevel discectomy and resection of the posterior inferior and superior corner of the adjacent vertebra to do a unisegmental anterior decompression. In cases where the compression of the spinal cord is mainly due to disc on several levels, then this technique can be applied on each individual level by maintaining the main part of the vertebral body. The latter is helpful to place intervertebral spacers and to restore the cervical lordosis. In case there is more compression due to relevant osteophytes, extension of the compression beyond the disc space and in case there is concomitant OPLL, one or even two level vertebrectomies may be necessary with an anterior reconstruction with (expandable or rigid) cages or bony struts (fibula or iliac crest) and plate fixation. If this stabilisation seems to be insufficient and specifically is not really restoring lordosis, a combined posterior fixation with tension-banding and re-aligning of the cervical spine in lordosis may be necessary. There is of course the option left of posterior surgery through laminectomy, laminotomy on several levels or laminoplasty. In case there is insufficient physiological lordosis (in fact kyphosis), then a simultaneous fixation of the decompressed cervical spine along with the decompression may be necessary. In this case, today, most of the time lateral mass screws combined with rod systems is the technique of choice. This surgery is combined with a posterolateral fusion, either by bone substitutes or with cancellous bone from the iliac crest. Since the cervical spine surgery is not as invasive as the lumbar spine surgery, also elderly people with significant co-morbidities can be treated specifically by anterior surgery under neuromonitoring, since there is relatively little blood loss to be expected and the surgical trauma is more or less "local", not involving the whole homeostasis of the body as in a surgery of the lumbar spine in prone position over longer time period.

Degenerative Spondylolisthesis

Degenerative spondylolisthesis occurs usually at the level of L4/5, less frequently at the level of L3/4 and L5/S1. Very often, this degenerative spondylolisthesis is combined with spinal stenosis. The spondylolisthesis is a consequence of a disc degeneration and insufficiency of the facet joints to maintain the stability of the segment. In these cases very often the facet joint effusion can be demonstrated, as well as air inclusion in the disc as well as in the facet joints. The spondylolisthesis can also be combined with a facet joint synovial cyst, which may add to the compressive effect of the spondylolisthesis with a secondary narrowing of the spinal canal. It is still debated whether this pathology needs to be decompressed and stabilised or whether simple decompression is sufficient [1, 27, 32a]. If instability can be demonstrated in functional X-rays with maximal bending and maximal extension over a hypomotion of the lumbar spine in supine position and accompanying low back pain in combination with irradiation into the legs, a stabilisation may well be indicated. Here again, there is a debate whether this should be a pedicle fixation alone or in combination with an interbody fusion, like PLIF or TLIF [9, 27, 32a, 36, 41].

According to the guidelines of NASS [27], there is very little evidence, whether a spondylolisthesis is to be operated with decompression alone, in combination with fusion with or without implant (screws and cages) and whether a reduction is necessary or not.

Degenerative Deformity (Scoliosis and/or Kyphosis)

The degenerative deformity mainly of the lumbar spine and the thoracolumbar spine is a typical disease of the elderly, specifically women.

This is basically a disc disease with the whole cascade described before: disc degeneration as the initial starting point, usually unilateral or asymmetrical, incongruence of the facet joints with subluxation and rotatory deformity, which appears in the AP-view as a translational dislocation, mostly at the level of L2/3 or L3/4 [4]. The deformity in the frontal plane (scoliosis) is practically always combined with a lumbar kyphosis, and this deformity very frequently is combined with recessal or foraminal stenosis, occasionally appearing as a so-called dynamic stenosis, only being clinically relevant when the patient is in upright position or in a certain position while lying or sitting (de novo scoliosis) [4]. The clinical appearance of the degenerative deformity is pain, mostly back pain, with frequent irradiation into the legs, be it a so-called pseudoradicular irradiation or as a real radicular irradiation and claudication symptomatology. Therefore, the clinical problem to be addressed is the progressing deformity, the instability of one or several segments, the neurocompression in the spinal canal, be it centrally or laterally, and very frequently the combination with osteoporosis. These patients are usually unbalanced, not only in the frontal plane but more importantly in the sagittal plane. There is very little substantial non-surgical treatment for these patients. Occasionally, a brace can be tried and a walker or canes may be used to maintain balance.

These patients are generally much better while walking in water, since the water carries them by the buoyant force of the water. The only efficient treatment, however, although tainted by complications and relevant risks, is the surgical treatment.

Surgical treatment is almost always indicated when progression of the curve can be demonstrated over time, and in case of relevant central, recessal and/or foraminal stenosis with significant radicular pain and/or neurological deficit. There is not only a segmental instability, visible in many of these deformities, but there is also a global instability of the spine which means that the spine is collapsing along the sagittal axis which increases the deformity when upright and decreases the deformity when the patient is prone [4].

In general, this surgery is demanding, not only for the patient but also for the surgeon. Since many of these patients are beyond 65 and usually have several risk factors due to polymorbidity, such a surgery needs to be well prepared and thoroughly discussed with the patient and the family, also pointing out risks and consequences in further life. The patients have to understand, together with their family, that such a surgery could finally end up lethally. For this exact reason, a lot has been done in the last few years to facilitate and to reduce the risk of this surgery for these elderly patients. One of the key issues is the blood loss and therefore there are different techniques to be applied to reduce the blood loss, to return the blood with cell saver and to lower the blood pressure as far as possible. Also the staging of the incision during a surgical procedure from the back can help to diminish the blood loss [36], i.e. the parts of the spine are opened portion by portion, then instrumented and finally corrected and stabilised. This reduces the exposure field of the wound and therefore the potential blood loss. In most of these degenerative scoliosis or deformities, if they need surgery, a pedicle fixation is indicated to develop the power to correct to a certain degree the deformity, specifically in the sagittal plane.

Whether cages need to be placed intervertebrally in these elderly people, usually with concomitant osteoporosis, is certainly a question of debate [Lit]. By correct restoration of the lordosis and establishing the plumb-line out of C7 behind the hip joint, the force transmission goes through the posterior elements and therefore a disc anterior support with cage may not be necessary. To avoid cage surgery in these elderly patients is a major element to reduce blood loss and surgical risk. As a result, depending on the problem of the patient, the demands of these patients and of course the co-morbidities, different surgical options in terms of invasiveness may be applicable. Again, in recent years, the application of the far lateral trans-psoas approach with selected correction of the most severely involved segments may be a solution to diminish the surgical trauma in these frail patients [6, 14, 15, 35].

Vertebral Compression Fractures

In recent years different options have been proposed to treat vertebral compression fractures in elderly people and there is still continuous controversy about these different methodologies. Essentially, several technologies have been developed to augment compressed vertebrae as a consequence of osteoporotic fractures. The simplest one is the so-called vertebroplasty, where transpedicular injection of cement into a fractured vertebral body can stabilise this vertebral body. There is, however no relevant potential to reduce a fracture with this technique, except by positioning of the patient. There are several risks involved in this treatment and there is still an on-going debate whether in randomised clinical trials the surgical augmentation really has a benefit over conservative treatment of these fractures [11, 22]. The major risk of this treatment is cement leak, most relevantly leak of cement into the spinal canal through the posterior wall, less problematically leak to the side or to the front, as long as it is only a small amount of cement. The second relevant risk is that cement can go into the venous sinuses of the vertebral body and from there into the venous system with cement thrombosis and/or embolism in the lung [19]. There has been significant progress in cement technology to diminish cement risk to a minimum. Performance of vertebroplasty includes a third risk, which is the placement of the working tubes through the pedicle into the vertebral body. Obviously, there is the risk that this tube can be placed into the spinal canal or outside the pedicle into the lateral paravertebral area with vascular damage. Just as in pedicle screw placement, however, with today's X-ray technology, percutaneous placement of a cannula into a pedicle has become a standard procedure and it should not be a major obstacle to do this procedure when adhering to the proper recommendations of the technique. The pedicle projection has to be visualized carefully in the AP-view and the guiding K-wire has to be placed in a way that it is projected completely within the oval contour of the pedicle in the frontal plane. The K-wire is slightly convergent towards the mid-line and it can cross the inner wall of the pedicle projection contour when at this point in the lateral view the K-wire tip is already in the vertebral body. Therefore, it is important to observe the forward drilling K-wire in the pedicle projection in the AP-view by checking quickly at each step the lateral view to understand the progress of the tip in the depths of the vertebral body. Once the K-wire is placed properly, the Jamshidi needle or a similar instrument can be introduced over the K-wire and progressed into the vertebral body. This opens the pedicle for the working tube, which is then introduced after removing the Jamshidi needle. Once the working cannula is positioned properly into the posterior one third of body, the vertebral body can be drilled in preparation of the seat for the balloon catheter or the cement applicator (in case of simple vertebroplasty). Through this working channel also biopsies can be taken. In case of an additional kyphoplasty, the balloon catheter can be driven into the working cannula and the balloon can be placed in the prepared seat in the vertebral body. The same is true for the balloon catheter, which is armed with a stent, which then is inflated by the balloon and expanded as vertebral body supporter and partial corrector of the compression fracture. It is obvious that with the simple vertebroplasty there is almost no correction which can be done directly with the cement. In an early stage of fractures with the kyphoplasty balloon as well as the kyphoplasty balloon combined with a stent, a certain reduction of the impressed end-plate can sometimes be acheived. The introduction of the balloon kyphoplasty and stent kyphoplasty technology has made this procedure of cement augmentation safer. According to some meta-analysis, the morbidity as well as the mortality and the cement complications are significantly lower with kyphoplasty procedure compared to the simple vertebroplasty [19]. The augmentation technology, however, has failed until today to prove superior to conservative treatment in randomised clinical trials [11, 22]; however, there are several flaws in these prospective trials which are basically contradictory to the everyday clinical experience [5]. From prospective case series it has been learned, that this augmentation surgery is very beneficial and successful for patients in severe pain in combination with vertebral body compression fractures. The indication for such augmentation surgery should be primarily pain in still active fractures, i.e. fractures, which are not healed and are represented in the so-called STIR sequences in the MRI as white vertebrae. Usually, the concept is to apply an augmentation surgery not before 6 weeks after the fracture, with all the correct attempts of conservative treatment.

The second benefit, namely the correction of the vertebral body wedge shape and indirect correction of a secondary kyphosis, is less well supported. However, if there are several fractures with wedge deformity of vertebral bodies, it can lead to a significant kyphosis with a significant disturbance of the sagittal balance, which is detrimental in a long term for an elderly patient. In such cases, the surgical treatment with augmentation of the vertebral body to avoid further progression of kyphosis may be extremely beneficial and important for the patient (Fig. 7).

Other Typical Disorders of the Spine in Elderly Patients

As the treatment options for cancer pathology are getting more and more sophisticated with an increase of survival time, there is also a higher probability that elderly patients develop metastases in the spine [3]. Many of those metastases due to chemotherapy and local irradiation can be managed today without surgical treatment. However,

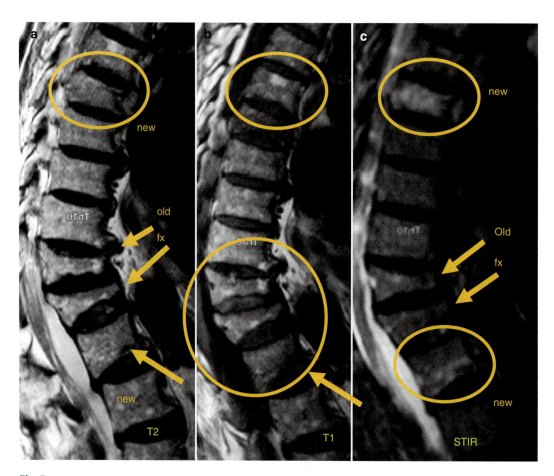

Fig. 7

Fig. 7 (continued)

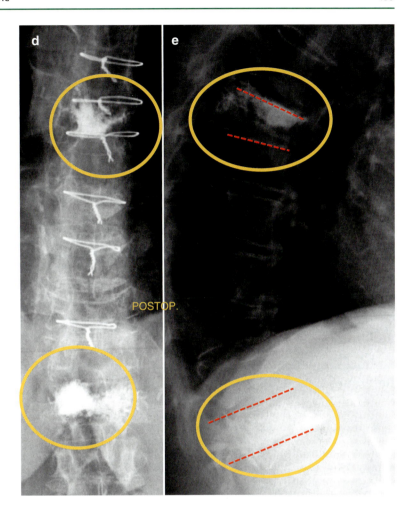

there are still patients left with significant pain due to metastatic pathological fractures of the spine or compression of the spinal canal due to tumour expansion into the spinal canal. The most frequent tumours are metastasis of breast cancer in women and prostate cancer in men as well as the multiple myeloma disease of the spine [3].

With today's available minimally-invasive technology, there is often a combination possible of so-called augmentation technologies described above with less invasive stabilisation technology, as palliative procedures in this kind of elderly patients who suffer from the consequences of spinal metastasis.

Spinal infections in elderly people are again getting more frequent, too. The spondylodiscitis and the spondylitis can be quite a destructive disease with an interruption of the anterior column and secondary kyphosis. The early stage of spondylodiscitis can be treated with antibiotics and partial immobilisation. The indication for surgical treatment is unrelieved pain in spite of proper pain medication, persistent high infection parameters in the blood (CRP, blood sedimentation rate, leucocytes) and increasing secondary deformity and neurological deficit. The procedures are very similar as for tumour surgery. The risks of surgery in frail elderly patients with an infection of the spine, which is mostly a secondary infection of an infection somewhere else in the body (bladder, lungs, lower limbs, skin), is high for septic complications and surgery should only be considered when the above-mentioned criteria are fulfilled.

Summary

Spinal disorders in elderly and usually frail patients with polymorbidity have become a major challenge in spinal surgery. It is not only a major challenge in terms of technical and surgical demands, but also a major challenge in terms of increasing numbers of these patients and the consequences for the treatment. The medical infrastructures are heavily loaded by these pathologies and an interdisciplinary approach to these patients is unavoidable. More and more the surgeon plays here the role of a highly specialised consultant for the specific spinal problem, which needs to be treated in the context of the whole medical care. Therefore, complex spinal problems in elderly patients belong in major medical centres to make sure that these cases can be handled together in an interdisciplinary team.

References

1. Abdu WA, Lurie JD, Spratt KF et al (2009) Degenerative spondylolisthesis: does fusion method influence outcome? Four-year results of the spine patient outcomes research trial. Spine 34(21):2351–2360
2. Adams MA, Roughley PJ (2006) What is intervertebral disc degeneration, and what causes it? Spine 31(18):2151–2161
3. Aebi M (2003) Spinal metastasis in the elderly. Eur Spine J 12(Suppl 2):202–213
4. Aebi M (2005) The adult scoliosis. Eur Spine J 14(10):925–948
5. Aebi M (2009) Vertebroplasty: about sense and non-sense of uncontrolled "controlled randomized prospective trials". Eur Spine J 18(9):1247–1248
6. Anand N, Baron EM (2013) Minimally invasive approaches for the correction of adult spinal deformity. Eur Spine J 22(Suppl. 2):232–241
7. Anandjiwala J, Seo JY, Ha KY, Oh IS, Shin DC (2011) Adjacent segment degeneration after instrumented posterolateral lumbar fusion: a prospective cohort study with a minimum five-year follow-up. Eur Spine J 20(11):1951–1960
8. Battié MC, Videman T, Parent E (2004) Lumbar disc degeneration: epidemiology and genetic influences. Spine 1:29(23):2679–2690 (8a. Heine J (1926) Ueber die arthritis deformans. Virch Arch Pathol Anat 260: 521–663. Cited 8)
9. Battié MC, Videman T, Levälahti E, Gill K, Kaprio J (2008) Genetic and environmental effects on disc degeneration by phenotype and spinal level: a multivariate twin study. Spine 33(25):2801–2808
10. Bibby SR, Jones DA, Ripley RM, Urban JP (2005) Metabolism of the intervertebral disc: effects of low levels of oxygen, glucose, and pH on rates of energy metabolism of bovine nucleus pulposus cells. Spine 30(5):487–496
11. Buchbinder R et al (2009) A randomized trial of vertebroplasty for painful osteoporotic vertebral fractures. N Engl J Med 361(6):557–568
12. Chen BL, Wei FX, Ueyama K, Xie DH, Sannohe A, Liu SY (2011) Adjacent segment degeneration after single-segment PLIF: the risk factor for degeneration and its impact on clinical outcomes. Eur Spine J 20(11):1946–1950
13. Cheung KM, Samartzis D, Karppinen J et al (2012) Are "patterns" of lumbar disc degeneration associated with low back pain?: new insights based on skipped level disc pathology (SLDD). Spine 37(7):E430–E438
14. Cho KJ, Suk SI, Park SR, Kim JH, Choi SW, Yoon YH, Won MH (2009) Arthrodesis to L5 versus S1 in long instrumentation and fusion for degenerative lumbar scoliosis. Eur Spine J 18(4):531–537
15. Crawford CH 3rd, Carreon LY, Bridwell KH et al (2012) Long fusions to the sacrum in elderly patients with spinal deformity. Eur Spine J 21:2165–2169
16. Ekman P, Möller H, Shalabi A, Yu YX, Hedlund R (2009) A prospective randomised study on the long-term effect of lumbar fusion on adjacent disc degeneration. Eur Spine J 18(8):1175–1186
17. Harding IJ, Charosky S, Vialle R, Chopin DH (2008) Lumbar disc degeneration below a long arthrodesis (performed for scoliosis in adults) to L4 or L5. Eur Spine J 17(2):250–254
18. Horner HA, Urban JP (2001) Volvo Award Winner in Basic Science Studies: effect of nutrient supply on the viability of cells from the nucleus pulposus of the intervertebral disc. Spine 26(23):2543–2549
19. Hulme PA, Krebs J, Ferguson SJ, Berlemann U (2006) Vertebroplasty and kyphoplasty: a systematic review of 69 clinical studies. Spine 36(17):1983–2001
20. IIASA/ERD Database (2002) International Institute for Applied Systems Analysis, Laxenburg. www.IIASA.ac.at/research/ERD/. Accessed 27 Apr 2003
21. Isaacs RE, Hyde I, Goodrich JA et al (2010) A prospective, nonrandomized, multicenter evaluation of extreme lateral interbody fusion for the treatment of adult degenerative scoliosis: perioperative outcomes and complications. Spine 35(26 Suppl):S322–S333
22. Kallmes DF et al (2009) A randomized controlled trial of vertebroplasty for osteoporotic spine fractures. N Engl J Med 361(6):569–579
23. Kinsella K, Velkoff V (2001) An aging world. U.S. Census Bureau, vol series p95/01-1. U.S. Government Printing Office, Washington, D.C
24. Labrom RD, Tan JS, Reilly CW et al (2005) The effect of interbody cage positioning on lumbosacral vertebral endplate failure in compression. Spine 30(19):E556–E561
25. Le TV, Baaj AA, Dakwar E et al (2012) Subsidence of polyetheretherketone intervertebral cages in minimally

invasive lateral retroperitoneal transpsoas lumbar interbody fusion. Spine 37(14):1268–1273
26. Lee CS, Hwang CJ, Lee SW, Ahn YJ, Kim YT, Lee DH, Lee MY (2009) Risk factors for adjacent segment disease after lumbar fusion. Eur Spine J 18(11): 1637–1643
27. NASS (North American Spine Society) (2008) Evidence-based clinical guidelines on diagnosis and treatment of degenerative lumbar spondylolisthesis. http://www.spine.org/Documents/Spondylolisthesis_Clinical_Guideline.pdf
28. NASS (North American Spine Society) 2011 (revised version): Evidence-based clinical guidelines on diagnosis and treatment of spinal stenosis. http://www.spine.org/Documents/Lumbar stenosis 11.pdf
29. National Center for Chronic Disease Prevention and Health Promotion, CDC (1999) Chronic disease notes and reports, special focus. Healthy Aging 12:3
30. Ohshima H, Urban JP (1992) The effect of lactate and pH on proteoglycan and protein synthesis rates in the intervertebral disc. Spine 17(9):1079–1082
31. Pluijm SM, Tromp AM, Smit JH, Deeg DJ, Lips P (2000) Consequences of vertebral deformities in older men and women. J Bone Miner Res 15(8):1564–1572
32. Resnick et al (2005) Guidelines for the performance of fusion procedures for degenerative disease of the lumbar spine. (a) Part 9: fusion in patients with stenosis and spondylolisthesis and (b) Part 10: fusion following decompression in patients with stenosis without spondylolisthesis. J Neurosurg: Spine 2: 679–691
33. Rodgers WB, Gerber EJ, Patterson J (2011) Intraoperative and early postoperative complications in extreme lateral interbody fusion. An analysis of 600 cases. Spine 36(1):26–32
34. Roughley PJ (2004) Biology of intervertebral disc aging and degeneration: involvement of the extracellular matrix. Spine 29(23):2691–2699
35. Schulte TL, Leistra F, Bullmann V, Osada N, Vieth V, Marquardt B, Lerner T, Liljenqvist U, Hackenberg L (2007) Disc height reduction in adjacent segments and clinical outcome 10 years after lumbar 360° fusion. Eur Spine J 16(12):2152–2158
36. Schwarzenbach O, Rohrbach N, Berlemann U (2010) Segment-by-segment stabilization for degenerative disc disease: a hybrid technique. Eur Spine J 19(6): 1010–1020
37. Sengupta DK, Herkowitz HN (2005) Degenerative spondylolisthesis: review of current trends and controversies. Spine 30(6 Suppl):S71–S81
38. Suratwala SJ, Pinto MR, Gilbert TJ et al (2009) Functional and radiological outcomes of 300 fusions of three or more motion levels in the lumbar spine for degenerative disc disease. Spine 34(10):E351–E358
39. Szpalski M, Gunzburg R (2003) Lumbar spinal stenosis in the elderly: an overview. Eur Spine J 12(Suppl 2):S170–S175
40. Szpalski M, Gunzburg R, Mélot C, Aebi M (2003) The aging of the population: a growing concern for spine care in the twenty-first century. Eur Spine J 12(Suppl 2):S81–S83
41. Tsahtsarlis A, Wood M (2012) Minimally invasive transforaminal lumbar interbody fusion and degenerative lumbar spine disease. Eur Spine J 21:2300–2305
42. Urban JP, Smith S, Fairbank JC (2004) Nutrition of the intervertebral disc. Spine 29(23):2700–2709

Part VI

Shoulder and Elbow

New Trends in Shoulder Arthroplasty

Anders Ekelund

Shoulder arthroplasty is today a routine procedure with reproducible good outcome. The standard total shoulder arthroplasty has a stemmed humeral component with modular head and an all polyethylene glenoid component. Increased knowledge of the anatomy of the shoulder and the importance of anatomical reconstruction have lead to a variety of different shoulder arthroplasty design tailored to different pathologies of the shoulder. One of the most important developments during the last decades has been the reverse arthroplasty design by Grammont and Baulot [22]. Previously non-treatable conditions can now be successfully treated. The goal for all these changes is to improve the results of the procedure and the longevity of the implants.

Pre-operative Evaluation

It is important to have a detailed knowledge about the bone deformities as well as the quality of the rotator cuff in order to choose the optimal implant and to perform an anatomical reconstruction with a shoulder arthroplasty. The glenoid deformities can be difficult to analyze on plain radiographs and therefore computed tomography (CT) is recommended, allowing analyses of bone and soft tissues. The glenoid in degenerative conditions has been classified by Walch and posterior erosion and bone loss are often seen and can be very challenging to treat [60] (Fig. 1).

Ianotti et al. have developed a CT system with 3-D reconstructions which creates a virtual model of the glenoid to determine the location and amount of bone loss (Fig. 2) [10, 18, 26, 46]. This system allows the surgeon to select the optimal glenoid component and position it correctly. Combining this technique with patient specific instrument can improve the surgeon's ability to place the prosthetic component in the pre-determined location. It can become a valuable tool for the surgeon in the future. The best way to treat cases with severe retroversion or significantly posterior bone loss remains to be defined. We

A. Ekelund, MD, PhD
Department of Orthopaedics,
Capio St Görans Hospital,
Stockholm 112 81, Sweden
e-mail: anders.ekelund@capiostgoran.se

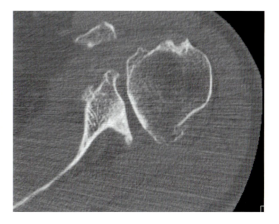

Fig. 1 Computed tomography image showing a bi-concave glenoid with posterior bone loss and posterior subluxation of the humeral head

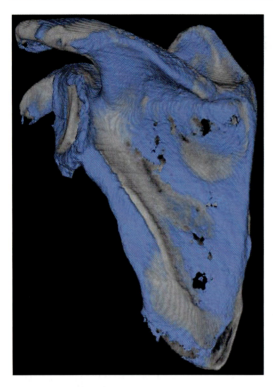

Fig. 2 Overlapping three-dimensional CT-scan model that illustrates the bone loss in the pathological shoulder (normal in *grey*, pathologic in *blue*)

routinely perform plain radiographs and CT scan pre-operatively in all our elective shoulder arthroplasties.

Surgical Approach and Technique

The classical deltopectoral approach is the most common incision used for performing a total shoulder arthroplasty. However, the development of the reverse arthroplasty concept has created an interest in the superior deltoid-splitting approach [37]. The anterior part of the deltoid is released from the anterior acromion (with or without a small bony chip) and then the deltoid is split in the antero-lateral direction in the direction of its fibres for about 4 cm. That will give excellent access to the shoulder joint to perform a reverse arthroplasty or a hemi-arthroplasty for fractures. The advantage is that there is no need, if a reverse arthroplasty is performed, to take down any of the remaining rotator cuff tendons and glenoid exposure is easier.

In the classic deltopectoral approach the subscapularis tendon is cut and reconstructed at the end of the procedure with tendon-to-tendon or tendon-to-bone sutures. Subscapularis insufficiency is a recognized complication and may lead to poor outcome [36, 48]. In order to avoid subscapularis failure Gerber has advocated that a lesser tuberosity osteotomy should be performed in order to avoid having to cut the tendon [19, 20]. Good results in 39 shoulders were reported with no failure. In 2010 Scalise et al. reported the results of a randomized study comparing tenotomy of the subscapularis and ostetomy of the lesser tuberosity [47]. Better clinical outcome was seen in the lesser tuberosity osteotomy group.

Lafosse has developed a new technique to avoid subscapularis problems [32]. The total shoulder arthroplasty was performed through the rotator interval without touching the subscapularis. An approach inferior to the subscapularis tendon can be added in order to more easily remove the rim osteophytes of the humeral head. The results in 17 of 22 patients were reported in 2010. Subjective outcome was excellent in 12 and good in 5. Since the subscapularis is not taken down the technique allows very early active rehabilitation.

The majority of arthroplasties are still done through a deltopectoral approach, but these trends and developments reflect the awareness of the importance of subscapularis repair in order to have a good outcome.

Computed-assisted surgery in total knee arthroplasty has been shown to improve component position [11, 12]. Similar system has been developed for the implantation of shoulder arthroplasty [29, 59] (Fig. 3). Nguyen et al. showed that computed-assisted technique was more accurate in achieving correct glenoid implantation [38]. However, the impact on long term outcome remains to be seen and the technique is still in a developing phase and rarely used today.

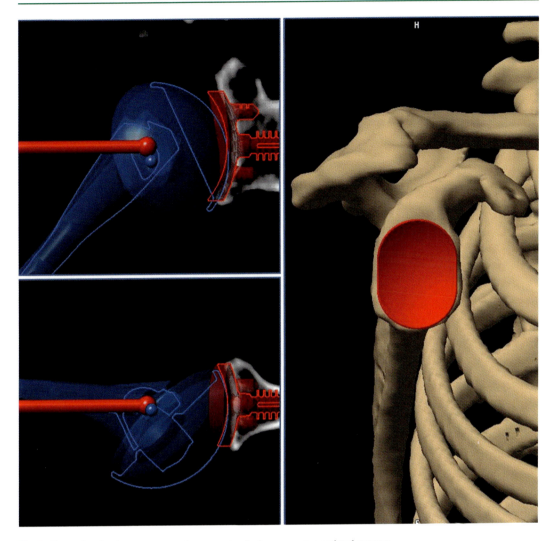

Fig. 3 Example of an image seen on the computer during computer-assisted surgery

Anatomical Arthroplasties

Humeral Component

Shoulder replacement started with stemmed hemi-arthroplasty for complex fractures of the proximal humerus (Neer). Since then the stemmed humeral component has been the gold standard in shoulder arthroplasty without any strong scientific evidence that the stem is necessary. A stemless resurfacing design was popularized by Copeland and excellent results have been published using the resurfacing device as a hemi-arthroplasty [35, 57]. It proved that the standard stem was not necessary. However, the re-surfacing technique has some drawbacks; it cannot be used if there is no humeral head left or in acute fracture cases. Furthermore, it is more difficult to expose the glenoid when the head is preserved. Therefore, the re-surfacing technique is primarily used as a hemi-arthroplasty, even though exposure of the glenoid and inserting a glenoid component is possible. Another stemless design that is used more and more frequently is the metaphyseal

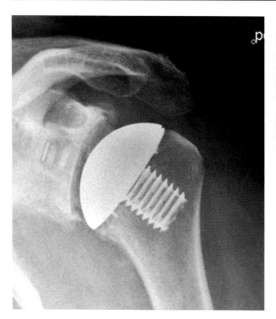

Fig. 4 An example of a stemless, metaphyseal fixed total shoulder arthroplasty (Eclipse, Arthrex)

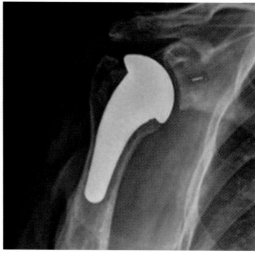

Fig. 5 Radiograph showing a short stem humeral component

fixed components (Fig. 4). The humeral head is removed by cutting along the anatomical head and the humeral component is fixed in the metaphyseal bone by various techniques. Today there are many different designs of this type on the market, but still few publications. In 2010 Huguet et al. reported on 72 total shoulders with a stemless humeral component (TESS, Biomet) with a mean follow-up of 45 months [24]. Constant score was 75 at follow-up and no radiolucencies or component migration was seen. Since the head is removed the exposure of the glenoid is done exactly the same way as for traditional stemmed implants. If the bone quality of the proximal humerus is poor or if there is an acute fracture a stemmed implant is still necessary.

During recent years the stemmed implants have also changed and short stems have been introduced, but little data regarding these implants is available (Fig. 5). The trend is the move away from stemmed implants to stemless or short stem designs. However, more studies are needed to evaluate whether these new designs have the same excellent outcome as the traditional total shoulder arthroplasty.

The humeral components have become more and more modular. It has been shown that the proximal humeral anatomy is highly variable with different neck-shaft angles, retroversion and head size [1, 23, 25, 27, 43]. Most modern humeral components therefore have a modularity making it possible for the surgeon to adapt the implant to the patient-specific anatomy. Furthermore, the centre of rotation has a medial and posterior offset in relation to the shaft. Asymmetrical heads have been developed to compensate for this off set making it possible to cover the cut surface, resulting in a more anatomical reconstruction. Using asymmetrical heads resulted in less micromotion of the glenoid component [41]. With a stemless design there is no need for having different inclination angles, retroversion, asymmetrical heads and it can be used in mal-united fractures. There is also a relationship between head diameter and head thickness, which many prosthetic systems on the market are taking into account, i.e. the number of heads can be reduced [1, 23, 25]. It helps the surgeon to perform an anatomical reconstruction without overstuffing the joint.

In summary, today we see a trend towards more stemless metaphyseal components being used. However, stemmed implants are still necessary and in these implants the stem is being shortened. Few studies have been published on these new stemless designs and therefore they should be used with caution. The traditional stemmed humeral component, cemented or uncemented, remains the gold standard.

The Glenoid

The glenoid component is the weak link in anatomical shoulder arthroplasty and a high percentage of radiolucencies around the component have been reported [33, 53]. The cemented keeled all polyethylene design has been the standard for many years. Due to the risk for glenoid loosening hemi-arthroplasty has been advocated, but then there is a risk for glenoid erosion. There is growing evidence that total shoulder arthroplasty results in better functional outcome compared to hemi-arthroplasty [44]. In order to enhance fixation and longevity of the glenoid component new designs have been tested. The keel has been replaced by pegs of various configurations. Edwards et al. reported on a randomized study (53 shoulders) where they compared pegged and keeled glenoid components [14]. At a mean follow up of 26 months significantly more radiolucencies were seen around keeled compared to pegged components. Nuttall et al. compared a five pegged glenoid with keeled design using radiostereometric analysis [40]. The relative motion of the glenoid component with respect to the scapula was measured. Using this sensitive method all components moved, but keeled components moved more at 2 years follow up. However, in another study using stereometric analysis glenoid component with three pegs inline behaved no differently than a keeled design [45]. Thus, it is not only a question of pegs or keel, but also the number of pegs, and shape and position of the pegs. Throckmorton et al. compared 50 patients with a keeled glenoid component with 50 patients with a pegged design [58]. No clinical or radiographic differences were found. A recent design (Anchor peg, DePuy Orthopaedics, Warsaw, USA) combines peripheral pegs for cementing with a central fluted peg for cementless fixation. Wirth et al. reported on 44 shoulders with this minimally cemented pegged glenoid component with a mean follow up of 4 years [63]. Radiodensity was seen among 30 of the central uncemented peg and it was positively associated with radiolucency scores. The trend today is to use more pegged glenoid designs than keeled. However, further studies are needed to prove that these designs are superior. The author is concerned with the components with pegs in the

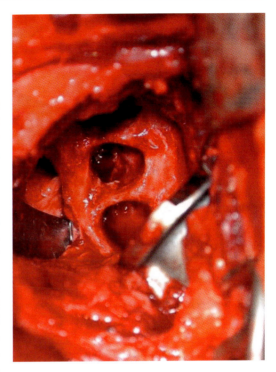

Fig. 6 Intra-operative photograph showing severe bone loss around the pegs of a removed glenoid component

periphery. In revision cases a loosening process can create large non-contained defects which are more difficult to manage compared to a central defect after a loose keeled component (Fig. 6).

Non-cemented metal backed designs have been tried, but these have so far not proved to be better than the cemented all polyethylene designs [8, 16, 54, 55]. However, it would be attractive to have a reliable cementless fixation of a glenoid component to reduce the incidence of radiographic or clinical loosening. Recently, Castagna et al. reported on 35 consecutive total shoulder arthroplasties with a metal backed glenoid component [8]. No loosening or implant related complications were seen at a mean follow up of 75 months. Taunton et al. found a high failure rate of a metal backed bony-ingrowth glenoid component [55]. After a mean follow up of 9 years 33 of the 83 shoulders studied had radiographic signs of glenoid loosening. The 10 year survival rate was calculated to be 52 %. The authors raised concern regarding the use of metal-backed components.

The trend today is to use a cemented all poly glenoid component with pegs and convex posterior

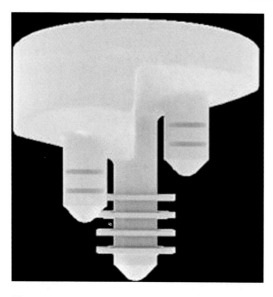

Fig. 7 New design of a posterior augmented glenoid component (STEP-TECH, DePuy Orthopaedics)

surface and to prepare the glenoid with specific reamers and guides to optimize the position of the component.

Glenoid erosion is frequently seen in degenerative conditions with posterior bone loss [60] (Fig. 1). These cases are very challenging. In elderly patients the author uses the reverse arthroplasty in some of these difficult glenoids. Reaming down the high side or adding a posterior bone graft has been recommended, but limited studies are available [39, 52]. Recently, an all polyethylene augmented step glenoid has been introduced to restore anatomy with limited bone removal and without the need for a bone graft (Fig. 7) [28]. This is an attractive way to restore anatomy, but no studies have been published to prove that it is a reliable technique.

Anatomical Fracture Arthroplasty

For many years the same arthroplasty was used for degenerative conditions and acute fractures. The outcome of hemi-arthroplasty in complex fractures has been very unpredictable and the main difficulty has been to achieve anatomical tuberosity healing [2]. Therefore, specific fracture arthroplasties have been designed to facilitate placement and fixation of the tuberosities. Despite these designs the outcomes, particularly in the elderly, remains poor. When the tuberosities do not heal the rotator cuff function is not restored, which results in poor function and sometimes pain. The only solution in these cases is revision to a reverse arthroplasty. To improve the results in complex fractures the reverse arthroplasty is used more and more frequently in acute proximal humeral fractures in the elderly (see under "Reverse Arthroplasty") [6, 7, 9, 17, 30].

The introduction of locked plating of proximal humeral fractures has reduced the number of hemi-arthroplasties. The published overall results for locked plating in three to four part fractures are superior compared to the results after hemi-arthroplasties [31, 56]. However, the locked plating is associated with more complications and revision surgeries, particularly in the elderly [42]. When anatomical reduction of an acute fracture is not possible the surgeon has to switch to use a hemi-arthroplasty or a reverse arthroplasty.

One of the latest designs of a fracture arthroplasty is the Global Unite (DePuy Orthopaedics, Warsaw, USA) which can be used cementless and cementless (Fig. 8). The size of the proximal part can be adapted to the thickness of the tuberosities and the reduction of the tuberosities is facilitated by a collar where sutures can be placed, followed by placing these sutures through the cuff insertion. When these sutures are tied the cuff insertion will automatically be at the humeral head rim, thus avoiding malpositioning. Another feature is the capacity to revise this to a reverse arthroplasty without removing the stem (Platform system).

Platform Systems

Failed fracture hemi-arthroplasties or failed anatomical arthroplasties are usually managed by revision to a reverse Grammont type arthroplasty. Removing a well fixed cemented humeral component is challenging and splitting the humerus is often necessary. To facilitate this growing number of revisions, "platform" systems have been introduced. The humeral component can be converted from an anatomical design to a reverse design without stem removal (Fig. 9). The same trend is seen on the glenoid side where there are some systems on the market where a cementless metal-backed glenoid component can be converted from an anatomical to a reverse design.

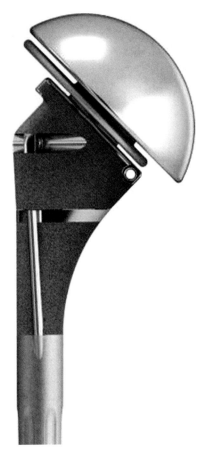

Fig. 8 Fracture hemi-arthroplasty that can be used as a platform arthroplasty (Global Unite, DePuy Orthopaedics)

Reverse Arthroplasty

The Delta reverse arthroplasty concept developed by Grammont has proven to be very successful. His idea of a large hemisphere on the glenoid side and a humeral component with a non-anatomical inclination angle has revolutionized shoulder arthroplasty during the last decades [3, 22]. The previous reverse designs were associated with high failure rate and hardly used. Today the new Grammont type reverse arthroplasty is used for different pathologies, such as cuff tear arthropathy, massive rotator cuff tears, failed anatomical arthroplasties, chronic dislocations, mal-united fractures, non-unions, acute fractures, and tumours [15, 51, 61, 62]. The first series reported a high incidence of complications such as instability and infections. However, with modern implants and modern techniques the number of complications has dropped significantly. The reverse arthroplasty is now routinely used to treat cuff- deficient shoulders to restore function and relieve pain. The author has also used it routinely for acute three to four part fractures in patients over 75 years since 1998 with very satisfactory results (Fig. 10). It is now used more and more for trauma indications and will probably become standard treatment for complex fractures in the elderly [6, 7, 9, 30].

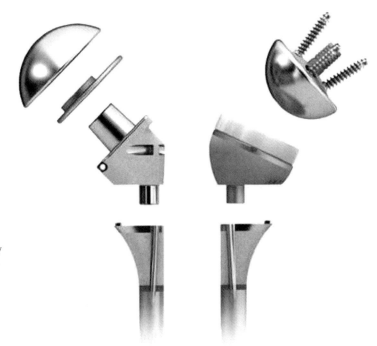

Fig. 9 Fracture hemi-arthroplasty that can be converted to a reverse arthroplasty by changing the proximal epiphyseal component to a Delta Xtend reverse component, but without need for stemrevision (Global Unite, DePuy Orthopaedics)

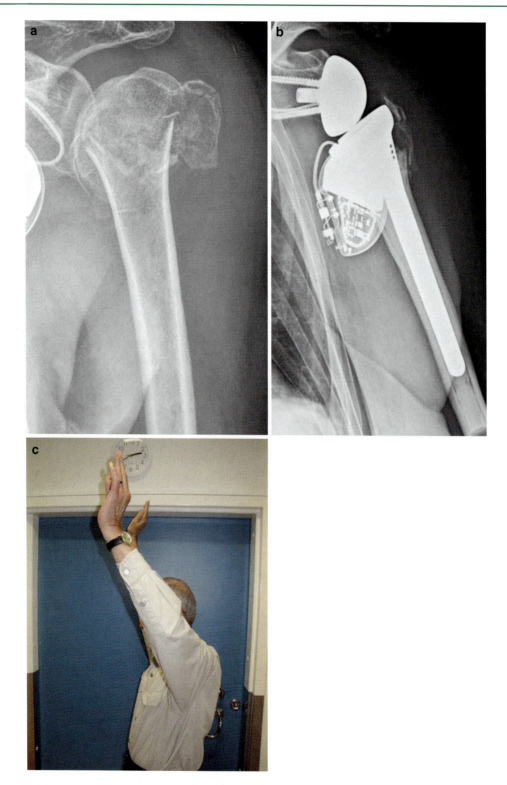

Fig. 10 Comminuted proximal humeral fracture (**a**) treated with a Delta Xtend reverse arthroplasty (**b**). Excellent outcome 6 months after surgery (**c, d**)

Fig. 10 (continued)

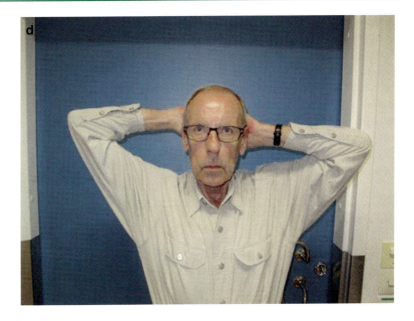

One concern with the reverse arthroplasty is the development of an erosion on the scapula inferior to the glenoid component i.e. notching (Fig. 11) [34, 50]. If the glenoid component is placed as low as possible on the glenoid and the glenosphere has an inferior overhang the risk of notching is reduced [13]. Notching can also be reduced by having a lateralized centre of rotation, but such design increases the load on the glenoid component [15]. Boileau has suggested adding a bone graft on the glenoid surface in order to increase the length of the scapular neck (BIO-RSA) in order to reduce the impingement of the humeral component against the scapula [5]. The tension of the remaining rotatorcuff is also increased which has a favourable effect on stability and may improve rotational forces.

Even though the reverse arthroplasty primarily relies on the deltoid muscle for function and stability, it has been shown that the results are superior if there is a remaining functional teres minor present [49]. Lack of external rotation is the main problem if the entire posterior rotator cuff is missing. In such cases it has been suggested that the reverse shoulder arthroplasty should be combined with a latissimus dorsi transfer in order to restore functional external rotation. In 2007 Gerber et al. reported on 12

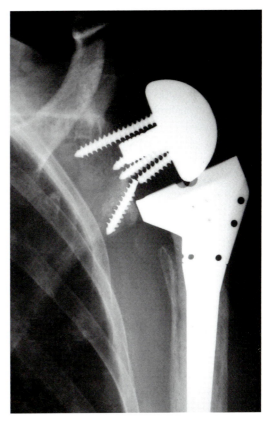

Fig. 11 Radiograph showing scapular notching after implantation of a reverse total shoulder arthroplasty with breakage of inferior screw. The glenoid component was stable

patients treated with a reverse arthroplasty combined with a latissimus dorsi transfer [21]. Functional external rotation measured according to Constant score (maximum 10 points) increased from 4, 6 to 8 points. In 2010 Boileau found significantly improvement in external rotation in 17 patients with a combination of a reverse arthroplasty and transfer of latissimus dorsi and teres major (modified L´Episcopo procedure) [4].

New Materials

Wear is a main concern in all arthroplasties. Improved polyethylene (cross-linked) has been introduced that has better wear characteristics. New materials will be tried in the future to reduce wear and improve longevity of the implants.

An interesting material is pyrocarbon. It has similar structure to graphite, but improved durability. It has been used in artificial heart valves since the 1960s. It has been used for many years in small joints like carpo-metacarpal and radial head implants, but is now being introduced also for shoulder arthroplasties. The bio-elasticity of pyrocarbon is similar to bone, the friction coefficient is very low, and pyrocarbon is very resistant to wear and tear. Thus, it has favourable biological properties. Pyrocarbon implants have no mechanical or biological fixation to bone. They are stabilized by press-fit.

Clinical studies are now being performed for a re-surfacing design and also for a pyrocarbon sphere, which will be placed as an interposition arthroplasty (Fig. 12). It will be very interesting to see the results from these studies and to compare them with the outcome seen after a traditional total shoulder arthroplasty.

Summary

Shoulder arthroplasty is a reliable technique to restore function of the shoulder and the number of procedures is increasing. The surgical

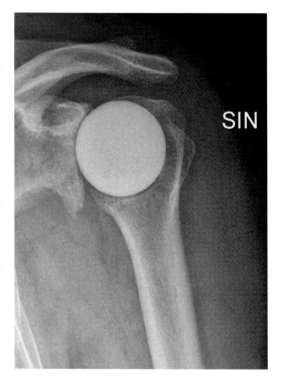

Fig. 12 Radiograph showing a pyrocarbon sphere as an interposition arthroplasty of the shoulder

technique has improved with better instrumentation and increased focus on managing the soft tissue, particularly the subscapularis. There has been a tremendous evolution of these implants over the last decades. The anatomical arthroplasties can be adapted to the patient-specific anatomy to optimize outcome. The trend is to move away from the stemmed implants to more stemless designs. Specific fracture arthroplasties have been developed to facilitate tuberosity reconstruction and healing. The reverse arthroplasty introduced by Grammont has proven to be an important tool to restore function in rotator cuff deficient shoulders and will be used more and more, particularly in trauma. To facilitate the revision from an anatomical arthroplasty to a reverse arthroplasty different platform systems have been developed and introduced on the market. The results of these systems remain to be seen. It is a risk that such a design makes the revision easier but compromises on the biomechanics.

References

1. Boileau P, Walch G (1997) The three-dimensional geometry of the proximal humerus. J Bone Joint Surg 79-B:857–865
2. Boileau P, Krishnan SG, Tinsi L et al (2002) Tuberosity malposition and migration: reasons for poor outcomes after hemiarthroplasty for displaced fractures of the proximal humerus. J Shoulder Elbow Surg 11:401–412
3. Boileau P, Watkinson DJ, Hatzidakis AM et al (2005) Grammont reverse prosthesis: design, rationale, and biomechanics. J Shoulder Elbow Surg 14:147S–160S
4. Boileau P, Chuinard C, Rousanne Y et al (2008) Reverse shoulder arthroplasty combined with a modified latissimus dorsi and teres major transfer for the shoulder pseudoparalysis associated with dropping arm. Clin Orthop Relat Res 466:584–593
5. Boileau P, Moineau G, Roussanne Y et al (2011) Bony increased-offset reversed shoulder arthroplasty: minimizing scapular impingement while maximizing glenoid fixation. Clin Orthop Relat Res 469:2558–2567
6. Boyle MJ, Youn SM, Frampton CM et al (2013) Functional outcomes of reverse shoulder arthroplasty compared with hemiarthroplasty for acute proximal humeral fractures. J Shoulder Elbow Surg 22:32–37
7. Bufquin T, Hersan A, Aubert L et al (2002) Reverse shoulder arthroplasty for the treatment of three and four part fracture of the proximal humerus in the elderly: a prospective review of 43 cases with short term follow up. J Bone Joint Surg 89-B:516–520
8. Castagna A, Randelli M, Garofalo R et al (2010) Midterm results of a metal-backed glenoid component in total shoulder replacement. J Bone Joint Surg 92-B:1410–1415
9. Cazeneuve JF, Cristofari DJ (2006) Grammont reversed prosthesis for acute complex fracture of the proximal humerus in an elderly population with 5 to 12 years follow up. Rev Chir Orthop Reparatrice Appar Mot 92:543–548
10. Codsi MJ, Bennets C, Gordiev K et al (2008) Normal vault anatomy and validation of a novel glenoid implant shape. J Shoulder Elbow Surg 17:471–478
11. Confalonieri N, Chemello C, Cerveri P et al (2012) Is computer-assisted total knee replacement for beginners or experts? Prospective study among three groups of patients treated by surgeons with different levels of experience. J Orthop Traumatol 13:203–210
12. Dattani R, Patnaik S, Kantak A et al (2009) Navigation knee replacement. Int Orthop 33:7–10
13. DeWilde LF, Poncet D, Middemacht B et al (2010) Prosthetic overhang is the most effective way to prevent scapular conflict in a reverse total shoulder prosthesis. Acta Orthop 81:719–726
14. Edwards TB, Labriola JE, Stanley RJ et al (2010) Radiographic comparison of pegged and keeled glenoid components using modern cementing techniques: a prospective randomized study. J Shoulder Elbow Surg 19:251–257
15. Frankle M, Siegal S, Pupello D et al (2005) The reverse shoulder prosthesis for the glenohumeral arthritis associated with severe rotator cuff deficiency. J Bone Joint Surg 87-A:1697–1705
16. Fucentese SF, Costouros JG, Kuhnel SP et al (2010) Total shoulder arthroplasty with an uncemented soft-metal-backed glenoid component. J Shoulder Elbow Surg 19:624–631
17. Gallinet D, Clappaz P, Garbuio P et al (2009) Three or four parts complex proximal humerus fractures: hemiarthroplasty versus reverse prosthesis: a comparative study of 40 cases. Orthop Traumatol Surg Res 95:48–55
18. Ganapathi A, McCarron JA, Chen X et al (2011) Predicting normal glenoid version from pathological scapula: a comparison of 4 methods in 2- and 3-dimensional models. J Shoulder Elbow Surg 20:234–244
19. Gerber C, Yian EH, Pfirrmann AW et al (2005) Subscapularis muscle function and structure after total shoulder replacement with lesser tuberosity osteotomy and repair. J Bone Joint Surg 87-A:1739–1745
20. Gerber C, Pennington SD, Yian EH et al (2006) Lesser tuberosity osteotomy for total shoulder arthroplasty. Surgical technique. J Bone Joint Surg 88-A:170–177
21. Gerber C, Pennington SD, Lingenfelter EJ et al (2007) Reverse Delta-III total shoulder replacement with latissimus dorsi transfer. A preliminary report. J Bone Joint Surg 89-A:940–947
22. Grammont PM, Baulot E (1993) Delta shoulder prosthesis for rotator cuff rupture. Orthopedics 16:65–68
23. Hertel R, Knothe U, Ballmer FT (2002) Geometry of the proximal humerus and implications for prosthetic design. J Shoulder Elbow Surg 11:331–338
24. Huquet D, DeClercq G, Rio B et al (2010) Results of a new stemless shoulder prosthesis: radiologic proof of maintained fixation and stability after a minimum of three years follow-up. J Shoulder Elbow Surg 19:847–852
25. Iannotti JP, Gabriel JP, Schneck SL et al (1992) The normal glenohumeral relationships. J Bone Joint Surg 74-A:491–500
26. Iannotti JP, Greeson C, Downing D et al (2012) Effect of glenoid deformity on glenoid component placement in primary shoulder arthroplasty. J Shoulder Elbow Surg 21:48–55
27. Jeong J, Bryan J, Iannotti J (2009) Effect of a variable prosthetic neck-shaft angle and the surgical technique on replication of normal humeral anatomy. J Bone Joint Surg 91-A:1932–1941
28. Kirane YM, Lewis GS, Sharkey NA et al (2012) Mechanical characteristics of a novel posterior-step prosthesis for biconcave glenoid defects. J Shoulder Elbow Surg 21:105–115
29. Kircher J, Wiedermann M, Magosch P et al (2009) Improved accuracy of glenoid positioning in total shoulder arthroplasty with intraoperative navigation: a prospective-randomized clinical study. J Shoulder Elbow Surg 18:515–520
30. Klein M, Juschka M, Hinkenjann B et al (2008) Treatment of comminuted fractures of the proximal

humerus in the elderly patients with the Delta III reverse shoulder arthroplasty. J Orthop Trauma 22:698–704
31. Kontakis G, Tosounidis T, Galanakis I et al (2008) Prosthetic replacement for proximal humeral fractures. Injury 39:1345–1358
32. Lafosse L, Schnaser E, Haag M et al (2009) Primary total shoulder arthroplasty performed entirely thru the rotator interval: technique and minimum two-year outcomes. J Shoulder Elbow Surg 18:864–873
33. Lazarus MD, Jensen KL, Southworth C et al (2002) The radiographic evaluation of keeled and pegged glenoid component insertion. J Bone Joint Surg 84-A:1174–1182
34. Lévigne C, Garret J, Boileau P et al (2011) Scapular notching in reverse shoulder arthroplasty: is it important to avoid it and how? Clin Orthop Relat Res 469:2512–2520
35. Levy O, Copeland SA (2004) Cementless surface replacement arthroplasty (Copeland CSRA) for osteoarthritis of the shoulder. J Shoulder Elbow Surg 13:266–271
36. Miller SL, Hazrati Y, Klepps S et al (2003) Loss of subscapularis function after total shoulder replacement: a seldom recognized problem. J Shoulder Elbow Surg 12:29–34
37. Molé D, Wein F, Dézaly C et al (2011) Surgical technique: the anterosuperior approach for reverse shoulder arthroplasty. Clin Orthop Relat Res 469: 2461–2468
38. Nguyen D, Ferreira LM, Brownhill JR et al (2009) Improved accuracy of computed assisted glenoid implantation in total shoulder arthroplasty: an in-vitro randomized controlled trial. J Shoulder Elbow Surg 18:907–914
39. Nowak DD, Bahu MJ, Gardner TR et al (2009) Simulation of surgical glenoid resurfacing using three-dimensional computed tomography of the arthritic glenohumeral joint: the amount of glenoid retroversion that can be corrected. J Shoulder Elbow Surg 18:680–688
40. Nuttall D, Haines JF, Trail IA (2007) A study of the micromovement of pegged and keeled glenoid components compared using radiostereometric analysis. J Shoulder Elbow Surg 16:65S–70S
41. Nuttall D, Haines JF, Trail IA (2009) The effect of the offset humeral head on the micromovement of pegged glenoid components: a comparative study using radiostereometric analysis. J Bone Joint Surg 91-B:757–761
42. Owsley KC, Gorczyca JT (2008) Displacement/screw cutout after open reduction and locked plate fixation of humeral fractures. J Bone Joint Surg 90-A:233–240
43. Pearl M (2005) Proximal humeral anatomy in shoulder arthroplasty: implications for prosthetic design and surgical technique. J Shoulder Elbow Surg 14:99S–104S
44. Radnay CS, Setter KJ, Levine WN et al (2007) Total shoulder replacement compared with humeral head replacement for the treatment of primary glenohumeral osteoarthritis: a systematic review. J Shoulder Elbow Surg 16:396–402
45. Rahme H, Mattson P, Wikblad L et al (2009) Stability of cemented in-line pegged glenoid component with keeled glenoid components in total shoulder arthroplasty. J Bone Joint Surg 91-A:1965–1972
46. Scalise JJ, Bryan J, Polster J et al (2008) Quantitative analysis of glenoid bone loss in osteoarthritis using a three-dimensional computed tomography scans. J Shoulder Elbow Surg 17:328–335
47. Scalise JJ, Ciccone J, Iannotti JP (2010) Clinical, radiographic, and ultrasonographic comparison of subscapularis tenotomy and lesser tuberosity osteotomy for total shoulder arthroplasty. J Bone Joint Surg 92-A:1627–1634
48. Scheibel M, Habermeyer P (2008) Subscapularis dysfunction following anterior surgical approaches to the shoulder. J Shoulder Elbow Surg 17:671–683
49. Simovitch RW, Helmy N, Zumstein MA et al (2007) Impact on fatty infiltration of teres minor muscle on the outcome of reverse total shoulder arthroplasty. J Bone Joint Surg 89-A:934–939
50. Simovitch RW, Zumstein MA, Lohri E et al (2007) Predictors of scapular notching in patients managed with the Delta III reverse total shoulder replacement. J Bone Joint Surg 89-A:588–600
51. Sirveaux F, Favard L, Oudet D et al (2004) Garmmont inverted total shoulder arthroplasty in the treatment of glenohumeral osteoarthritis with massive rupture of the cuff. J Bone Joint Surg 86-B:388–395
52. Steinmann SP, Cofield RH (2000) Bone grafting for glenoid deficiency in total shoulder replacement. J Shoulder Elbow Surg 9:361–367
53. Strauss EJ, Roche C, Flurin P-H et al (2009) The glenoid in shoulder arthroplasty. J Shoulder Elbow Surg 18:819–833
54. Tammachote N, Sperling JW, Vathana T et al (2009) Long-term results of cemented metal backed glenoid components for the osteoarthritis of the shoulder. J Bone Joint Surg 91-A:160–166
55. Taunton MJ, McIntosh AL, Sperling JW et al (2008) Total shoulder arthroplasty with metal-backed, bone ingrowth glenoid component. Medium to long-term results. J Bone Joint Surg 90-A:2180–2188
56. Thasanas C, Kontakis G, Angoules A et al (2009) Treatment of proximal humerus fractures with locking plates: a systematic review. J Shoulder Elbow Surg 18:837–844
57. Thomas SR, Wilson AJ, Chambler A et al (2005) Outcome of Copeland replacement shoulder arthroplasty. J Shoulder Elbow Surg 14:485–491
58. Throckmorton TW, Zarkadas PC, Sperling JW et al (2010) Pegged versus keeled glenoid components in total shoulder arthroplasty. J Shoulder Elbow Surg 19:726–733
59. Verborgt O, De Smedt T, Vanhees M et al (2011) Accuracy of placement of the glenoid component in reversed shoulder arthroplasty with and without navigation. J Shoulder Elbow Surg 20:21–26
60. Walch G, Badet R, Boulahia A et al (1999) Morphologic study of the glenoid in primary glenohumeral osteoarthritis. J Arthroplasty 14:756–760

61. Wall B, Nové-Josserand L, O'Connor DP et al (2005) Treatment of painful pseudoparesis due to irreparable rotator cuff dysfunction with the Delta III reverse-ball-and-socket total shoulder prosthesis. J Bone Joint Surg 87-A:1476–1486
62. Werner CML, Steinmann PA, Gilbart M et al (2005) Treatment of painful pseudoparesis due to irreparable rotator cuff dysfunction with the Delta III reverse-ball-and-socket total shoulder prosthesis. J Bone Joint Surg 87-A:1476–1486
63. Wirth MA, Loredo R, Garcia G et al (2012) Total shoulder arthroplasty with an all-polyethylene pegged bone-ingrowth glenoid component: a clinical and radiographic outcome study. J Bone Joint Surg 94-A:260–267

Surgery of the Elbow: Evolution of Successful Management

Bernard F. Morrey

In general, the evolution of elbow surgery can be considered in a temporal fashion and is expressed by advances in technique or of product over time (Fig. 1). The earliest dramatic improvement in fracture management began with the contributions of the AO group in developing the concept of rigid fixation in the 1960's. In the 1970's the widespread use of polymethylmethacrylate (PMMA) allowed reliable prosthetic replacement of other major joints and served as a beginning for an eventual reliable solution for the elbow. Arthroscopy was developed in Canada, United States and worldwide in the early 1970's and this technique has also given rise to substantial improvement in the management of elbow pathology particularly elbow stiffness. Finally, with the ever-evolving interest in and performance of prosthetic replacement, the ability to revise and salvage disastrous pathology has evolved allowing the elbow to be effectively managed even in the most extreme conditions. This presentation reviews the salient advances that are responsible for the current level of success when managing elbow pathology.

Because the elbow is a subcutaneous joint it is certainly well known to be vulnerable to infection both as a result of underlying disease such as rheumatoid arthritis or due to the subcutaneous nature,

---

B.F. Morrey, MD
Mayo Clinic,
200 First St., SW, Rochester, MN 55905, USA

University of Texas Health Science Center,
San Antonio, TX, USA
e-mail: morrey.bernard@mayo.edu

it is particularly vulnerable to open fracture. The recognition that antibiotics can be effectively administered as a prophylaxis in both trauma and reconstructive settings has resulted in a substantive decrease in the alarmingly high early infection rate. While still much greater than other joints, the generally accepted 2–5 % infection rate is considerably less than was present prior to the advent of antibiotics. The reduction in the infection rate has allowed a more aggressive approach to operative fracture management and reconstruction options.

For the remainder of the discussion I will portray the evolution of successful elbow management according to the underlying pathology. This includes discussions regarding trauma, sepsis, primary osteoarthritis, rheumatoid arthritis, and post-traumatic arthritis.

Trauma

The modern management of trauma is truly a success story that has its origins in the AO group in Switzerland. Beginning in the late 1950s and 1960s the principles of rigid fixation was synergistic with the increasing use of antibiotics to avoid infection (Fig. 2). An equally important contribution of the AO group was the precise methodology and instrumentation was the introduction of an education system that allowed hands-on experience lessening the likelihood of technical problems and failures with the new opportunities for fixation. These contributions along with concepts of technique allowed rigid

Fig. 1 The introduction of various treatment as a function of time. *Circled* are those contributions that have had a significant impact on our current management. The *arrows* on the x-axis indicate the modern era that began in the 1950s with the introduction of the AO fracture management philosophy and education. The author's involvement began in 1980

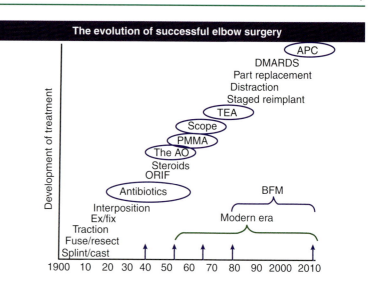

Fig. 2 Highlights of successful management of elbow surgery over the last 110 years

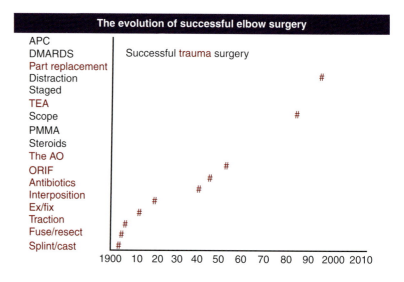

fixation even for significantly comminuted fractures.

The arthroscope has also proven to be very helpful in the management of problems, particularly the sequelae of trauma. Today one can reliably allow a severely traumatized elbow to heal recognizing that a secondary procedure, often with a scope, can be offered that will address the number one complication of elbow trauma, that of joint stiffness.

Finally, with the development of successful elbow joint replacement implants the acute AO classified C3 injury is now well accepted to be managed in the older patient with severe comminution with an acute joint replacement. In addition, those elbows that have developed post-traumatic arthritis after an effort at open reduction and internal fixation are also reliably treated with elbow joint replacement. Unfortunately in the latter group that results do deteriorate with time usually due to mechanical features of use including implant loosening and articular wear. The success of these interventions has resulted in surgical fusion being rarely indicated as a salvage to the post-traumatic elbow joint.

Fig. 3 The successful management of sepsis began in the early 1940s with the introduction of penicillin which has culminated today in the introduction of techniques to manage excessive bone loss in patients with elbow sepsis

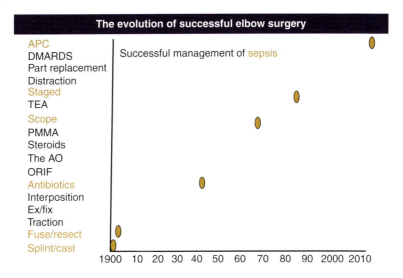

Fig. 4 Treatment of osteoarthritis is a relatively recent development. Today this is effectively performed arthroscopically. This is not a condition that typically requires joint replacement

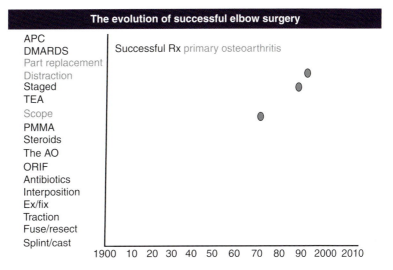

Successful Management of Sepsis

As noted earlier the true initial break-through for the management of sepsis of the elbow originated with the introduction of penicillin in 1942–1943 in Great Britain (Fig. 3). The increasing understanding of the value of prophylactic antibiotics has rendered many of the surgical procedures much more reliable. Hence, the arthroscope is effective in the management of the acute septic joint allowing visualization, lavage, and debridement. The continued high infection rate following joint replacement particularly that of the rheumatoid disease-remitting agents has been documented to be successfully addressed with staged re-implantation similar to that which is documented for the hip and the knee. It has been demonstrated that the infected elbow may be salvaged with the reliability of about 80–90 % with the use of staged revision implantation.

Osteoarthritis

It is interesting and surprising to realize that primary osteoarthritis was appreciated at the elbow only in the 1960s. One of the earliest descriptions of the management of primary arthritis of the elbow was a debridement procedure (Fig. 4). Using a posterior arthrotomy a trephine removed the osteophytes from the olecranon and coronoid fossae. The introduction of the arthroscope has allowed the majority of patients with degenerative arthritis to be managed in a less invasive manner with the use of arthroscopic debridement. The key pathological feature of this disease is that of osteophyte reaction at the margin of the articular surface. The actual articular cartilage is preserved in most instances. This condition, therefore, lends itself ideally to a debridement procedure such as offered by the arthroscope. In the Mayo's experience of over 1,000 primary total elbows, only six had been performed before primary osteoarthritis of the elbow.

Inflammatory Arthritis

Fortunately the burden of this disease is decreasing with time. Unfortunately the reason for the gradual demise of the inflammatory arthritis as a surgical condition is a result of the use of disease-remitting agents which have an adverse effect on those that do require surgical intervention. In any event in the 1920's and 1930's interposition arthroplasty was offered to patients suffering an inflammatory disease (Fig. 5). The interposition arthroplasty was unfortunately found to be unpredictable and, although the elbow was more amenable than the hip or the knee, due to its difficulty and marginal functional improvement, it never became widely accepted. The use of steroids dramatically improved the symptomatic disease in the 1960s. Once again the introduction of arthroscopy in the 1970s allowed a less invasive synovectomy of this joint and lessened the likelihood of losing motion which was not uncommon after an open synovectomy.

The real break-through in the management of the inflammatory elbow, however, was the introduction of reliable elbow joint replacements in the 1970s largely due to the ability to attain secure fixation with polymethylmethacrylate (PMMA). The inflammatory elbow is the most reliably managed with prosthetic replacement. Unpublished data from Mayo reveals that in over 450 patients treated in a 25 year period at the time of final review averaging approximately 15 years, over 90 % of the implants are in place without having had a revision.

In addition to prosthetic replacement, interest in interposition arthroplasty particularly for the young rheumatoid patient has been revisited. Similar to that of total joint replacement, improved techniques both of preparation, and application of the interposition tissue and the enhanced performance of tissue such as the Achilles tendon allograft and the adjunctive use of distraction to allow reliable reconstruction of the collateral ligaments and allow the interposed membrane to heal to the bone prior to sustaining the forces of

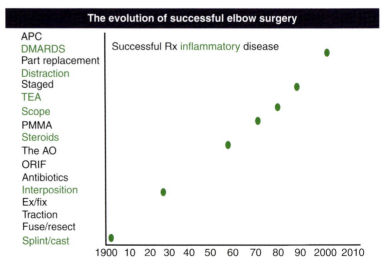

Fig. 5 The successful management of rheumatoid arthritis began with immobilization and migrated to interposition. The use of steroids and medications have dramatically served as the underpinning for the management of this disease. However, joint replacement has proven to be reliable and effective in this patient population

an articulation, seems to have increased the reliability of that option as well.

Finally, the use of disease-remitting agents such as methotrexate has dramatically changed the management of the rheumatoid patient. The patient with a refractory synovitis has almost disappeared from the practice, even in end-stage destruction of the joint is uncommonly seen. Unfortunately, if intervention is required in the patient who is on these medications, the infection rate is definitely increased and such infections seem to be much more refractory to effective management.

Reconstruction Procedures to Salvage the Post-traumatic Elbow and Failed Arthroplasty

In the author's opinion the greatest challenge in the management of elbow arthritis is addressing the needs of the young patient. These most always relate to a post-traumatic condition in which the sequelae have resulted in stiffness and often joint destruction. The key to this type patient is to recognize clearly that the initial treatment offers the best opportunity for successful management. Hence, once again, the introduction of AO principles for the management of the acute fracture is the first step in the enhanced management of these patients, that is decreasing the number of individuals requiring post-traumatic arthritic joint salvage. However, in those patients in whom a post-traumatic condition has resulted in stiffness, the distraction interposition arthroplasty has proven reliable (Fig. 6). A mean improvement in motion allowing a functional arc of 100° is typical. The vast majority of patients have little or no pain.

In the older individual, joint replacement arthroplasty has proven to be effective. We have found a 5 year satisfactory rate of 90 %, which does deteriorate over time due to mechanical failure of loosening and bushing wear. A special case that deserves mention is that of distal humeral non-union. This condition frequently results in a distal fragment that is not salvageable. Not uncommonly the ulna and the articular segment become arthritic or may become ankylosed to the ulna. The un-united fragment is usually relatively small which has contributed to the establishment of the non-union. The management of these in the older patient, that is, over the age of 55 or 60, is to remove the segment and to replace the elbow joint. This has proven once again to be quite effective in the short term, however, as with post-traumatic arthritis, the results do deteriorate over a period of time.

In recent years the advances in the concept of prosthetic replacement has advanced the notion of the use of hemi- or partial replacements. Thus, more anatomical designs have been developed

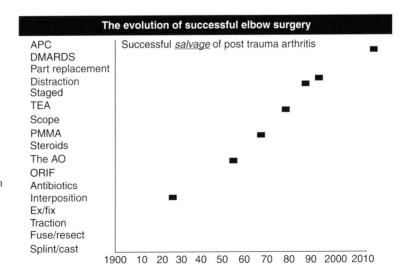

Fig. 6 The use of prosthetic replacement and interposition arthroplasty as well as augmentation procedures with allograft have been the mainstays of recent developments for the salvage of a host of elbow conditions

that allow replacement of the distal humerus when the radial and ulnar articulations are still essentially normal. There is limited indication and application for such implants and in the United States the FDA has not approved their use. Nonetheless, this does represent an important advance in our thinking and in the management of these patients.

Allograft/Prosthetic Composites

Finally, the salvage of the unsalvageable elbow appears to be at hand. The application of the principles learned from the hip and knee experience have allowed the development of a system of reconstructions using allograft prosthetic composites in any one of three applications. A type 1 is one in which an expanded canal is filled with an allograft that has an implant inserted within it.

A type 2 reconstruction addresses extensive bone loss but calls for the implant stem to traverse the allograft and enter host bone. The construct is stabilized by the allograft continuing distally or proximally as a strut.

Finally, in those patients with massive bone loss the simple introduction of an allograft bone to replace that which is lost using a side-to-side fixation strategy has proven effective in the majority of cases. As a matter of fact, in 18 patients with aseptic conditions, 90 % were successfully managed at a mean of 4 years surveillance with the use of the allograft prosthetic constructs described above.

Summary and Conclusions

Over the years the spectrum of elbow pathology has been addressed by several advances in understanding and technique. Today elbow pathology can be reliable and effectively managed. It is felt that the future is bright for further improvement in large measure is not so much because of the development of further technique, but because of basic research which is targeting an understanding of the genetic basis of host variation.

Part VII

Forearm

The Forearm Joint

Christian Dumontier and Marc Soubeyrand

Introduction

The forearm has three main functions: to allow prono-supination and therefore appropriate hand positioning, to transfer longitudinal loads between the wrist and the elbow, and to serve as an attachment site for the muscles that move the wrist and fingers. The forearm is made of two bones, the radius and the ulna, which are joined at the proximal and distal radio-ulnar joints (PRUJ and DRUJ, respectively). Both joints are located at the ends of the forearm and are therefore often considered either part of the elbow (PRUJ) or wrist (DRUJ). The largest part of the forearm, between the DRUJ and PRUJ, is composed of the radial and ulnar shafts linked by the interosseous membrane (IOM) and is classically viewed as a transition segment between the elbow and wrist.

However anatomical works and biomechanical studies have shown that both the PRUJ and DRUJ are not independent of the forearm and cannot function if the forearm is either locked, unstable or destroyed and we introduced the "three locker" concept in 2007 [60]. This also had led some authors to consider the radial and ulnar shafts

C. Dumontier (✉)
Department of Hand and Plastic Surgery,
Hôpital St Roch, 5 rue Pierre Devoluy,
BP 1319, 06006 Nice, France
e-mail: dumontier.c@chu-nice.fr

M. Soubeyrand
Service de Chirurgie Orthopédique,
Hôpital du Kremlin-Bicêtre, 78 rue du général Leclerc,
94275 Le Kremlin-Bicêtre, France

linked by the IOM as an authentic joint, just as are the scapulo-thoracic junction or subacromial space. Because this joint is intercalated between the PRUJ and DRUJ, an appropriate designation is 'middle radio-ulnar joint' (MRUJ), as suggested by LaStayo and Lee [27]. Comparison of species have shown that the forearm joint (zeugopodium) has evolve differently among mammalian species and is part of the evolution of primates for whom prono-supination was useful to live in trees [61]. Most of the muscles involved in prono-supination (i.e., pronator teres, brachial biceps, and supinator) insert at the MRUJ. Studies focussed on the IOM (and therefore the MRUJ) establish that the IOM is not merely a fibrous band filling the interosseous space, but instead a multicomponent ligamentous structure that has a complex behaviour and plays an essential role in forearm stability and physiology [2]. This also suggests that the conventional description of the forearm as a simple segment intercalated between the wrist and the elbow may be outdated and that a more relevant concept may be that of a tri-articular complex in which the MRUJ plays a crucial role [12, 16, 17]. Therefore it seems appropriate to describe the forearm unit as the "forearm joint" to better understand its pathology.

Anatomy and Biomechanics

Both the PRUJ and DRUJ have been widely described and are well known. The stability of the PRUJ is achieved by the annular ligament

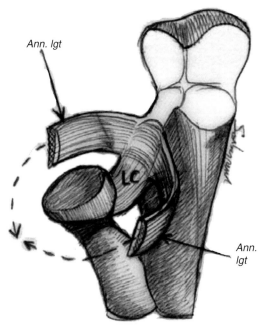

Fig. 1 Three-quarters anterior view of the ligamentous system that stabilizes the radial head. *AL* annular ligament, *LC* quadrate ligament of Denucé. The collateral ligament is not represented (Redrawn from Soubeyrand et al. [62])

attached to the anterior and posterior margin of the radial notch of the ulna and which encircles the radial head (Fig. 1). This ligament is tunnel-shaped, with a smaller diameter in the distal aspect than the proximal border. This condition allows approximately 1–5 mm distal migration of the radius and maintains radial head stability through the entire range of motion. The annular ligament has a close relationship with the lateral radial collateral ligament and they are important stabilizers acting against postero-lateral dislocation/instability. The quadrate ligament (of Denucé) lies between the inferior margin of the annular ligament and the ulna. The oblique ligament or Weitbrecht's ligament extends from the ulna below the radial notch and ends at the radius below the biceps tuberosity. It becomes taut when the radius is in supination.

The DRUJ is inherently unstable as the articular surface of the radius is flatter than that of the ulna. This implies that rotation in the DRUJ must include translation as well as rotation with less than 10 % of surface in contact at extremes of rotation. The TFCC is the most important stabilizer of the DRUJ and has two main components (Fig. 2). The articular disc, a biconcave fibrocartilage whose thickness is variable and depends of the relative length of the ulna; Anterior and posterior re-inforcements of the articular disc are known as the radio-ulnar ligaments [66]. Recently, anatomical dissections have shown that some people (about 40 %) have a thickening of the distal part of the IOM called the distal oblique bundle (DOB) [26, 44] (Fig. 3). The DOB is an obvious thick fibre running within the distal IOM that originates from the distal one-sixth of the ulnar shaft and runs distally to insert on the inferior rim of the sigmoid notch of the radius. The mean width is 4.4 mm (range, 2–6 mm) and mean thickness is 1.5 mm (range, 0.5–2.6 mm). The fibres blend into the capsular tissue of the DRUJ. The DOB, when present, seems to be important stabilizer of the DRUJ. Biomechanical studies have shown that the DOB changed minimally in length during forearm rotation; therefore, it was suggested to be an isometric stabilizer of the forearm. The presence of a DOB was also shown to have a significant impact on DRUJ stability ($P<.05$). The TFCC is the primary soft tissue DRUJ stabilizer, and in normal situations, the influence of the distal IOM on DRUJ stability is relatively inconsequential. However, after TFCC injury, ulnar head resection, or Sauvé-Kapandji procedure, it is likely that the distal IOM has a more important role in the stability of the ulnar head or ulnar stump [39].

The MRUJ is composed of the radial and ulnar shafts linked by the IOM and oblique cord (Fig. 4). While the ulnar shaft axis is almost linear, the radial shaft exhibits a supinator curvature and a pronator curvature that are essential to prono-supination [32, 51]. IOM length is 10.6 cm- on average [73]. The interosseous tubercle, where most of the fibres originate, is on the ulnar aspect of the radius, approximately 8 cm from the elbow joint. Poitevin [49] calls this tubercle "the assemblage nucleus of the IOM." The IOM is formed by two groups of fibres [38, 49, 60]. Fibres of the first group course proximally toward the ulna, while those of the second group run proximally toward the

The Forearm Joint

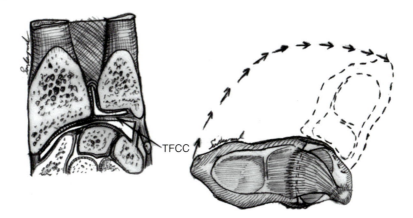

Fig. 2 Schematic representation of the TFCC the main stabilizers of the DRUJ (From Soubeyrand et al. [62] with permission)

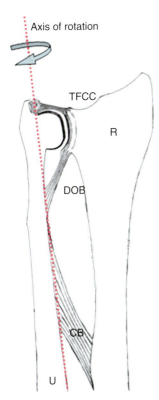

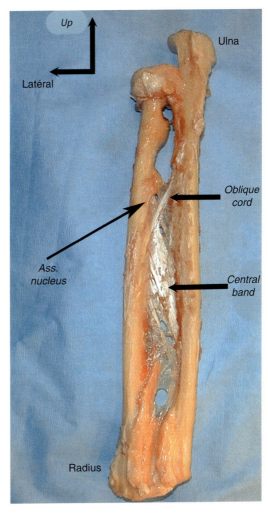

Fig. 3 The distal oblique bundle (DOB), which is a reinforcement of the distal interosseous membrane, is present in 40 % of cadaver dissections and is part of the stabilizing system of the DRUJ. *CB* central band of the IOM (Re-drawn from Moritomo et al. [38])

radius. The second group is the most important in terms of thickness and function. It can be separated into at least three parts according to morphology and function. The most important part is the middle part, known as the central band, which is a strong coherent structure about

Fig. 4 Anatomical dissection of the forearm (posterior view). One can see that the interosseous membrane has variable thickness, the thickest and most important part being the central band. Ass. nucleus: the assemblage nucleus where all the fibres tend to insert

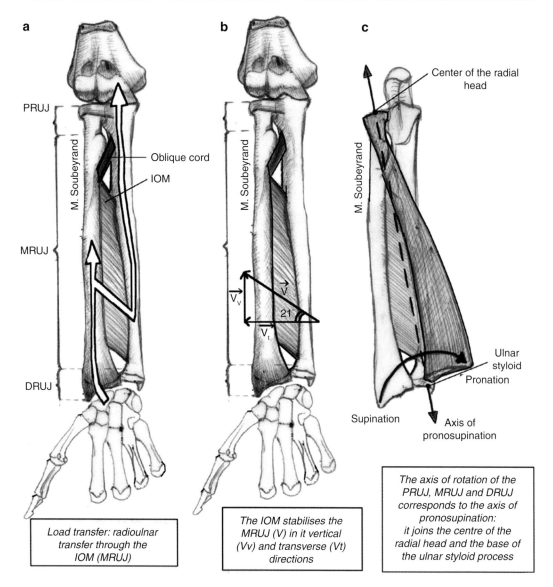

Fig. 5 (**a**) Load transfer occurs mostly at the radio-capral joint at the wrist, and at the ulno-humeral joint at the elbow dus to load transmission through the IOM at the forearm. (**b**) The IOM has two functions represented by two vectors: it contributes both to transverse and longitudinal stability. (**c**) The axis of rotation of the PRUJ, MRUJ and DRUJ corresponds to the axis of prono-supination: it joins the centre of the radial head and the base of the ulnar styloid process (Re-drawn from Soubeyrand et al. [62])

17 mm long and 2 mm thick [19, 56] with intermediate characteristics between a ligament and a membrane with 84 % of collagen [33]. It is inserted on the ulna at an angle of 21° on average to the longitudinal axis of the ulna [56]. The central band fibres are the thickest fibres in the IOM, whereas the distal fibres are the thinnest.

The IOM plays an important role in the longitudinal and transverse stability of the forearm [15], to which the PRUJ and DRUJ also contribute (Fig. 5). The transverse vector reflects the role of the IOM in limiting interosseous space expansion, like the annular ligament proximally maintains the radial head in the lesser sigmoid notch of the ulna and the TFCC distally prevents expansion of the space between the distal ulnar and radial epiphyses.

The vertical vector limits the proximal migration of the radius and contributes to maintain the distal radio-ulnar variance along with the joint between the radial head and the capitellum, as does the TFCC at the DRUJ [50, 53]. At the wrist, longitudinal loads pass chiefly through the radiocarpal joint and to a lesser extent from the carpus to the ulna [29, 30, 46, 47]. At the elbow, this ratio is inverted, with most of the longitudinal loads transmitted between the forearm and humerus passing through the humero-ulnar joint. This ratio difference implies that a load transfer occurs between the radius and the ulna by the MRUJ via the IOM and mostly the central band [2, 19, 29, 30, 36, 46, 48, 53–55, 57, 68, 69] (Fig. 5).

The IOM also absorbs part of the loads protecting the proximal upper limb from the effects of longitudinal impacts on the wrist such as occur, for instance, during a fall on the outstretched hand. An example is the Essex-Lopresti syndrome [8], in which the longitudinal stabilizers (i.e., radial head, IOM, and TFCC) are injured but the proximal upper limb is usually intact.

The specific movement of the forearm joint is prono-supination, in which the radius rotates around the ulna (Fig. 5c). This rotation occurs around a constant axis that is independent of elbow flexion and extension and joins the centre of the radial head and the base of the styloid ulnar process at the insertion of the triangular fibrocartilage complex (TFCC) [18, 37]. Fibre tension is greatest in neutral rotation in the central band and in full supination in the distal fibres [38, 41, 42, 44]. As supination or pronation increases, progressive recruitment of the distal or central band fibres, respectively, occurs. Changes in the positional relationship between this axis and the IOM modify MRUJ kinematics, thereby inducing loss of prono-supination [74], as illustrated by the contribution of IOM fibre retraction to the loss of prono-supination in children with brachial plexus birth palsy, in whom IOM release is required to restore passive rotation of the radius [45, 52]. Thus, the stabilizing role of the various IOM components depends on forearm position.

Pathophysiology: The "Three Lockers" Concept

The PRUJ and the DRUJ share with the MRUJ the above-described axis of rotation. We described the forearm joint as the association of three lockers [61]: The PRUJ is the proximal locker, the MRUJ the middle locker and the DRUJ the distal one. All these lockers should be mobile and stable. Any pathological condition can be seen either as a locked, an unstable or an absent locker (Table 1).

With this conception, it is easy to understand that:

- The range of motion of each joint in the tri-articular complex of the forearm joint depends directly on the range of motion of the other two joints. Either a synostosis at any level between the radius and ulna or stiffness involving the PRUJ or DRUJ can lead to loss of pronation/

Table 1 The three-lockers concept. Either locker may be absent, unstable or lock. Some example of pathologies

	Absent	Locked	Unstable
PRUJ	Radial head resection	Proximal radio-ulnar synostosis	Postero-lateral instability
		Severe ankylosis (post-fracture)	Monteggia's fracture
			Essex-Lopresti's lesion
MRUJ	Probably do not exist	Forearm fracture malunion	Leung's criss-cross injury
		Middle forearm synostosis	Essex-Lopresti's lesion
		IOM retraction (children)	
DRUJ	Ulnar head resection (Darrach's and variants)	DRUJ arthritis	Isolated DRUJ dislocation
		Distal radio-ulnar synostosis	Galeazzi's fracture

supination of the entire forearm [24]. An example of forearm stiffness due to MRUJ disease is angular or rotational mal-union of the radial or ulnar shaft [32, 67]. MRUJ stiffness can also be caused by IOM contracture in patients with brachial plexus birth palsy [45, 52].

- Absence of a single locker has little if any consequence on longitudinal stability. For example Darrach's procedure does not impair prono-supination if the two others lockers are intact [5]. However ulnar head resection can lead to transverse instability with radio-ulnar abutment. Radial head resection does not impair prono-supination if the IOM is intact [11, 21]. An intact IOM limits proximal migration of the radius; with long-term follow-up only a 1.9 mm migration has been reported after radial head resection [40]. Our anatomical dissections have shown that isolated section of the IOM has no influence on the longitudinal stability. However, transverse instability in more severe lesion can lead to impairment of prono-supination. Examples of transverse instability include radial head dislocation at the PRUJ, for instance in Monteggia's fracture [7], ulnar head dislocation at the DRUJ, as in Galeazzi's fracture [13], and isolated ulnar head dislocation. In these situations, inadequate stabilization of either the PRUJ or the DRUJ is sufficient to induce loss of prono-supination, even if the other forearm joints are intact. Leung et al. [28] have described a pattern of lesion called 'criss-cross injury' in which both the PRUJ and the DRUJ are dislocated, whereas the MRUJ is intact (intact IOM, radial shaft, and ulnar shaft). The dislocations prevent forearm rotation.
- When two lockers are unstable, the third cannot compensate: A radial head resection when the IOM is disrupted will lead to a global destabilization of the forearm with progressive proximal migration of the radius and a poor clinical result [64]. A DRUJ dislocation implies, experimentally, the disruption of the IOM [14, 25, 72]. Longitudinal instability occurs in the Essex-Lopresti syndrome [8], in which all three forearm joints are damaged: the PRUJ (radial head fracture), the MRUJ

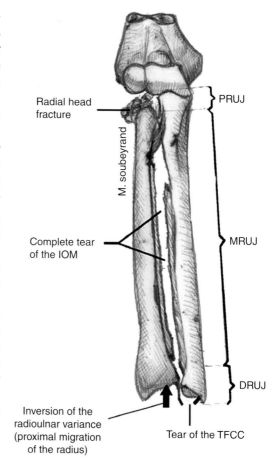

Fig. 6 Schematic drawing of Essex-Lopresti's lesion in which all three radio-ulnar joint are disrupted (Re-drawn from Soubeyrand et al. [62])

(tear of the IOM), and the DRUJ (TFCC tear and inversion of the radioulnar variance with ulnocarpal abutment) (Fig. 6).

How to Diagnose Traumatic Lesions of the Forearm Joint?

Plain X-rays, and CT scan will help the Orthopaedic surgeon to define the bony lesions observed after trauma to the forearm and many published classifications (Mason, AO,…) will help in deciding the choice of treatment. However the most difficult is to understand whether or not associated soft-tissue lesions (i.e. the IOM) will modify the treatment plan.

IOM disruptions are usually the consequences of a longitudinal trauma, such as a fall on the outstretched hand with the wrist in extension, as shown by cadaveric studies [35]. The injury is usually severe, experimental studies showing a peak load at 1,038 N [71]. Both the intensity of the load and the rotational position of the forearm explained the observed lesions [33]. In full supination, one will observe forearm fractures while as rotation moves to pronation the fracture of the radial head becomes more and more comminuted. An Essex-Lopresti lesion is observed around neutral or pronation [33].

To make the diagnosis of IOM disruption, the surgeon will rely on clinical assessment, per-operative evaluation and imaging techniques.

- Clinical Assessment: The mechanism of injury is frequently not known by the patients. However are signs of IOM lesions:
  - A painful wrist in association with a elbow injury
  - Complex fractures of the radial head as they share the same mechanism;
  - Two injuries at the forearm i.e. bone fracture+dislocation, as in Monteggia or, Galeazzi fractures,... should raise suspicion of an associated longitudinal tear of the IOM [9];
  - Both DRUJ and PRUJ lesions in the same patient are highly suspicious for a longitudinal injury of the IOM [8].
- Per-operative evaluation:
  - During surgery, one can rely on stress x-Rays, trying to move the radius up and down. Smith et al. [58], described the 'radius pull test'; after radial head resection, one pulls the radius proximally. The patient lays supine, shoulder abducted to 90° and internally rotated so that the extremity lies flat on the table. The elbow is flexed to 90°, and the forearm and wrist are placed in neutral rotation. A bone-reduction holder is then used to grasp the proximal part of the radius and a longitudinal pull of approximately 20 lb is applied manually in line with the radius. Fluoroscopy is used to measure ulnar variance and proximal radial migration. A proximal migration over 6 mm is diagnostic of a disruption of both the TFCC and IOM;
  - We also describe a simple clinical test to be perform during radial head resection "the intra-operative radius joystick test". During surgery, after radial head resection (or reconstruction) one places a clamp on the radius neck and tries to pull on the radius. In full pronation, it is impossible to move the radial neck if the IOM is intact [63]. If the radius can be pulled out, then the IOM is disrupted (Fig. 7). Sensitivity of this test is 100 % (95 % CI 97–100), specificity 88 % (95 % CI 81–93), positive predictive value 90 % (95 % CI 83–94), and negative predictive value 100 % (95 % CI 97–100), respectively.
- Imaging techniques
  - Plain X-rays are rarely informative but a high index of suspicion must exist as a positive ulnar variance is associated with a radial head fracture. To not miss such lesions, facing a forearm injury six incidences must be made over the elbow, the wrist and the forearm. A ulnar styloid fracture is evocative of a TFCC injury.
  - Sonography is a very promising technique. The IOM appears as a hyperechoic band between the two bones and its rupture can be seen with an accuracy of 96 %, in cadavers... [9, 10, 20, 31]. However static evaluation is sometimes difficult, especially in the traumatized patient with haematoma of the forearm. Soubeyrand described a dynamic sonographic evaluation in which the muscles of the posterior compartment of the forearm are pushed anteriorly and appear as a "muscular hernia" in the anterior compartment which indicates the IOM disruption [59] (Fig. 8).
  - MRI is considered to be the gold standard and sensibility and specificity over 90 % have been reported. The IOM can be evaluated best by axial T2-weighted fast spin echo images with fat suppression [10, 34, 42, 43, 65]. However in a traumatized forearm, and in the presence of metallic devices, artifacts may limit its diagnostic potential and we prefer to rely on sonography.

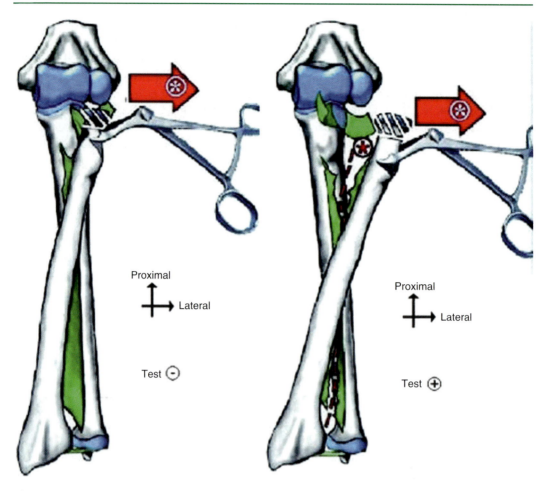

Fig. 7 The radius "joystick pull test". During surgery, with the forearm in full pronation, one cannot pull off the radius which remains immobile under the humeral capitellum despite the lateral traction (*asterisk* in *red arrow*) (*Left*). When the radius can displace laterally, the test is positive and the interosseous membrane is disrupted (Re-drawn from Soubeyrand et al. [63])

However the main explanation for missing such lesions in the Emergency Room is the surgeon who focuses on the most easily seen lesion (the radial head fracture for instance) and forgets to make a thorough examination of the entire forearm joint.

The Essex-Lopresti Lesion as an Example of a "Forearm Joint" Injury

The first description of an IOM lesion was made by Curr and Coe in 1946 [4], a few years before the description by Essex-Lopresti [8] of two cases of a forearm complex injury with dislocation of both the PRUJ and DRUJ, one case with, the other without, a radial head injury. A literature review shows that the Essex-Lopresti syndrome is only part of the forearm joint instability [15, 61]; Delayed diagnosis produces the worst results; Surgical treatment of chronic injuries often gives only average or poor results with both wrist and elbow limitations.

In Essex-Lopresti lesions, all "lockers" (PRUJ, DRUJ and MRUJ) are disrupted and instability occurs both longitudinally (comminuted radial head fracture and positive ulnar variance) and transversally (dislocation of the

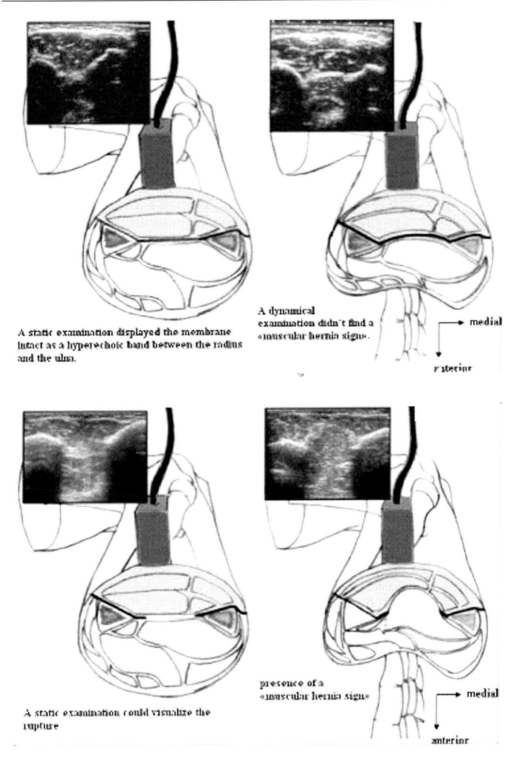

Fig. 8 Dynamic sonography as proposed by Soubeyrand et al. The device is placed on the dorsal side of the forearm (*upper left*). If one presses on the anterior compartment, the IOM will become slightly convex but the anterior muscles are not seen herniating between the two bones (*upper right*). When the IOM is torn, the muscles herniate between the two bones when one presses on the anterior compartment (Re-printed from Soubeyrand et al. [61] with permission)

DRUJ and/or the PRUJ). All should be repaired but treatment differs in acute and chronic cases. Although it may be easy to separate the components of the injury into a fractured radial head, torn IOM, and disrupted DRUJ, it is essential to consider the injury as a disruption of the "forearm 'joint" [6].

In acute cases, one should remember that the radial head is the main stabilizer of the forearm [19] and it should always be either repaired or replaced to prevent proximal migration of the radius [70]. Prosthetic replacement of the radial head is often necessary but may lead to elbow pain and prosthesis subluxation, because of the IOM tear. The radius is pulled proximally by muscles such as the biceps. When the IOM fails to ensure longitudinal stability, the radiocapitellar joint is exposed to excessive loads that damage the capitellar cartilage [23]. This mechanism may explain the development of elbow pain after prosthetic replacement of a fractured radial head that is actually one manifestation of missed Essex-Lopresti syndrome [22, 23].

At the wrist the DRUJ must be stabilized. As the TFCC has a potential for healing, percutaneous pinning of the DRUJ in an anatomical position is usually preferred, although some authors have proposed a TFCC re-attachment.

IOM suture has been proposed [9] with poor results and no one knows if the IOM has the potential to heal. If both the PRUJ and DRUJ are repaired it may not be necessary to do an immediate ligamentoplasty. Rehabilitation of elbow flexion-extension should be started immediately (the three elbow articular surfaces are included in a single capsule) while rehabilitation of prono-supination is delayed until TFCC healing (about 6 weeks).

In chronic cases, the longitudinal instability will be responsible for a radio-capitellar abutment syndrome with pain, limitation of prono-supination and development of radio-capitellar arthrosis.

At the wrist, pain, limitation of mobility and progressive posterior dislocation of the ulnar head are observed. Often, deformities are fixed and cannot be reduced without surgical debridement of the joints. The combined damage to the PRUJ, MRUJ, and DRUJ explains why most authors recommend treatment of all three joints and why several IOM ligamentoplasty techniques have been developed [3, 15, 60, 61]. We believe that the most important factor is to re-establish the appropriate longitudinal relationship between the radius and the ulna. The proximal and distal radio-ulnar joints must be fully reduced in order to stabilize the forearm. This may either be achieved by replacement of the head of the radius, which corrects the proximal migration, and/or by shortening of the distal ulna.

At the elbow, reconstruction of the radial head is mandatory as already pointed out by Essex-Lopresti [8]. Radial head reconstruction with radial head prosthesis is usually necessary. However the prosthesis must be stabilized by reconstruction of both the IOM and the annular and lateral collateral ligaments, sometimes with tendinous grafts. In a cadaver study, Pfaeffle et al. [48] demonstrated that IOM ligamentoplasty decreased the loads applied by the prosthesis to the capitellum (Fig. 9).

At the wrist, it is sometimes necessary to perform an ulnar shortening to restore the radio-ulnar variance. In cases of chronic ulnar head dislocation, removal of the fibrosis in the joint is necessary to obtain reduction. Stabilisation is performed by reconstruction of the TFCC, mainly the radio-ulnar ligaments using either sutures or a ligamentoplasty [1]. The Sauve-Kapandji procedure may be useful when the distal radio-ulnar joint remains unstable, despite the restoration of normal radio-ulnar alignment [22].

IOM reconstruction is very difficult. Many techniques have been described [6, 57, 69, 70]. They usually try to reproduce the central band anatomy but loads are so high that they cannot resist the normal stresses. We believe that a good ligamentoplasty should be in the axis of rotation of the forearm and we described such a technique in 2007 [60] (Fig. 1). Our cadaveric experiments have shown that with this ligamentoplasty, we obtained a complete axial stabilisation. Our clinical experience has confirmed our work but we had some failures in the first cases, not addressing the DRUJ lesions. We believe now that they must always be addressed as even if the TFCC was not torn in some cases, disruption of the distal oblique bundle of the IOM as shown by Moritomo [39] may explain some persisting DRUJ instability in our patients.

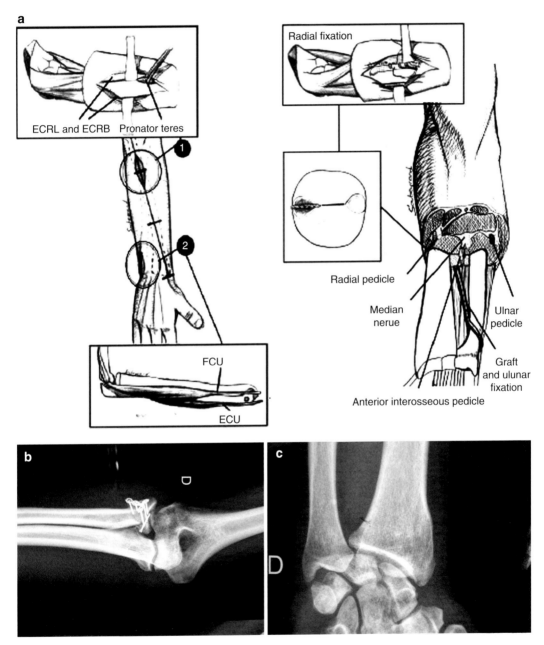

Fig. 9 Surgical treatment of Essex-Lopresti's lesion. (**a**) Schematic drawing of our ligamentoplasty. (**b**) Severe radial head fracture (motocross) with failure of osteosynthesis at 4 months. (**c**) Associated DRUJ lesion was initially missed and proximal migration of the radius occurred. (**d**) Surgical repair associated radial head prosthesis and a synthetic ligamentoplasty. (**e**) A TFCC repair was also done (**f**)

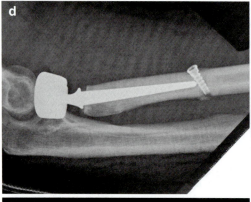
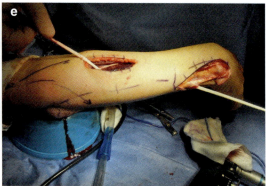
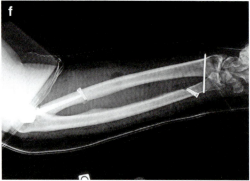

Fig. 9 (continued)

Conclusion

The "forearm joint", the "three lockers" concept,... is one way to realize that all structures in the forearm contribute to the prono-supination movement. If bony injuries are well-known, soft-tissues lesions are most difficult to diagnose and treat. This is especially true for the interosseous membrane which is an important anatomical structure whose injuries may lead to a global forearm instability which will preclude normal rotation of the forearm.

References

1. Adams BD, Berger RA (2002) An anatomic reconstruction of the distal radioulnar ligaments for post-traumatic distal radioulnar joint instability. J Hand Surg Am 27(2):243–251
2. Birkbeck DP, Failla JM, Hoshaw SJ et al (1997) The interosseous membrane affects load distribution in the forearm. J Hand Surg Am 22:975–980
3. Chloros GD, Wiesler ER, Stabile KJ et al (2008) Reconstruction of Essex-Lopresti injury of the forearm: technical note. J Hand Surg Am 33:124–130
4. Curr JF, Coe WA (1946) Dislocation of the inferior radioulnar joint. Br J Surg 34:74
5. DiBenedetto MR, Lubbers LM, Coleman CR (1991) Long-term results of the minimal resection Darrach procedure. J Hand Surg Am 16(3):445–450
6. Dodds SD, Yeh PC, Slade JF III (2008) Essex-Lopresti injuries. Hand Clin 24:125–137
7. Eathiraju S, Mudgal CS, Jupiter JB (2007) Monteggia fracture- dislocations. Hand Clin 23:165–177, v
8. Essex-Lopresti P (1951) Fractures of the radial head with distal radio-ulnar dislocation; report of two cases. J Bone Joint Surg Br 33:244–247
9. Failla JM, Jacobson J, van Holsbeeck M (1999) Ultrasound diagnosis and surgical pathology of the torn interosseous membrane in forearm fractures/dislocations. J Hand Surg Am 24:257–266
10. Fester EW et al (2002) The efficacy of magnetic resonance imaging and ultrasound in detecting disruptions of the forearm interosseous membrane: a cadaver study. J Hand Surg 27(A)(3):418–424
11. Fuchs S, Chylarecki C (1999) Do functional deficits result from radial head resection? J Shoulder Elbow Surg 8(3):247–251
12. Gabl M, Zimmermann R, Angermann P et al (1998) The interosseous membrane and its influence on the

distal radio-ulnar joint. An anatomical investigation of the distal tract. J Hand Surg Br 23:179–182
13. Giannoulis FS, Sotereanos DG (2007) Galeazzi fractures and dislocations. Hand Clin 23:153–163, v
14. Gofton WT, Gordon KD, Dunning CE, Johnson JA, King GJ (2004) Soft-tissue stabilizers of the distal radioulnar joint: an in vitro kinematic study. J Hand Surg Am 29(3):423–431
15. Green JB, Zelouf DS (2009) Forearm instability. J Hand Surg Am 34:953–961
16. Hagert CG (1987) The distal radioulnar joint. Hand Clin 3:41–50
17. Hagert CG (1992) The distal radioulnar joint in relation to the whole forearm. Clin Orthop Relat Res 275:56–64
18. Hollister AM, Gellman H, Waters RL (1994) The relationship of the interosseous membrane to the axis of rotation of the forearm. Clin Orthop Relat Res 298:272–276
19. Hotchkiss RN et al (1989) An anatomic and mechanical study of the interosseous membrane of the forearm: pathomechanics of proximal migration of the radius. J Hand Surg 14-A(2 Pt 1):256–261
20. Jaakkola JI et al (2001) Ultrasonography for the evaluation of forearm interosseous membrane disruption in a cadaver model. J Hand Surg 26-A(6):1053–1057
21. Janssen RP, Vegter J (1998) Resection of the radial head after Mason type-III fractures of the elbow: follow-up at 16 to 30 years. J Bone Joint Surg Br 80(2):231–233
22. Jungbluth P, Frangen TM, Arens S et al (2006) The undiagnosed Essex-Lopresti injury. J Bone Joint Surg Br 88:1629–1633
23. Jungbluth P, Frangen TM, Muhr G et al (2008) A primarily overlooked and incorrectly treated Essex-Lopresti injury: what can this lead to? Arch Orthop Trauma Surg 128:89–95
24. Kamineni S, Maritz NG, Morrey BF (2002) Proximal radial resection for posttraumatic radioulnar synostosis: a new technique to improve forearm rotation. J Bone Joint Surg Am 84:745–751
25. Kihara H, Short WH, Werner FW, Fortino MD, Palmer AK (1995) The stabilizing mechanism of the distal radioulnar joint during pronation and supination. J Hand Surg Am 20(6):930–936
26. Kitamura T, Moritomo H, Arimitsu S, Berglund LJ, Zhao KD, An KN et al (2011) The biomechanical effect of the distal interosseous membrane on distal radioulnar joint stability. J Hand Surg 36A:1626–1630
27. LaStayo PC, Lee MJ (2006) The forearm complex: anatomy, biomechanics and clinical considerations. J Hand Ther 19:137–144
28. Leung YF, Ip SP, Ip WY et al (2005) The crisscross injury mechanism in forearm injuries. Arch Orthop Trauma Surg 125:298–303
29. Markolf KL, Lamey D, Yang S et al (1998) Radioulnar load-sharing in the forearm. A study in cadavera. J Bone Joint Surg Am 80:879–888
30. Markolf KL, Dunbar AM, Hannani K (2000) Mechanisms of load transfer in the cadaver forearm: role of the interosseous membrane. J Hand Surg Am 25:674–682
31. Matsuoka J et al (2003) Ultrasonography for the interosseous membrane of the forearm. Hand Surg 8(2):227–235
32. Matthews LS, Kaufer H, Garver DF et al (1982) The effect on supination–pronation of angular malalignment of fractures of both bones of the forearm. J Bone Joint Surg Am 64:14–17
33. McGinley JC, Heller JE, Fertala A, Gaughan JP, Kozin SH (2003) Biochemical composition and histologic structure of the forearm interosseous membrane. J Hand Surg Am 28(3):503–510
34. McGinley JC, Roach N, Gaughan JP, Kozin SH (2004) Forearm interosseous membrane imaging and anatomy. Skeletal Radiol 33(10):561–568
35. McGinley JC, Roach N, Hopgood BC, Limmer K, Kozin SH (2006) Forearm interosseous membrane trauma: MRI diagnostic criteria and injury patterns. Skeletal Radiol 35(5):275–281
36. Miura T, Firoozbakhsh K, Cheema T, Moneim MS, Edmunds M, Meltzer S (2005) Dynamic effects of joint-leveling procedure on pressure at the distal radioulnar joint. J Hand Surg Am 30(4):711–718
37. Mori K (1985) Experimental study on rotation of the forearm – functional anatomy of the interosseous membrane. J Jpn Orthop Assoc 59:611–622
38. Moritomo H, Noda K, Goto A et al (2009) Interosseous membrane of the forearm: length change of ligaments during forearm rotation. J Hand Surg Am 34:685–691
39. Moritomo H (2012) The distal interosseous membrane: current concepts in wrist anatomy and biomechanics. J Hand Surg Am 37(7):1501–1507
40. Morrey BF, Askew LJ, Chao EY (1981) A biomechanical study of normal functional elbow motion. J Bone Joint Surg Am 63A:872–877
41. Nakamura T, Yabe Y, Horiuchi Y (1999) Functional anatomy of the interosseous membrane of the forearm – dynamic changes during rotation. Hand Surg 4:67–73
42. Nakamura T, Yabe Y, Horiuchi Y (1999) In vivo MR studies of dynamic changes in the interosseous membrane of the forearm during rotation. J Hand Surg Br 24:245–248
43. Nakamura T, Yabe Y, Horiuchi Y, Seki T, Yamazaki N (2000) Normal kinematics of the interosseous membrane during forearm pronation-supination – a three-dimensional MRI study. Hand Surg 5(1):1–10
44. Noda K, Goto A, Murase T et al (2009) Interosseous membrane of the forearm: an anatomical study of ligament attachment locations. J Hand Surg Am 34:415–422
45. Ozkan T, Aydin A, Ozer K et al (2004) A surgical technique for pediatric forearm pronation: brachioradialis rerouting with interosseous membrane release. J Hand Surg Am 29:22–27
46. Pfaeffle HJ, Fischer KJ, Manson TT et al (1999) A new methodology to measure load transfer through the forearm using multiple universal force sensors. J Biomech 32:1331–1335

47. Pfaeffle HJ, Fischer KJ, Manson TT et al (2000) Role of the forearm interosseous ligament: is it more than just longitudinal load transfer? J Hand Surg Am 25:683–688
48. Pfaeffle HJ, Stabile KJ, Li ZM, Tomaino MM (2006) Reconstruction of the interosseous ligament unloads metallic radial head arthroplasty and the distal ulna in cadavers. J Hand Surg Am 31(2):269–278
49. Poitevin LA (2001) Anatomy and biomechanics of the interosseous membrane: its importance in the longitudinal stability of the forearm. Hand Clin 17:97–110, vii
50. Rabinowitz RS, Light TR, Havey RM et al (1994) The role of the interosseous membrane and triangular fibrocartilage complex in forearm stability. J Hand Surg Am 19:385–393
51. Schweizer A, Furnstahl P, Harders M et al (2010) Complex radius shaft malunion: osteotomy with computer-assisted planning. Hand (NY) 5(2):171–178
52. Seringe R, Dubousset JF (1977) Attitude of the paralytic supination of the forearm in children. Surgical treatment in 19 cases. Rev Chir Orthop Reparatrice Appar Mot 63(7):687–699
53. Shaaban H, Giakas G, Bolton M, Williams R, Scheker LR, Lees VC (2004) The distal radioulnar joint as a load-bearing mechanism – a biomechanical study. J Hand Surg Am 29(1):85–95
54. Shaaban H, Giakas G, Bolton M, Williams R, Wicks P, Scheker LR, Lees VC (2006) The load-bearing characteristics of the forearm: pattern of axial and bending force transmitted through ulna and radius. J Hand Surg Br 31(3):274–279
55. Shepard MF, Markolf KL, Dunbar AM (2001) The effects of partial and total interosseous membrane transection on load sharing in the cadaver forearm. J Orthop Res 19(4):587–592
56. Skahen JR 3rd, Palmer AK, Werner FW et al (1997) The interosseous membrane of the forearm: anatomy and function. J Hand Surg Am 22:981–985
57. Skahen JR 3rd, Palmer AK, Werner FW, Fortino MD (1997) Reconstruction of the interosseous membrane of the forearm in cadavers. J Hand Surg Am 22((6): 986–994
58. Smith AM, Urbanosky LR, Castle JA et al (2002) Radius pull test: predictor of longitudinal forearm instability. J Bone Joint Surg Am 84:1970–1976
59. Soubeyrand M, Lafont C, Oberlin C et al (2006) The 'muscular hernia sign': an original ultrasonographic sign to detect lesions of the forearm's interosseous membrane. Surg Radiol Anat 28:372–378
60. Soubeyrand M, Oberlin C, Dumontier C, Belkheyar Z, Lafont C, Degeorges R (2006) Ligamentoplasty of the forearm interosseous membrane using the semitendinosus tendon: anatomical study and surgical procedure. Surg Radiol Anat 28(3):300–307
61. Soubeyrand M, Lafont C, De Georges R et al (2007) Traumatic pathology of antibrachial interosseous membrane of forearm. Chir Main 26:255–277
62. Soubeyrand M, Wassermann V, Hirsch C, Oberlin C, Gagey O, Dumontier C (2011) The middle radioulnar joint and triarticular forearm complex. J Hand Surg Eur Vol 36(6):447–454
63. Soubeyrand M, Ciais G, Wassermann V, Kalouche I, Biau D, Dumontier C, Gagey O (2011) The intraoperative radius joystick test to diagnose complete disruption of the interosseous membrane. J Bone Joint Surg Br 93(10):1389–1394, Erratum in: J Bone Joint Surg Br. 2011;93(12):1679
64. Sowa DT, Hotchkiss RN, Weiland AJ (1995) Symptomatic proximal translation of the radius following radial head resection. Clin Orthop Relat Res 317:106–113
65. Starch DW, Dabezies EJ (2001) Magnetic resonance imaging of the interosseous membrane of the forearm. J Bone Joint Surg Am 83:235–238
66. Stuart PR, Berger RA, Linscheid RL, An KN (2000) The dorsopalmar stability of the distal radioulnar joint. J Hand Surg Am 25(4):689–699
67. Tarr RR, Garfinkel AI, Sarmiento A (1984) The effects of angular and rotational deformities of both bones of the forearm. An in vitro study. J Bone Joint Surg Am 66:65–70
68. Tejwani SG, Markolf KL, Benhaim P (2005) Reconstruction of the interosseous membrane of the forearm with a graft substitute: a cadaveric study. J Hand Surg Am 30(2):326–334
69. Tejwani SG, Markolf KL, Benhaim P (2005) Graft reconstruction of the interosseous membrane in conjunction with metallic radial head replacement: a cadaveric study. J Hand Surg Am 30(2): 335–342
70. Tejwani NC, Mehta H (2007) Fractures of the radial head and neck: current concepts in management. J Am Acad Orthop Surg 15:380–387
71. Wallace AL, Walsh WR, van Rooijen M et al (1997) The interosseous membrane in radio-ulnar dissociation. J Bone Joint Surg Br 79(3):422–427
72. Watanabe H, Berger RA, Berglund LJ et al (2005) Contribution of the interosseous membrane to distal radioulnar joint constraint. J Hand Surg Am 30: 1164–1171
73. Wright TW (2001) Interosseous membrane of the forearm. J Am Soc Surg Hand 1(2):123–134
74. Yasutomi T, Nakatsuchi Y, Koike H et al (2002) Mechanism of limitation of pronation/supination of the forearm in geometric models of deformities of the forearm bones. Clin Biomech (Bristol, Avon) 17: 456–463

Part VIII

Hip

Current Evidence on Designs and Surfaces in Total Hip Arthroplasty

Theofilos Karachalios

Introduction

Since its introduction in the 1960's, total hip arthroplasty (THA) has proved to be an excellent and reliable mode of treatment for the end stages of hip pathology, with satisfactory clinical outcomes at 15–20 years [1–4]. Following the initial problems which the pioneers reported in the 1960's and 1970's (such as surgical technique, structural design failures and infection), in the 1980's. Orthopaedic surgeons faced problems of choice of designs of both acetabular and femoral components and the selection of cemented or cementless implant fixation. Soon afterwards, it was proved that the above dilemmas had been misleading since the long-term survival of an implant relates also to the diagnosis, the patient, the surgeon and surgical technique (Fig. 1). However, until now, the implant has been easy to blame for failures. A possible explanation is the fact that we do not have strong evidence supporting implant design and fixation principles. Instead, we have evidence of good and bad surgical regimes, surgeons having learnt by experience from devastating clinical failures and patients having often been "fashion victims" [5].

In the modern era of THA, it seems that bearing surfaces are a crucial issue for the long-term survival of the artificial joint, and in all international hip fora, implant design and implant fixation issues are considered by many to have been solved. Can we therefore reply to the question, "What is the optimal design and fixation of the implant?" This question is of importance especially nowadays when Economic Health Providers are asking challenging questions.

In an attempt to throw light on the latter question, data from basic science studies, experimental in vivo and in vitro biological and mechanical models, autopsy specimens and long-term clinical studies, have been critically evaluated. It is obvious that a huge effort has been put in both by individual research centres and the implant industry sometimes

T. Karachalios, MD, DSc
Department of Orthopaedic Surgery,
School of Health Sciences, Faculty of Medicine,
University of Thessalia and CERETETH,
University General Hospital of Larissa,
Mezourlo Region, 41110 Larissa, Hellenic Republic
e-mail: kar@med.uth.gr

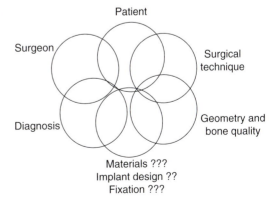

Fig. 1 Parameters affecting the long-term survival of a THA

without considering the cost-effectiveness of this research. It has also become apparent that theoretical and laboratory studies do not always hold up in the "cold light" of long-term clinical studies and there are few quality Level I and II clinical studies. In contrast, there are numerous Level III studies in which the factors such as mid-term follow-up, patient selection criteria, one centre or one surgeon experience, implant modifications and a high rate of drop-out after 15 years, reveal serious defects.

Achieving Implant Incorporation

The lifetime of a THA can be divided into three phases: the initial months during which the implant must become rigidly fixed (early stable phase), and the remainder of the implant's life, during which fixation may be either maintained (late stable phase) or lost (late unstable phase). An early unstable phase may also be seen, although infrequently these days, due mainly to surgical technique errors. The qualities of the arthroplasty that facilitate short-term fixation (such as cement mantle and implant surface texture) may not be the ones most important for long-term fixation (such as implant geometry and stiffness). Three methods are now routinely used to achieve initial fixation:
1. cementing the implant in the bone using polymethylmethacrylate (PMMA),
2. creating a porous or rough implant surface into which bone can grow, and
3. stimulating bone apposition by covering the implant surface with a bio-active substance such as hydroxyapatite (HA) [6].

Bone-Cement Interface

PMMA that has been utilized since the early 1960s has stood the test of time. Cement is not glue and there is no adhesion between cement and bone; it merely forms a micromechanical interlock with bone (Fig. 2). If the bone surface is smooth, the mechanical interlock is poor. To

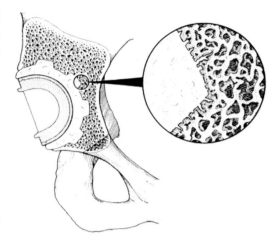

Fig. 2 Cement-bone micro-interlock

achieve fixation, therefore, the bony surfaces must be rough and irregular. Intimate contact between cement and bone can only be achieved when the bone surface is clean (removal of bone debris and blood clots is an advantage) and the trabecular space is open. Thus, cleaning of the bone bed with pressure lavage and pressurization of the cement are very important. The initial bone reaction can be described as an infarct with necrosis of the bone marrow. The dead marrow tissue is replaced with fibrous tissue and repair of the fractured trabeculae is accomplished via removal by osteoclastic resorption, and new bone formation within the fibrous tissue. Osteoid and later mineralized bone may fill the irregular surface of the bone. In other areas, foreign body giant cells can be seen together with connective tissue membrane. Bone or an intact haematopoietic marrow can be found beyond this membrane. Bone re-modelling of the underlying bone occurs due to an alteration in the stress pattern occasioned by use of an implant [7–11]. Willert has categorized the response of bone to the insertion of cement into three phases [12]. In phase I, the first 2–3 weeks after surgery, tissue necrosis is the dominant finding. In phase II there is a reparative stage (fibrous, cartilaginous and osseous tissue) which lasts up to 2 years. During phase III a stable bed forms. Direct contact between cement and bone can occur but the usual interface at the mid-term stages is a fibrohistiocytic

Cement-Femoral Stem Interface

It has been shown that the optimal shape of a stem should transmit torsional as well as axial load to the cement and to the bone without creating damaging peak stresses and without excessive micro-movement. Mechanical factors, cement type and creep, implant type, alloy material, hip stem design, cross-sectional geometry, stem surface finish and heat generation during the exothermic polymerization of cement can all affect the interface (Fig. 4). The stem should remain mechanically stable in the long term despite being subjected to repetitive loading. Two methods have been adopted to achieve these goals: 'loaded-taper' or 'force-closed' fixation and 'composite-beam' or 'shaped-closed' fixation [14, 15]. In the loaded-taper model epitomised by the Exeter implant and its modern counterparts, the stem is tapered in two or three planes and becomes lodged as a wedge in the cement mantle during axial loading, reducing peak stresses in the proximal and distal cement mantle. The stem is allowed to subside at early stages without compromising long term clinical outcome. Polished stems with a loaded-taper design are preferred since they allow stepwise subsidence to a stable position, with the associated micro-movement producing less metal and cement debris at the cement-stem interface. They are very sensitive to a rough surface finish and are incompatible with the use of a collar as a positioning device, an anatomical shape or canal-filling design of the stem, since these features prevent subsidence within the cement mantle.

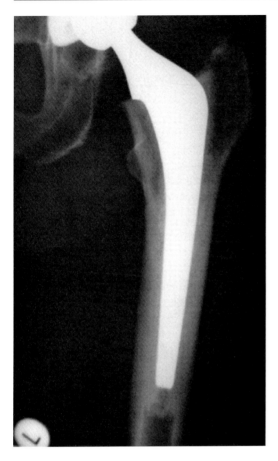

Fig. 3 Third generation of cementing technique. Satisfactory clinical and radiological outcome at 18 years follow-up

membrane [7–12]. With old generations of cement techniques (thumb and finger insertion), only 20 % of cement was in direct contact with the bone, while with second generation (medullary canal plug) and third generation (plug, pulsatile lavage, and pressure device) an estimated 40–60 % of direct contact can be expected (Fig. 3). Cemented femoral components are well tolerated by the skeleton over a long period of use, and fibrous tissue is sparsely formed at the femoral cement-bone interface of those well fixed and clinically successful prostheses. The cement-mantle can be well supported by extensive medullary bone remodeling and the formation of a dense shell of new bone that resembles a new cortex, is attached to the outer cortex by new trabecular struts [13].

In the composite-beam concept, the stem needs to be rigidly bound to the cement since subsidence or impairment of the stem-cement interface may result in damage to the cement, with the generation of PMMA and/or metal debris, and ultimately failure of the implant. These implants are not intended to subside at the early stages, and in order to optimise stability, roughening or cement pre-coating of the surface has been shown to increase cement-stem bonding. Implants with a strong cement stem bond are more sensitive to the presence of incomplete and thin cement mantles with a

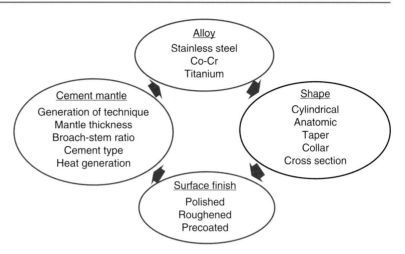

Fig. 4 Implant related parameters affecting the long-term survival of cemented THA

poor cement-bone interface than are polished stems. Discussion about the behaviour of the cement-stem interface was initiated by Harris who observed that cement failure begins at the stem-cement interface [16]. In his opinion the cement-stem interface can be made stronger by fixing the cement to the stem. Rough stems need a thick, continuous cement mantle of good quality with a strong cement-bone interface and should be made of wear resistant materials, whereas polished stems may be more tolerant to sub-optimal cementing and manufactured from less wear-resistant materials. It has been recommended that a cement mantle which is subjected to high stresses should be between 2 and 5 mm thick, especially in the proximal-medial part of the implant and around the tip of the distal stem [17]. Several features of the shape of the stem influence the in vivo behaviour of femoral components, including the overall shape (straight or anatomical), the cross-section (oval or square), the presence of a collar, the shape of the tip of the stem, the length of the stem and whether the edges are rounded to a greater or lesser degree [14, 15]. A stem relying on the composite-beam principle can be either straight or anatomical. Composite beams can be achieved with the interposition of a thick or a thin layer of cement, depending on whether the implant is undersized compared with the broach or not. A canal-filling stem (stems related to the "French paradox" principle) is cemented line-to-line with the size of the last broach used and stem cortex contact points as well as areas of thin cement supported by cortical bone help to stabilise the implant.

The Test of Time

Cemented surgical techniques and the design of implants have evolved dramatically. Some of these changes have resulted in improved survival rates (good regimes) while others have not (bad regimes) and registry data have shown that not all cemented cups and stems are the same [18]. It should be understood that satisfactory cemented designs are at least 15–20 years ahead of cementless designs, lessons have been learnt, and reliable long-term data exists. Cement has been implicated as a major cause of failure responsible for large lytic and foreign body reactions around both acetabular and femoral implants [19]. Later it was understood that these reactions were the result of a biological response to wear debris.

Cemented Cups

We have learned that cemented cups require exposure to cancellous bone, the bone bed must be clean and dry and adequate bony coverage of the cup is necessary. Wear and septic loosening appear late after the tenth post-operative year and survival rates are inferior in younger patients. We are still not able to fully control radiolucent lines at the bone cement interface and cemented cups still produce inconsistent results [20]. Cemented cups have shown a 97 % survival rate at 10 years and 85 % at 20 years [21, 22]. A survival rate of 98 % at 10 years and 90 % at 16 years (based mainly on the Charnley and Exeter cup) has been reported in the 2007 annual report of the Swedish Registry. However, survival rates of 78 % at 10 years and 68 % at 20 years were reported in younger patients [23–25].

Cemented Stems

It has been reported (long-term studies and registry data) that improved cementing techniques have resulted in improved clinical outcomes [26, 27]. However, even a small change in a satisfactory design can have a substantial effect on long-term outcome. Young age does not affect femoral long-term survival (Swedish, Norwegian and Danish Registries, 2007 annual reports). Third generation cementing techniques are affected by stem pre-coating problems. Survival rates vary, at a high level, but satisfactory designs tend to produce a constant 1–1.5 % aseptic loosening rate of the femoral stem at 15 years. Good loaded-taper recipes are: The Charnley stem with survival rates of over 90 % at 10 years with losses of 10 % per decade and a final 77–81 % at 20–30 years [25, 28, 29], and the Exeter stem with an exceptional survival rate of 93.5 % at 33 years [30, 31]. Good composite-beam recipes are: the Lubinus SP II stem [32–34] and the original Muller straight stem with a 94 % survival rate at 15 years [35, 36]. The French paradox regime (by far the most inexperienced user-friendly technique) including different polished rectangular canal filling stems cemented line-to-line, has produced excellent long-term results [37–40]. Although in vivo both concepts of stem fixation have proved to be effective, they cannot work together. It is important to understand on which principle a particular stem relies.

Bone-Implant Interface

Despite unsatisfactory early attempts at cementless fixation, in the early 1980s. it became evident that lamellar bone can be attached to specific implant surfaces without intervening fibrous tissue, a phenomenon called "osteo-integration" [41]. Since osteo-integration was considered to be a more biological mode of implant fixation, numerous biological, biomechanical and human retrieval studies were performed in order to throw light on this biological process. We now know that this is a fracture healing-like process which occurs approximately 4–12 weeks after implantation and may continue for up to 3 years [42, 43]. During the stages of this "interface healing" process cartilaginous, fibrous and osseous tissue are formed (primary stable membrane, 4–6 weeks) and at the end, the surface of the prosthesis is covered, to a varying degree, by bone (stable interface, 4 months). The initial stages of this process are direct contact and micro-motion sensitive and early stability (press-fit technique) of the interface is mandatory [44, 45]. Several factors affect the osseo-integration of implants, with their relative importance being unknown (Fig. 5). Ingrowth occurs when bone grows inside a porous surface, a phenomenon which depends on the surface characteristics of the implant. Surfaces for ingrowth include sintered beads, fibre mesh, and porous metals (Fig. 6). Sintered beads are microspheres of either cobalt chromium or titanium alloy attached by the use of high temperatures (excellent bond strength, high resistance to abrasion) [46]. Fibre mesh coatings are titanium metal pads attached by diffusion bonding [46]. Porous metals (a recent development) have a uniform three dimensional network, with high interconnectivity of the voids and high porosity (75–85 %) compared with that of sintered beads and fibre metal coatings (30–50 %) [47]. Ingrowth requires a pore size between 50 and 400 mm, and the percentage of voids within the coating should be between 30 and 40 % to maintain mechanical strength [48].

Ongrowth occurs when bone grows onto a roughened surface. Ongrowth surfaces are created by grit blasting or plasma spraying (Fig. 6). Grit blasting creates a textured surface by bombarding the implant with small abrasive particles. The surface roughness ranges from 3 to 5 mm [43, 49]. Plasma spraying involves mixing metal powders with an inert gas that is pressurized and ionized, forming a high-energy

Fig. 5 Implant-related parameters affecting the long-term survival of cementless THA

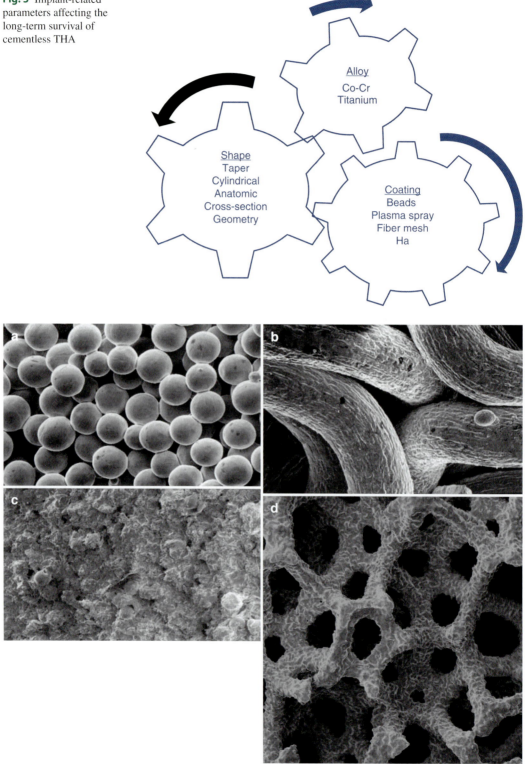

Fig. 6 (**a**) Sintered beads coating. (**b**) Fiber mesh coating. (**c**) Plasma spray coating. (**d**) Porous metal surface

flame. The molten material is sprayed onto the implant, creating a textured surface (weaker mechanical bond, abrasion and wear). There is less interconnecting porosity than with the ingrowth surfaces; however, 90 % of implant fatigue strength is retained, whereas only 50 % is retained after diffusion bonding and sintering [50]. Hydroxyapatite is a calcium phosphate compound that is plasma sprayed directly on the implant alone or over a porous coating. It is osteoconductive and enhances the growth of mineralized bone onto the implant [51, 52]. HA bone interface is more tolerant to interface gaps and micromotion. Interface strength, interface degradation and HA particle third-body wear are of concern [53, 54]. The good "regime" for HA coated implants is titanium alloy substrate, plasma spray technique, high crystallinity HA of 50–75 μm thickness, which does not compromise its strength or biological behaviour [54, 55].

It is generally accepted that fixation surfaces need to be circumferential and continuous. Metaphyseal osseo-integration and proximal stress transfer are enhanced and coating provides a seal which stops wear particle migration preventing interface osteolysis [56, 57]. Cobalt-chromium-molybdenum alloys and titanium-aluminum-vanadium alloys are most commonly used for cementless femoral stem designs. The modulus of elasticity of titanium alloys is closer to that of bone than is that of cobalt-chromium alloys. Theoretically, this should produce less thigh pain and stress-shielding [58]. Thigh pain, however, is believed to be a result of not only the stiffness of the metal, but also the stem geometry and recent long-term clinical data have shown that proximal stress shielding phenomena have been overestimated from the clinical point of view [59, 60]. In a modern cementless implant direct bone formation can be seen on 70–80 % of porous surfaces, fibrous tissue (with well-organized dense collagen network) on 20 % of porous surfaces and amorphous fibrous tissue on smooth surfaces. Improved direct bone formation is seen in HA coated prostheses. Proximal femoral morphology and bone quality also seems to affect fixation [61]. Early cementless stems were classified as straight or curved. Current stems are referred to as proximally porous-coated tapered or fully-coated cylindrical. While these simplifications are acceptable in general terms, they miss important design characteristics and make comparisons misleading. A comprehensive classification system is needed, with that proposed by Khanuja being useful for comparisons, although not complete [62].

The Test of Time

Cementless surgical techniques and the design of implants have also evolved dramatically. Some of these changes have also resulted in improved survival rates (good regimes) while others have not (bad regimes) and mid-term and long-term clinical and registry data have also shown that not all cementless cups and stems are the same. No data exist to support the idea that the use of super alloys and improved surfaces, as a single factor, affect clinical results at 15 years. Despite improvements in manufacturing, structural failures of implants still appear [63]. The long-term results of the first generation of cementless cups are heavily affected by problems of the locking mechanism, "back side" wear and osteolysis. Cups made of porous materials, approaching the 10-year time interval, present promising clinical data [64, 65]. Additionally, high failure rates were observed with the use of HA coated hemispherical cups [66]. There is also evidence that femoral stem geometry is more important than alloy and surface characteristics [59, 67–69].

There are several good "regimes" which combine different alloy, geometry and surface finish principles [62]. Numerous reports of the CLS Spotorno femoral stem, which is a grit blasted single wedge for tapered proximal fixation, show a 98.8 % survival rate at 15–20 years [70]. Taper-Lock and Tri-Lock, two versions (plasma spray and porous coated) of a single wedge for proximal tapered fixation, showed a 99 % survival rate at 22 years [71]. Two versions of the Omnifit stem, a double wedge for metaphyseal filling and proximal HA fixation, showed a 99 % survival rate at 17–24 years [66, 69, 72]. Another similar design, the Corail HA coated stem, showed a

97 % survival rate at 20 years [73]. In the same category, the HA coated Furlong stem showed 97–99 % survival at 15–20 years [74]. The Mallory tapered round stem, for tapered proximal fixation, showed a 95.5 % survival rate at 20 years [75]. The small Wagner stem, a tapered spline-cone for distal fixation, showed a 95–98 % survival rate at 15 years [76]. The Zweymuller grit blasted tapered rectangular stem, for tapered distal fixation, showed a 96–98 % survival rate at 20 years [77]. The Anatomic cylindrical fully coated stem for distal fixation showed a 92 % survival rate at 22 years [78, 79]. Generally, all the above designs and several modern 3° taper stems (with follow up observation just above 15 years) present an average 1.5 % revision rate for aseptic loosening at 15 years.

Evidence-Based Data

In a systematic review and meta-analysis of cemented v/s cementless cups it was found that using contemporary techniques, both cemented and uncemented sockets can yield good long-term results, but the overall/all cause re-operation risk is lower for cemented fixation. It is suggested until and unless crosslinked polyethylene (PE) liners or alternative bearings can prove to yield a superior outcome in the future, the cemented PE cup remains the gold standard, for all age groups, and by which every acetabular component should be compared [4, 80].

There are two systematic reviews comparing cemented and cementless femoral stems. In the first one no difference was found [3]. In the second, cemented stems showed superior clinical and functional results in the short-term but cemented stems showed less clear superiority in the long-term and radiological results did not correlate with the clinical outcome [81]. In a RCT (Level I) study with a 20 years follow-up cemented THA showed lower survival rates compared to cementless; the cementless tapered stem was associated with a survival rate of 99% [82]. Age younger than 65 years and male gender were predictors of revision surgery [82]. Finally, in a recent report from the Swedish Register, it was found that the survival of uncemented THA is inferior to that of cemented, mainly related to poorer performance of uncemented cups. Uncemented stems perform better than cemented stems but unrecognized intra-operative femoral fractures may be an important reason for early failure of uncemented stems [83].

Conclusions

Long term survival of THA is multi-factorial. The patient, diagnosis and surgeon factors are perhaps more important than the implant per se. There are several good and bad regimes for both cemented and cementless arthroplasty. It seems that a 1.5 % revision rate (for both cemented and cementless stem fixation) for aseptic loosening at 15 years follow-up is a target for future comparisons. Financial investment in the development of new materials and designs has not been translated in improved survival rates at 15 years followup. The weak link of contemporary THA remains the bearing surfaces.

References

1. Learmonth ID, Young C, Rorabeck C (2007) The operation of the century: total hip replacement. Lancet 370(0597):1508–1519
2. Laupacis A, Bourne R, Rorabeck C, Feeny D, Wong C, Tugwell P, Leslie K, Bullas R (1993) The effect of elective total hip replacement on health-related quality of life. J Bone Joint Surg 75-A:1619–1626
3. Morshed S, Bozic KJ, Ries MD, Maclau H, Colford JM Jr (2007) Comparison of cemented and uncemented fixation total hip replacement: a metaanalysis. Acta Orthop Scand 78(3):315–326
4. Pakvis D, van Hellemondt G, de Visser E, Jacobs W, Spruit M (2011) Is there evidence for a superior method of socket fixation in hip arthroplasty? A systematic review. Int Orthop 35:1109–1118
5. Muirhead-Allwood SK (1998) Lessons of a hip failure. BMJ 316(7132):644
6. Bauer TW, Schils J (1999) The pathology of total joint arthroplasty. I. Mechanisms of implant fixation. Skeletal Radiol 28:423–432
7. Charnley J (1970) The reaction of bone to self-curing acrylic cement. A long-term histological study in man. J Bone Joint Surg 52-B:340–353
8. Lindwer J, Van Den Hooff A (1975) The influence of acrylic cement on the femur of the dog: a histological study. Acta Orthop Scand 46:657–671

9. Petty W (1978) The effect of methylmethacrylate on bacterial phagocytosis and killing by human polymorphonuclear leukocytes. J Bone Joint Surg 60-A: 752–757
10. Rhinelander FW, Nelson CL, Stewart RD, Stewart CL (1979) Experimental reaming of the proximal femur and acrylic cement implantation: vascular and histologic effects. Clin Orthop Relat Res 141:74–89
11. Slooff TJ (1971) The influence of acrylic cement. Acta Orthop Scand 42:465–481
12. Willert HG, Ludwing J, Semlitsch M (1974) Reaction of bone to polymethacrylate after hip arthroplasty: a long term gross, light microscopic and scanning electron microscopic study. J Bone Joint Surg 56-A:1368–1382
13. Jasty M, Maloney WJ, Bragdon CR, Haire T, Harris WH (1990) Histomorphological studies of the long term skeletal responses to well fixed cemented femoral components. J Bone Joint Surg 72-A:1220–1229
14. Scheerlinck T, Casteleyn PP (2006) The design features of cemented femoral hip implants. J Bone Joint Surg 88-B:1409–1418
15. Shah N, Porter M (2005) Evolution of cemented stems. Orthopedics 28(8S):819–825
16. Harris WH (1998) Long-term results of cemented femoral stems with roughened precoated surfaces. Clin Orthop Relat Res 355:137–143
17. Ramaniraka NA, Rakotomanana LR, Leyvraz PF (2000) The fixation of the cemented femoral component: effects of stem stiffness, cement thickness and roughness of the cement-bone interface. J Bone Joint Surg 82-B:297–303
18. Espehaug B, Furnes O, Engesaeter LB, Havelin LI (2009) 18 years of results with cemented primary hip prostheses in the Norwegian Arthroplasty Register: concerns about some newer implants. Acta Orthop Scand 80:402–412
19. Jones LC, Hungerford MA (1990) Cement disease. Clinical Orthopaedics Relat Res 225:192–195
20. Ritter MA, Thong AE (2004) The role of cemented sockets in 2004: is there one? J Arthroplasty 19(4S): 92–94
21. Garcia-Cimberelo E, Munuera L (1992) Late loosening of the acetabular cup after low friction arthroplasty. J Bone Joint Surg 74-A:1119–1129
22. Berry DJ, Harmsen WS, Cabanela ME, Morrey BF (2002) Twenty five year survivorship of two thousand consecutive primary Charnley total hip replacements: factors affecting survivorship of acetabular and femoral components. J Bone Joint Surg 84-A:171–177
23. Georgiades G, Babis GC, Hartofilakidis G (2009) Charnley low friction arthroplasty in young patients with osteoarthritis: outcomes at minimum of twenty-two years. J Bone Joint Surg 91-A:2846–2851
24. Hartofilakidis G, Karachalios T, Zacharakis N (1997) Charnley low friction arthroplasty in young patients with osteoarthritis. A 12 to 24 year clinical and radiographic follow up study of 84 cases. Clin Orthop Relat Res 341:51–54
25. Hartofilakidis G, Karachalios T, Karachalios G (2005) The 20 year outcome of the Charnley arthroplasty in younger and older patients. Cin Orthop Relat Res 434: 177–182
26. Herberts P, Malchau H (2000) Long term registration has improved the quality of hip replacement: a review of the Swedish THR Register comparing 160,000 cases. Acta Orthop Scand 71:111–121
27. Halley DK, Glassman AH (2003) Twenty to twenty six year radiographic review in patients 50 years of age or younger with cemented Charnley low friction arthroplasty. J Arthroplasty 18(7S):79–85
28. Wroblewski BM, Siney PD, Fleming PA (2002) Charnley low-frictional torque arthroplasty in patients under the age of 51 years: follow-up to 33 years. J Bone Joint Surg 84-B:540–543
29. Wroblewski BM, Fleming PA, Siney PD (1999) Charnley low-frictional torque arthroplasty of the hip: 20-to-30 years results. J Bone Joint Surg 81-B: 427–430
30. Williams HD, Browne G, Gie GA (2002) The Exeter universal cemented femoral component at 8 to 12 years: a study of the first 325 hips. J Bone Joint Surg 84-B:324–334
31. Ling RS, Charity J, Lee AJ, Whitehouse SL, Timperley AJ, Gie GA (2009) The long term results of the original Exeter polished cemented femoral component: a follow up report. J Arthroplasty 24:511–517
32. Savilahti S, Myllyneva I, Pajamaki KJ, Lindholm TS (1997) Survival of Lubinus straight (IP) and curved (SP) total hip prosthesis in 543 patients after 4–13 years. Arch Orthop Trauma Surg 116:10–13
33. Partio E, von Bonsdorff H, Wirta J, Avikainen V (1994) Survival of the Lubinus hip prosthesis: an eight- to 12-year follow-up evaluation of 444 cases. Clin Orthop Relat Res 303:140–146
34. Soballe K, Christensen F, Luxhoj T (1987) Total hip replacement ad modum Lubinus: five- to seven-year follow-up. Arch Orthop Trauma Surg 106:108–112
35. Riede U, Luem M, Ilchmann T, Eucker M, Ochsner PE (2007) The ME Muller straight stem prosthesis: 15 year follow-up. Survivorship and clinical results. Arch Orthop Trauma Surg 127:587–592
36. Müller ME (1992) Lessons of 30 years of total hip arthroplasty. Clin Orthop Relat Res 274:12–21
37. Langlais F, Kerboull M, Sedel L, Ling RSM (2003) The 'French paradox'. J Bone Joint Surg 85-B:17–20
38. Langlais F, Howell JR, Lee AJC, Ling RSM (2002) The "French paradox". Hip Int 12:166–168
39. Kerboull L, Hamadouche M, Courpied JP, Kerboull M (2004) Long-term results of Charnley-Kerboul hip arthroplasty in patients younger than 50 years. Clin Orthop Relat Res 418:112–118
40. Hamadouche M, Boutin P, Daussange J, Bolander ME, Sedel L (2002) Alumina -on- alumina total hip arthroplasty: a minimum 18.5-year follow-up study. J Bone Joint Surg 84-A:69–77
41. Albrektsson T, Branemark PI, Hanssson HA, Lindstrom J (1981) Osseointegrated titanium implants. Requirements for ensuring a long lasting, direct bone to implant anchorage in man. Acta Orthop Scand 52: 155–170

42. Galante J, Rostoker W, Lueck R, Ray RD (1971) Sintered fiber metal composites as a basis for attachment of implants to bone. J Bone Joint Surg 53-A: 101–114
43. Zweymuller KA, Lintner FK, Semitsch MF (1988) Biologic fixation of a press fit titanium hip joint endoprosthesis. Clin Orthop Relat Res 235:195–206
44. Engh CA, O'Connor D, Jasty M, McGovern TF, Bobyn JD, Harris WH (1992) Quantification of implant micromotion, strain shielding, and bone resorption with porous coated anatomic medullary locking femoral prostheses. Clin Orthop Relat Res 285:13–29
45. Jasty M, Bragdon C, Burke D, O'Connor D, Lowenstein J, Harris WH (1997) In vivo skeletal responses to porous surfaced implants subjected to small induced motions. J Bone Joint Surg 79-A:707–714
46. Bourne RB, Rorabeck CH, Burkart BC, Kirk PG (1994) Ingrowth surfaces. Plasma spray coating to titanium alloy hip replacements. Clin Orthop Relat Res 298:37–46
47. Bobyn JD, Stackpool GJ, Hacking SA, Tanzer M, Krygier JJ (1999) Characteristics of bone ingrowth and interface mechanics of a new porous tantalum biomaterial. J Bone Joint Surg 81-B:907–914
48. Haddad RJ Jr, Cook SD, Thomas KA (1987) Biological fixation of porous-coated implants. J Bone Joint Surg 69-A:1459–1466
49. Hacking SA, Bobyn JD, Tanzer M, Krygier JJ (1999) The osseous response to corundum blasted implant surfaces in a canine hip model. Clin Orthop Relat Res 364:240–253
50. Callaghan JJ (1999) The clinical results and basic science of total hip arthroplasty with porous-coated prostheses. J Bone Joint Surg 75-A:299–310
51. Søballe K, Gotfredsen K, Brockstedt-Rasmussen H, Nielsen PT, Rechnagel K (1991) Histologic analysis of a retrieved hydroxyapatite-coated femoral prosthesis. Clin Orthop Relat Res 272:255–258
52. Nakashima Y, Hayashi K, Inadome T, Uenoyama K, Hara T, Kanemaru T, Sugioka Y, Noda I (1997) Hydroxyapatite-coating on titanium arc sprayed titanium implants. J Biomed Mater Res 35:287–298
53. Bloebaum RD, Zou L, Bachus KN, Shea KG, Hofmann AA, Dunn HK (1997) Analysis of particles in acetabular components from patients with osteolysis. Clin Orthop Relat Res 338:109–118
54. Søballe K, Overgaard S (1996) The current status of hydroxyapatite coating of prostheses. J Bone Joint Surg 78-B:689–691
55. Søballe K, Hansen ES, Brockstedt-Rasmussen H, Bunger C (1993) Hydroxyapatite coating converts fibrous tissue to bone around loaded implants. J Bone Joint Surg 75-B:270–278
56. Emerson RH Jr, Sanders SB, Head WC, Higgins L (1999) Effect of circumferential plasma-spray porous coating on the rate of femoral osteolysis after total hip arthroplasty. J Bone Joint Surg 81-A:1291–1298
57. Bobyn JD, Jacobs JJ, Tanzer M, Urban RM, Aribindi R, Sumner DR, Turner TM, Brooks CE (1995) The susceptibility of smooth implant surfaces to periimplant fibrosis and migration of polyethylene wear debris. Clin Orthop Relat Res 311:21–39
58. Healy WL, Tilzey JF, Iorio R, Specht LM, Sharma S (2009) Prospective, randomized comparison of cobalt-chrome and titanium Trilock femoral stems. J Arthroplasty 24:831–836
59. Lavernia C, D'Apuzzo M, Hernandez V, Lee D (2004) Thigh pain in primary total hiparthroplasty: the effects of elastic moduli. J Arthroplasty 19(7S2):10–16
60. Karachalios T, Tsatsaronis C, Efraimis G, Papadelis P, Lyritis G, Diakomopoulos G (2004) The long-term clinical relevance of calcar atrophy caused by stress shielding in total hip arthroplasty: a 10-year, prospective, randomized study. J Arthroplasty 19:469–475
61. Dorr LD, Faugere MC, Mackel AM, Gruen TA, Bognar B, Malluche HH (1993) Structural and cellular assessment of bone quality of proximal femur. Bone 14(3):231–242
62. Khanuja HS, Vakil JJ, Goddard MS, Mont MA (2011) Cementless femoral fixation in total hip arthroplasty. J Bone Joint Surg 93-A:500–509
63. Magnissalis EA, Zinelis S, Karachalios T, Hartofilakidis G (2003) Failure analysis of two Ti-alloy total hip arthroplasty femoral stems fractured in vivo. J Biomed Mater Res 15:299–305
64. Macheras GA, Papagelopoulos PJ, Kateros K, Kostakos AT, Baltas D, Karachalios T (2006) Radiological evaluation of the metal bone interface of a porous tantalum monoblock acetabular component. J Bone Joint Surg 88-B:304–309
65. Malizos KN, Bargiotas K, Papatheodorou L, Hantes M, Karachalios T (2008) Survivorship of monoblock trabecular metal cups in primary THA: midterm results. Clin Orthop Relat Res 466:159–166
66. Capello WN, D'Antonio JA, Jaffe WL, Geesink RG, Manley MT, Feinberg JR (2006) Hydroxyapatite-coated femoral components: 15-year minimum followup. Clin Orthop Relat Res 453:75–80
67. Kim YH (2004) Titanium and cobalt-chrome cementless femoral stems of identical shape produce equal results. Clin Orthop Relat Res 427:148–156
68. Camazzola D, Hammond T, Gandhi R, Davey JR (2009) A randomized trial of hydroxyapatite-coated femoral stems in total hip arthroplasty: a 13-year follow-up. J Arthroplasty 24:33–37
69. Incavo SJ, Beynnon BD, Coughlin KM (2008) Total hip arthroplasty with the Secur-Fit and Secur-Fit Plus femoral stem design a brief follow-up report at 5 to 10 years. J Arthroplasty 23:670–676
70. Muller LA, Wenger N, Schramm M, Hohmann D, Forst R, Carl HD (2009) Seventeen year survival of the cementless CLS Spotorno stem. Arch Orthop Trauma Surg 130:269–275
71. McLaughlin JR, Lee KR (2008) Total hip arthroplasty with an uncemented tapered femoral component. J Bone Joint Surg 90-A:1290–1296
72. Epinette JA, Manley MT (2008) Uncemented stems in hip replacement—hydroxyapatite or plain porous: does it matter? Based on a prospective study of HA

Omnifit stems at 15-years minimum followup. Hip Int 18:69–74
73. Vidalain JP (2011) Twenty-year results of the cementless Corail stem. Int Orthop 35:189–194
74. Valera Pertegàs M, Vergara-Valladolid P, Crusi-Sererols X, Sancho-Navarro R (2010) Fully hydroxyapatite-coated total hip replacement: ten-year results. Hip Int 20(7S):79–85
75. Lombardi AV Jr, Berend KR, Mallory TH, Skeels MD, Adams JB (2009) Survivorship of 2000 tapered titanium porous plasma-sprayed femoral components. Clin Orthop Relat Res 467:146–154
76. Schuh A, Schraml A, Hohenberger G (2009) Long-term results of the Wagner cone prosthesis. Int Orthop 33:53–58
77. Suckel A, Geiger F, Kinzl L, Wulker N, Garbrecht M (2009) Long-term results for the uncemented Zweymuller/Alloclassic hip endoprosthesis. A 15-year minimum followup of 320 hip operations. J Arthroplasty 24:846–853
78. Engh CA Jr, Claus AM, Hopper RH Jr, Engh CA (2001) Long-term results using the anatomic medullary locking hip prosthesis. Clin Orthop Relat Res 393:137–146
79. Belmont PJ Jr, Powers CC, Beykirch SE, Hopper RH Jr, Engh CA Jr, Engh CA (2008) Results of the anatomic medullary locking total hip arthroplasty at a minimum of twenty years. A concise follow-up of previous reports. J Bone Joint Surg 90-A:1524–1530
80. Clement ND, Biant LC, Breusch SJ (2012) Total hip arthroplasty: to cement or not to cement the acetabular socket? A critical review of the literature. Arch Orthop Trauma Surg 132:411–427
81. Ni GX, Lu WW, Chiu KY, Fong DY (2005) Cemented or uncemented femoral component in primary total hip replacement? A review from a clinical and radiological perspective. J Orthop Surg 13:96–105
82. Corten K, Bourne RB, Charron KD, Au K, Rorabeck CH (2011) Comparison of total hip arthroplasty performed with and without cement: a randomized trial. A concise follow-up, at twenty years, of previous reports. J Bone Joint Surg 93-A:1335–1342
83. Hailer NP, Garellick G, Kärrholm J (2010) Uncemented and cemented primary total hip arthroplasty in the Swedish Hip Arthroplasty Register. Acta Orthop Scand 81:34–41

Risk Factors and Treatment of Dislocations of Total Hip Arthroplasty

Ullmark Gösta

Introduction

Dislocation after total hip arthroplasty (THA) is a difficult problem both for the patient, the treating surgeon and the health care system in general. The complication is associated with a considerable extra cost for the health care system [1]. Bozic et al. [2] found the most common causes of revision in the United States in 2005 and 2006 to be instability/dislocation (22.5 %). The true prevalence of post-operative dislocation varies because of different surgical, patient, and implant factors. Most reports from high-volume academic centres suggest a dislocation rate of 0.3–3 % of patients treated with primary THA for osteoarthritis (OA) [3]. THA dislocation compromises highly the quality of life in affected patients. Kotwal et al. [4] has studied the complication using the Oxford Hip Score and the EuroQol-5 Dimension (EQ-5D) questionnaire. A control group of patients who had not dislocated had a mean Oxford Hip Score of 17.4 (12–32). The score was 26.7 (15–47) after one episode of dislocation at a mean follow-up of 4.5 years (1–20). It was 27.2 (12–45) after recurrent dislocation, 34.5 (12–54) after successful revision surgery and 42 (29–55) after failed revision surgery.

This article outlines the aetiology of hip dislocation and provides the surgeon with an algorithm for the management of this common complication.

Aetiology

Incidence

A meta-analysis by Masonis and Bourne [5] involving 13,203 procedures found a dislocation rate of 3.23 % after a posterior approach compared with 2.18 % after an anterolateral, 1.27 % after a trans trochanteric, and 0.55 % after a direct lateral approach. Bigger head size and posterior soft tissue repair in case of a posterior approach might diminish those differences.

Most dislocations occur early after surgery. Bourne and Mehin [3] found that 60 % of dislocations occur within the first 5 weeks. No further dislocation occurred in about 2/3 of these patients. In the national Swedish hip register report 2010 [6], 32 % of revisions performed because of dislocations were done during the first year.

Patient Risk Factors

Important patient risk factors include female gender, prior surgery, neuromuscular disorders, dementia, inability to comply with activity restrictions and alcohol abuse. The risk for dislocation has been studied for patients with neuromuscular and cognitive disorders like cerebral palsy,

U. Gösta
Department of Orthopedics,
Center for Research and Development,
Gävle Hospital, Gävle 80187, Sweden

Ortopedmottagningen, Länssjukhuset,
Gävle 80187, Sweden
e-mail: gosta.ullmark@lg.se

dementia, muscular dystrophy, psychosis, and alcoholism [7]. Those disorders were present in 13 % of dislocating patients compared to 3 % (P=0.003) for non-dislocating. Woo and Morrey [8] found that compared to degenerative arthritis the dislocation rate was doubled for avascular necrosis, 3 times for congenital dislocation, fourfold for fracture, fivefold for non-union, malunion or a failed hip arthroplasty and 11 times increased for prosthetic instability. The national Swedish hip register [6] has reported an increasing risk for dislocation leading to revision surgery after repeated hip surgery. Dislocation resulting in revision was 8.7 % after primary THA, 14.7 % after first revision, 18.9 % after second and 29.1 % after more than two revisions. Wetters at al. [9] found 9.8 % to dislocate after revision THA. Risk factors were abductor deficiencies and a history of previous dislocation.

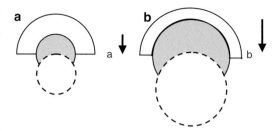

Fig. 1 (**a, b**) A smaller femoral head may dislocate after only a short distance (*a*) and is therefore theoretically less stable. A larger head must travel a greater distance (*b*) before dislocating and is therefore more stable

Surgical Risk Factors

Surgical factors leading to dislocation include component malpositioning, failure to restore leg length or offset, preserving the abductor mechanism and capsule, or using the posterior surgical approach.

Approach

In a meta-analysis involving 13,203 procedures Masonis and Bourne [5] found 3.23 % dislocation for the posterior approach (3.95 % without posterior repair and 2.03 % with posterior repair) and 2.18 % for the anterolateral approach.

Soft Tissue

Five independent studies of the posterior, posterolateral, and direct lateral approaches have reported equally good dislocation rates of less than 1 % when the approach includes a definitive posterior soft-tissue repair [10–14]. Soft tissue repair may reduce or together with a large head even eliminate the disadvantage of the posterior approach with respect to instability.

Soft-tissue tension is affected by femoral offset. Fackler and Poss [13] found a dislocating group of patients to have a notable loss of offset (average, 5.2 mm) compared to patients with stable hips (average, 0.02 mm).

Implant Factors

Several implant factors play an important role in dislocation. Factors that decrease the head-to-neck ratio will increase the risk for dislocation.

There are theoretical advantages in using larger head sizes with regard to stability. The improved head-to-neck ratio reduces component impingement and increases range of motion (ROM). The use of a skirted head component should be avoided, in order not to increase the tendency for impingement. Finally, larger heads are seated deeper within the acetabular liner, requiring greater translation before dislocation ("jump distance") (Fig. 1a, b). Nevelos et al. [15] has found the highest jump distance for all positions and activities to occur with the dual-mobility bearing. The use of heads >32 mm. has historically been limited by concerns about polyethylene wear. This shortcoming may be eliminated by ceramic femoral heads on cross-linked polyethylene or by ceramic head on ceramic liner.

Component Positioning

Harris stated that: "Cup anteversion should be 20°±5°, as measured about the axis of the cup (not the longitudinal axis of the body). To ensure proper positioning, close attention also must be paid to the orientation of the pelvis, especially when using a posterior approach. The pelvis of a patient in the decubitus position may be significantly adducted and anteverted relative to the table" [16]. Positioning of both the femoral and acetabular components is an important factor in stability. Excessive abduction of the acetabular component may result in lateral dislocation. Excessive retroversion or anteversion may result in posterior or anterior dislocation, respectively. For most cases, cup anteversion of 15°±10° and abduction of 40°±10° is considered to be the "safe zone" of lowest dislocation risk. Outside this safe range, dislocation has been shown to increased fourfold (6.1 % versus 1.5 %; P<0.05) [17]. Proper component positioning is a hazardous task and post-operative radiographs may be a surprising experience. In a study by Wera et al. [18] 75 cases suffering from repeat dislocation had a cup abduction angle varying from of 20–90° and an anteversion of 50° to −10°. Even more surprising is that also the angles after revision for dislocation varied substantially (abduction: 25–60°, anteversion: 0–35°). In a study by Biedermann et al. [19] using Einzel-Bild- Röntgen-Analysis to compare cup angles in a group of patients that dislocated after primary THA with a control group. In the control group the mean value of abduction was 44° and anteversion 15°. Patients with anterior dislocation showed significant differences in the mean angle of abduction (48°) and anteversion (17°), as did patients with posterior dislocation (abduction 42°, anteversion 11°). However two other studies were not able to detect a significant difference in cup angles between a dislocating group and a control group [20, 21]. Those results may simply be a reflection of the complex interplay of the other factors involved in dislocation. A safe stem rotation has been considered to be 20° anteversion±10° [18].

Impingement is another cause for dislocation. When the prosthetic femoral neck impinges against an osteophyte, the liner, cement, or heterotopic ossification a risk for dislocation is present. Components with higher head-to-neck ratio impinge less readily.

Liner Profile

A liner may cover more or less than 180° of the prosthetic head. A high degree of coverage means theoretically more range of movement before the head dislocates. At the same time the tendency for impingement of the prosthetic collar against the rim of the liner increases. The latter phenomenon counteracts hip stability. There are also liners with a posteriorly oriented elevated rim. Those liners have a greater contact portion of the femoral head posteriorly than do standard neutral liners. A study comparing neutral liners with 10° elevated-rim liners [22] reported respective probabilities of dislocation of 3.85 and 2.19 % (P=0.001). A disadvantage of the design, however, is increased impingement against the rim in extension and external rotation. Liner rim impingement may lead to liner wear, osteolysis, and loosening.

Management

The cause for instability may be either:
1. locally caused with explanatory radiographic findings,
2. locally caused without explanatory radiographic findings, or
3. non-locally caused, i.e. non-compliant patient with neuromuscular or cognitive disorders. Combinations of those three may also exist.

Post-dislocation Patient Assessment

A dislocation shortly after THA surgery has less chance of recurrence compared to a later dislocation. Ali Khan et al. [23] reported that dislocations occurring before 5 weeks had a 39.3 % chance of recurrence compared with 58.3 % for later dislocations (P<0.05). Woo and Morrey [8] found that patients without recurrence dislocated at an average of 54 days after surgery, whereas patients with recurrent dislocation had their first episode at an average of 122 days (0.05<P<0.10).

In analysing the cause of dislocation the history should include details of the current episode and any previous episodes of instability. The physical examination should include both lower extremities, with particular attention paid to position and leg length, neurovascular integrity, ROM, gait, and strength (particularly of the abductor muscles). Imaging should begin with plain radiographs, including an anteroposterior (AP) view of the pelvis, an AP view of the hip and a lateral view of the hip. Computed tomography is also useful for assessing version when used with software to reduce metallic artefacts.

When no obvious circumstances for instability are visible on radiography, manipulation under fluoroscopy is valuable to map out the direction and position of instability.

Reduction

When closed reduction is attempted, fluoroscopy is helpful in achieving and confirming reduction. Proper muscular relaxation of the patient is also helpful. Documentation of the fluoroscopic result concerning position for instability (lift out) is valuable, should a later revision for dislocation become necessary. Post-reduction radiographs and a neurovascular examination are always indicated.

After successful reduction of a posterior dislocation, the patient should be reminded to avoid provocative positions (a combination of >90° flexion, adduction and internal rotation). For noncompliant patients an orthosis may be used for some weeks post-dislocation to prevent the provocative position. However it includes an inherent discomfort and a risk for skin complications.

Three to six percent of dislocations are not reducible by closed manoeuvres and require open reduction [8, 13, 24]. If open reduction is planned, preparedness for revision must be present.

Revision

The failure and complication rate after surgery for THA instability is known to be high. Wera et al. [18] found the incidence for repeated dislocation after surgery for dislocation to be 14.6 % at a mean of 12 months and 21 % at a mean of 60 months post-operatively. They found the failure frequency to be even higher for both the pre-operative diagnosis abductor insufficiency and for using a constrained acetabular component, especially for the locking ringtype. The same study verifies the known high rate of deep infections (10 %) after this type of surgery. The total complication rate was 24 % after 2 years.

Revision strategies for instability are typically directed to correcting the underlying aetiology. In analysing the cause for instability and planning revision surgery, it is important to even if one of the three reasons mentioned above are found, continue to analyse and roll out each of the other two. Even when such a procedure has been followed, the surgeon should pre-operatively analyse additional causes for hip instability and be prepared to attend also to those.

All revision for instability should, despite other surgical measures, also strive for an upsizing of the head and liner and a proper soft tissue tension regarding off-set and leg length. Soft tissue tension can be achieved by exchange of modular components, capsulorrhaphy or trochanter advancement [25]. Those procedures must be weighed against the possibility of leg lengthening or altering hip kinetics. The posterior capsule might be incomplete or missing at time of revision surgery. A posterior pseudo-capsule, with preserved attachment to the lateral acetabular rim could sometimes be shaped from intra-articular posterior scar tissue. This flap of the pseudo-capsule can be attached to the posterior aspect of the major trochanter. Alternatively a fascia lata flap with preserved attachment to the greater trochanter can be mobilised and attached to the lateral rim of the acetabulum.

If impingement exists, osteophytes or cement should be resected and components can be exchanged to improve head-to-neck ratio.

A worn cemented cup or liner should be exchanged. A flat design could be exchanged to one with an elevated posterior rim. If a well-fixed uncemented metal shell is seated with an improper angle or a worn liner, a minor angle correction could be achieved by cementing in a new liner to the metal shell if accurate sizing of the liner, careful preparation of the substrate of the liner and the shell, and good cement technique is used [26].

Component Positioning

When mal-position of the acetabular or femoral component is the cause of instability, the component should be revised to a proper position. The prognosis for revision of that cause is relatively good [27].

Dual Mobility Cups

There are several reports of good results using dual mobility cups [28–32] (Fig. 2a, b). The dual mobility cup has an elevated lateral rim and an outer jumbo head resulting in a high lift-off distance. The components have gained increasing popularity and are an alternative to a constrained cup. A disadvantage can be large articulating poly ethylene (PE) surfaces including one convex with potency for increased wear. The use of cross-linked PE may diminish this disadvantage.

Constrained Cups

The use of constrained components for the unstable THA may be a solution [33]. The constrained cup is an acetabular component that uses a mechanism to restrain the femoral head within the liner. A constrained design inhibits ROM and transmits significant forces to the bone-prosthesis interface, which may lead to loosening. When dislocations do occur with a constrained design, they can be difficult to manage. Surgery is required in most cases to re-seat a disengaged locking ring, replace a broken one, or address a displaced liner or cup. In a review article [34] the mean rate of dislocation following revision with a constrained liner with a mean follow-up of 51 months was found to be 10 %. The mean re-operation rate for reasons other than dislocation was 4 %. There is however a recent report of much worse results using constrained cups [35].

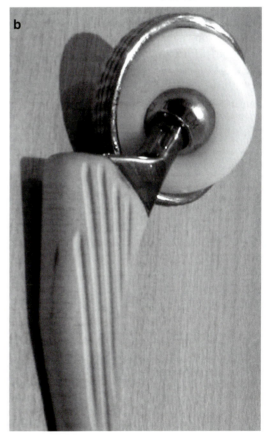

Fig. 2 (**a, b**) In a dual mobility socket, the femoral component head is pressed into the larger polyethylene head, by use of a screw clamp, before insertion in the patient. Properly coupled inside the polyethylene head, the smaller head is moving freely

Girdlestone Resection

The last resort for salvage is the Girdlestone resection arthroplasty. The remaining tissues form a scar, leaving the patient with a shortened limb and a significant limp.

Summary

Dislocation after THA is a difficult problem combined with a considerable extra cost for the health care system. It is one of the most common causes of re-operation. Revision surgery for dislocation is combined with a high incidence of both failure and deep infection.

Since prevention is the best approach, it is important for surgeons performing primary THA to have a deep knowledge of instability. An increased head neck ratio will diminish the risk. The posterior surgical approach has a higher risk for instability but a definitive posterior soft-tissue repair will however considerable reduce the risk. Since the individual patient risk factors vary by a factor 11 [8] it is important to before each primary THA to assess the individual risk.

In evaluating a recurrent dislocation, the problem may be structured in three causative fields, (1) locally caused with explanatory radiographic findings, (2) locally caused without explanatory radiographic findings, or (3) non-locally caused, i.e. no-compliant patient with neuromuscular or cognitive disorders or combinations of those three.

Revision strategies for instability are typically directed to correcting the underlying aetiology. In that respect a sufficient analysis of the causative factor or factors must be performed before surgery. All revisions for instability should despite other surgical measures, also strives for an upsizing of the head and liner and a proper soft tissue reconstruction and tension.

The use of a dual mobility cup may be a feasible alternative in revision THA for instability.

Algorithm

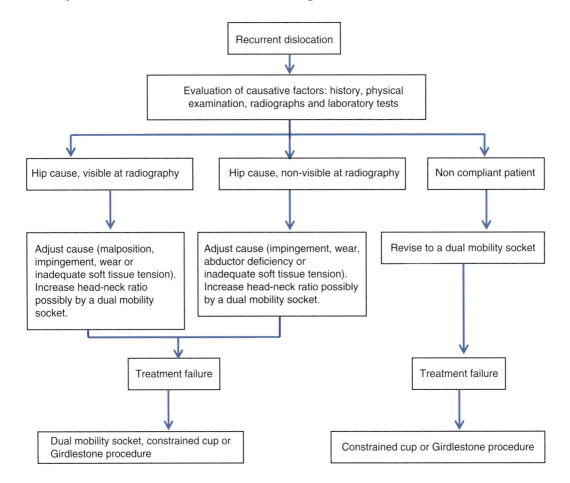

References

1. de Palma L, Procaccini R, Soccetti A, Marinelli M (2012) Hospital cost of treating early dislocation following hip arthroplasty. Hip Int 22(1):62–67. doi:10.5301/HIP.2012.9059
2. Bozic KJ, Kurtz SM, Lau E, Ong K, Vail TP, Berry DJ (2009) The epidemiology of revision total hip arthroplasty in the United States. J Bone Joint Surg Am 91(1):128–133
3. Bourne BB, Mehin R (2004) The dislocating hip: what to do, what to do. J Arthroplasty 19(4 Suppl 1):111–114
4. Kotwal RS, Ganapathi M, John A, Maheson M, Jones SA (2009) Outcome of treatment for dislocation after primary total hip replacement. J Bone Joint Surg Br 91(3):321–326
5. Masonis JL, Bourne RB (2002) Surgical approach, abductor function, and total hip arthroplasty dislocation. Clin Orthop Relat Res 405:46–53
6. Swedish Hip Arthroplasty Register Annual Report (2010). www.shpr.se
7. Woolston ST, Rahimtoola ZO (1999) Risk factors for dislocation during the first 3 months after primary total hip replacement. J Arthroplasty 14:662–668
8. Woo RYG, Morrey BF (1982) Dislocations after total hip arthroplasty. J Bone Joint Surg Am 64:1295–1306
9. Wetters NG, Murray TG, Moric M, Sporer SM, Paprosky WG, Della Valle CJ (2013) Risk factors for dislocation after revision total hip arthroplasty. Clin Orthop Relat Res 471:410–416
10. Pellicci PM, Bostrom M, Poss R (1998) Posterior approach to total hip replacement using enhanced posterior soft tissue repair. Clin Orthop 355:224–228
11. Goldstein WM, Gleason TF, Kopplin M, Branson JJ (2001) Prevalence of dislocation after total hip arthroplasty through a posterolateral approach with partial capsulotomy and capsulorrhaphy. J Bone Joint Surg Am 86:2–7
12. White RE Jr, Forness TJ, Allman JK, Junick DW (2001) Effect of posterior capsular repair on early dislocation in primary total hip replacement. Clin Orthop 393:163–167
13. Fackler CD, Poss R (1980) Dislocation in total hip arthroplasties. Clin Orthop 151:169–178
14. Ho KW, Whitwell GS, Young SK (2012) Reducing the rate of early primary hip dislocation by combining a change in surgical technique and an increase in femoral head diameter to 36 mm. Arch Orthop Trauma Surg 132:1031–1036
15. Nevelos J, Johnson A, Heffernan C, Macintyre J, Markel DC, Mont MA (2013) What factors affect posterior dislocation distance in THA? Clin Orthop Relat Res 471:519–526
16. Harris WH (1980) Advances in surgical technique for total hip replacement: without and with osteotomy of the greater trochanter. Clin Orthop 146:188–204
17. Soong M, Rubash HE, Macaulay W (2004) Dislocation after total hip arthroplasty. J Am Acad Orthop Surg 12(5):314–321
18. Wera GD, Ting NT, Moric M, Paprosky WG, Sporer SM, Della Valle CJ (2012) Classification and management of the unstable total hip arthroplasty. J Arthroplasty 27(5):710–715
19. Biedermann R, Tonin A, Krismer M, Rachbauer F, Eibl G, Stöckl B (2005) Reducing the risk of dislocation after total hip arthroplasty: the effect of orientation of the acetabular component. J Bone Joint Surg Br 87(6):762–769
20. Paterno SA, Lachiewicz PF, Kelley SS (1997) The influence of patient-related factors and the position of the acetabular component on the rate of dislocation after total hip replacement. J Bone Joint Surg Am 79:1202–1210
21. Pierchon F, Pasquier G, Cotten A, Fontaine C, Clarisse J, Duquennoy A (1994) Causes of dislocation of total hip arthroplasty: CT study of component alignment. J Bone Joint Surg Br 76:45–48
22. Cobb TK, Morrey BF, Ilstrup DM (1996) The elevated-rim acetabular liner in total hip arthroplasty: relationship to postoperative dislocation. J Bone Joint Surg Am 78:80–86
23. Ali Khan AMA, Brakenbury PH, Reynolds IS (1981) Dislocation following total hip replacement. J Bone Joint Surg Br 63:214–218
24. Joshi A, Lee CM, Markovic L, Vlatis G, Murphy JC (1998) Prognosis of dislocation after total hip arthroplasty. J Arthroplasty 13:17–21
25. Ekelund A (1993) Trochanteric osteotomy for recurrent of total hip arthroplasty. J Arthroplasty 8:629
26. Jiranek WA (2003) Acetabular liner fixation by cement. Clin Orthop Relat Res 417:217–223
27. Morrey BF (1992) Instability after total hip arthroplasty. Orthop Clin North Am 23:237–248
28. Philippot R, Adam P, Reckhaus M, Delangle F et al (2009) Prevention of dislocation in total hip revision surgery using a dual mobility design. Orthop Traumatol Surg Res 95(6):407–413, Epub 2009 Aug 4
29. Philippot R, Adam P, Farizon F, Fessy MH, Bousquet G (2006) Survival of cementless dual mobility sockets: ten-year follow-up. Rev Chir Orthop Reparatrice Appar Mot 92(4):326–331
30. Langlais FL, Ropars M, Gaucher F, Musset T, Chaix O (2008) Dual mobility cemented cups have low dislocation rates in THA revisions. Clin Orthop Relat Res 466(2):389–395
31. Levine RB, Della Valle CJ, Dermengian CA, Breien KM, Weeden SH, Sporer SM, Paprosky WG (2008) The use of a tripolar articulation in revision total hip arthroplasty: a minimum of 24 months' follow-up. J Arthroplasty 23:1182–1188
32. Stroh A, Naziri Q, Johnson AJ, Mont MA (2012) Dual-mobility bearings: a review of the literature. Expert Rev Med Devices 9(1):23–31. doi:10.1586/ERD.11.57
33. Shapiro GS, Weiland DE, Markel DC, Padgett DE, Sculco TP, Pellicci PM (2003) The use of a constrained acetabular component for recurrent dislocation. J Arthroplasty 18:250–258

34. Williams JT, Ragland PS, Clarke S (2007) Constrained components for the unstable hip following total hip arthroplasty: a literature review. Int Orthop 31(3): 273–277, Epub 2006 Aug 23

35. Noble PC, Durrani SK, Usrey MM, Mathis KB, Bardakos NV (2012) Constrained cups appear incapable of meeting the demands of revision THA. Clin Orthop Relat Res 470(7):1907–1916

Treatment of Early and Late Infection Following THA

José Cordero-Ampuero

Previous Considerations

When planning the treatment of an infected total hip arthroplasty (THA) a whole series of previous considerations must be analyzed in detail:
1. Temporal evolution: early or late infection
2. Geographical dissemination: superficial or deep infection
3. Bacteria infecting the THA (if they are known) and their ability to produce glycocalix
4. Antibiotic sensitivity of strains cultured
5. Co-morbidity and medical status of the patient (Cierny physiological status and classification)
6. Local status of soft tissues
7. Implant stability and degree of wear in friction surfaces
8. Bone stock, eventual bone defects
9. Technical abilities of the surgical team
10. Technical situation and support from hospital environment
11. Patient expectations

After judging and evaluating all these questions, there are a number of options available for treatment of infection in THA [24]:
- Suppressive antibiotic therapy with NO surgery
- Surgical debridement maintaining the infected implant
- Resection-arthroplasty (Girdlestone)
- One-stage exchange
- Two-stage exchange

Suppressive Antibiotics

This modality of treatment is based on maintaining patient with chronic antibiotics, at least for 6 months, without any surgery at all. Obviously two conditions are necessary: oral antibiotics are effective for the isolated bacteria, and patient is able to receive this long therapy without important secondary effects.

There are a short number of indications for this way of treatment: Tsukayama type IV THA infections, patient type C (Cierny), or repeated rejection of surgery by the patient.

Tsukayama Type IV

Tsukayama type IV is the name applied to a patient operated with a supposedly aseptic THA exchange but with multiple intra-operative positive cultures [59].

The classical recommendation for this situation is to maintain the implant (as long as it is right and the wound evolves satisfactorily) and to treat the patient with monotherapy of an effective intravenous antibiotic (selected according to cultures and antibiogram) for 6 weeks at least.

Alternatively, a different antibiotic protocol could be used taking advantage of late advances, applying a 6-month cycle of combined oral antibiotics [17, 19].

Tsukayama reported a 84 % healing of infection with intravenous antibiotics [59].

Cierny Type C Patient

According to the Cierny classification [12], type C patients are those with such a severe physiological compromise that surgical and/or anaesthetic risks are not acceptable. Then, the only possible treatment for these patients is the suppressive antibiotherapy.

So treated, the probability of healing infection is very poor, about 21 % [12, 29, 45, 65].

Repeated Rejection of Surgery

This is the case of patients rejecting repeatedly any surgical option, even after long and dedicated advice from the treating physicians.

Surgical Debridement

Surgical debridement, while maintaining the infected implant, is the preferred indication for early infections. This indication has been established since the 1970s, but several doubts have arisen lately. First of them is the temporal definition of "early", second the appropriateness of changing some components of the implant.

Indications

What is an "early" infection of a hip arthroplasty? In the 1970s. Fitzgerald defined it as the one presenting clinical signs and/or symptoms in the first 3 months after surgery or after haematogenous seeding from a distant focus. Later, along the 1980's and 1990's, that period was shortened to only 1 month after surgery or haematogenous seeding.

Some papers showed a dramatic difference in healing of infection because of the delay in debridement surgery [58]: 56 % healing when debridement was done in the first 48 h after diagnosis of infection, decreasing to 13 % if it was delayed more than 48 h. Along the past decade, new proposals from the European Bone and Joint Infection Society (EBJIS) supported a maximum period of 15 days after surgery for the definition of "early" arthroplasty infection. Moreover, some members proposed that debridement should be done urgently, as early as fractures, ideally in the first 24 h after diagnosis.

Nowadays research raises more doubts about the optimal period for debridement to be useful. Biofilm is formed on the surface of the implants in 24–48 h [25, 28], afterwards it evolves and matures. Once established, biofilm is not removed even with very aggressive debridement, so exchange of implants becomes compulsory. All these concepts could explain the high rate of failure of simple debridement.

Surgical Technique

As mentioned before, some aspects of classical surgical technique are changing lately:

First, debridement must be aggressive, meticulous, and systematic, nearly "tumoural". No suspicious tissue should be left behind. Failure in the appropriateness of debridement is one of the main causes for treatment failure.

Second, samples of all suspicious tissues must be sent to Microbiology for culture and antibiotic sensitivity. The number of samples must be 6 at least, and it is much better to send tissue pieces; liquids and swabs have a low number of bacteria, and microbiological performance is much worse. Of course, all fistulae and tissues with probable skin contamination should be avoided.

Third, irrigation should use at least 10 l of saline, and it may have added antiseptic or soap. After irrigation, it is very important to change the surgical field and the instruments with aseptic technique, as in cancer surgery, so as to diminish the number of bacteria as much as possible. For example, to use the same forceps, absolutely charged with bacteria, for initial debridement and for closing the wound, may ruin the procedure.

Fourth, and this is the most controversial point, the surgeon must decide which components should be changed. Classically all the implants were maintained. With the years and with the increasing knowledge about biofilm, recommendations are to exchange an increasing number of components. First was the polyethylene, afterwards the head, lately all the uncemented and loose components (it is supposed that in the first 2–4 weeks they are not biologically fixed, but this may be not true with hydroxyapatite-coated pieces)…The question arises immediately from a formal point of view: Is this a debridement, or this is a "one-stage" exchange? Possibly, in the future, early infections will be treated with "one-stage" and not with simple debridement.

Results

Published figures of healing of infection with debridement are very different, from only 30 % up to 71 % in the best scenario. Possibly this variability indicates great differences in delay, aggressiveness, exchanged components, and other confounding factors.

Some factors have been clearly associated with a worse prognosis, as is the case with delay for debridement or infection by *Staphylococcus aureus* [2, 55].

Girdlestone Pseudarthrosis

Results

Healing of Infection

Although commonly accepted as a sure method of healing infection, this is not always true: some series report from 80 to 90 % [6, 23, 36, 53, 54]. Moreover, figures are not so good in some clinical subsets: 61 % in rheumatoid arthritis patients [4], 76 % for enterococcal infections [21], or 84 % in methycillin-resistant *Staphylococci* [17, 48, 49]. Sometimes the cause for persistence of infection is residual cement [9].

Residual Pain

Also a classical teaching, but Girdlestone is not always a painless situation. Papers refer to pain as severe in 16–33 % of patients, moderate in 24–53 %, and mild in 76 % [6, 23, 36, 40, 53, 54, 57].

Oxygen Consumption

Resection-arthroplasty patients suffer an oxygen consumption 264 % greater than normal, even worse that persons with an above-knee amputation [35].

Walking Limitations

The problem increases dramatically in the geriatric population, where 45 % are unable to walk and only 29 % walk with crutches [40].

Global Functional Limitations

Published Harris Hip Scores (HHS) range from 25 to 64 [6, 11, 15, 17, 18, 40, 48, 49, 57], while Merle d'Aubigné only amounts to 3.5–6.7 points [23, 49].

Patient Satisfaction

An absolutely subjective evaluation, literature reports from only 13 % to quite good as 83 % [23, 48, 49, 53, 54, 57].

Indications

Considering published results, indications for resection-arthroplasty of the hip must be strictly limited [3, 15, 23, 48].

Non-ambulatory Patients

The most clear indication, there is a general consensus about non-ambulatory patients because of other problems or diseases (most of them neurologic comorbidities).

Dementia

Nowadays, one of the most discussed indications. Girdlestone drastically reduces functional status and walking ability, compromising social and nursing management [40]. Classical indication came from the high risk of dislocation, but modern solutions (bi-polar, tri-polar, constrained cups) will help to reduce this.

Immunocompromise
Again, a doubtful indication from a contemporary point of view. Immunocompromise is rather a quantitative or gradual characteristic. Whom do we condemn to Girdlestone? Those with HIV-infection? Organ-transplant? Corticoids or biological treatments for inflammatory arthritis? Diabetes/obesity?

The best recommendation is re-implantation after exhaustive informed consent and prophylaxis protocol.

Intravenous Drug Abuse
Possibly one of the more clear indications, but the problem arises with diagnosing this behaviour. Most patients will argue that they have long-time ago abandoned drugs.

Impossible Re-implantation
Sometimes the surgeon and patient desire re-implantation but the second-stage becomes impossible. This comes from new medical co-morbidities [3, 50, 53] or from technical difficulties in medically compromised patients (e.g., severe bone defects which require a too aggressive reconstruction) [53, 57].

Another cause continues to be patient rejection [10, 15], less frequent with the years, but still important [17, 18] because of cultural, clinical, psycho-social and/or economical reasons.

One-Stage Exchange

Problems

Physiopathological (Theoretical) Problems
One-stage revision surgery presents important conceptual problems [14, 16]:
- first, a new prosthesis is re-implanted, so partial devascularization of tissues and implants (first cause for chronicity of these infections) is maintained
- second, the negative effect of biomaterials on the immune system is not avoided (second cause for chronicity of implant infections)
- third, intracellular bacteria (fourth cause of chronicity) are only partially treated. To diminish this problem the surgeon is forced to perform very aggressive debridements, so compromising reconstruction techniques.

Practical Problems
Besides the described conceptual problems, one-stage revision also poses important practical difficulties:
- It is impossible to observe how bacteria are eliminated and how infection heals progressively
- It is impossible to use acrylic cement (PMMA) with specific antibiotics according to sensitivity of intra-operative cultures. Previous cultures from fistulae or intra-articular aspiration are much less reliable.
- It compels the surgeon to perform very aggressive debridements, and this implies very big components for re-implantation (worsening additionally the bone stock).

Contra-Indications

Considering all the above problems and clinical results (see below), most authors agree on a long list of contra-indications [10, 27, 32, 46, 50]:
- reumathoid arthritis
- diabetes
- obesity
- multiple previous surgeries
- generalized sepsis
- multiple fistulae
- polymicrobial infection
- bone defects
- necrotic bone
- osteomyelitis

Even traditional defenders of one-stage protocols establish some contra-indications nowadays, such as the presence of methicillin-resistant *Staphylococcus* [37].

Results

Published rates of healing of infection with one-stage protocols vary from 69 to 91 % [2, 19, 32, 37, 39, 46, 50, 55]. Recurrent infection is described in 8–22 % of patients [10, 50].

As previously explained, healing of infection is less than 60 % when methicillin-resistant Staphylococcus aureus are present, even when multiple repeated one-stage exchanges are performed [37].

Revision in Two Stages

Advantages

Theoretical Advantages

Two-stage revision surgery presents physiopathological and empirical advantages over one-stage. The theoretical or conceptual advantages are [14, 16]:
- after first surgery no devascularized implants or tissues remain locally (this is the first cause of bacterial resistance)
- biomaterials that may inhibit the immune system (second cause for bacterial resistance) are not present in the period between surgeries,
- implant removal eliminates adherent bacteria and biofilms (third cause for bacterial resistance and chronicity),
- antibiotics administered during this period are able to eliminate intracellular bacteria (fourth cause of bacterial resistance)

Practical Advantages

There are also practical (empirical) advantages with two-stage protocols [18]:
- intra-operative tissue cultures are much more reliable than fistula exudates or pre-operative intra-articular aspirates
- re-implantation is executed only when there is proof of healing of infection [17, 18, 56]

Disadvantages

Of course, two-stage revision surgery also presents disadvantages:

- traditional protocols are based on monotherapy with intravenous antibiotics between surgeries, usually from 3 to 6 weeks
- to maintain a permanent intravenous access means that the patient must remain in-hospital from the first to the second surgery (at least in many European countries). Alternatively the patient could be treated intravenously at home (usual in U.S.A., but is dependent on a complex nursing organization). Much more convenient are the modern protocols based on combinations of oral antibiotics [17–19]
- economical cost: very high because of the two surgeries and the long period in-hospital
- the last, but not the least, the suffering of the patient. It is very important because of the functional deficit between surgeries, the pain, the long period in-hospital, and the secondary effects from antibiotics.

Results

Healing of Infection

Results with conventional two-stage protocols are good. Healing of infection is expected in 85–100 % of patients [26, 27, 30, 32, 33, 39, 50–52, 56, 60, 64].

Nevertheless, it is convenient to remember an old concept for infectious diseases: healing is also dependent on the medical status of the patient (as graded by Cierny physiological type) [12, 43].

Recurrent Infection

According to literature, recurrent infection appears in 6–22 % of patients [13, 18, 38, 39, 42, 50, 59]. Supposedly, this variability may be explained by many differences among individual protocols [18, 50].

Alternative Modern Protocols

Two-stage protocols for arthroplasty infections, developed in the late 1970s, had been unchanged since the first series coming from the Hospital for Special Surgery in New York [50]. In 1993 Drancourt et al. [19] opened the possibility of treatment with combinations of oral antibiotics on an out-patient basis. The fusion of both ideas, a traditional two-stage surgical protocol and a long-term antibiotic treatment with oral combinations, was first communicated in 2007 [18]. This first series included 40 patients, 16 with hip arthroplasties, infected with 5- *S aureus* (2 methycillin-resistant), 30 *Staphylococcus* coagulase-negative (17 methicillin-resistant), 4 *Enterococcus*, 2 *Pseudomonas*, 2 *Proteus* and 1 *Serratia*.

These patients were treated with implant extraction, a combination of oral antibiotics (rifampin, ofloxacin/levofloxacin, ciprofloxacin, cotrimoxazol, clindamycin, fosfomicin, linezolid) for 6 months, and re-implantation with a cemented prosthesis (cement with gentamicin and clindamycin). Healing of infection was obtained in 15/16 patients (94 %), and functional results were also good, reaching an average HHS of 94/100 (from 84 to 98).

A second series was published in 2009 comparing infectious and functional results in methicillin-resistant *vs* methicillin-sensitive *Staphylococcus aureus* cases [17]. Healing of infection was accomplished in 16/19 resistant (84 %) *vs* 11/11 sensitive (100 %) isolations. Functional results were not so good, especially in resistant cases, because of a high proportion (10/19, 53 %) of definitive resection-arthroplasties. As expected, HHS reached 88 points in re-implanted patients and 52 in Girdlestone cases.

Controversies

Although two-stage protocols were begun more than 30 years ago, as explained, a number of controversies exist about them, especially with later developments [50].

Antibiotics

The period for antibiotic therapy may be fixed by protocol (usually 6 weeks), as in original descriptions [50], or may be variable. The variable period is based in some series on attainment of bactericidal levels in blood [39], in others series it is dependent on clinical and serological (erythrocyte sedimentation rate – ESR- and C-reactive protein – CRP-) normalization [17, 18].

The route of administration may be intravenous, as originally described [50]; alternatively it may be oral [17, 18], as referred to before; or antibiotics may be administered only in PMMA (without using any systemic therapy) [56, 62].

Spacers

Many surgeons use commercial spacers with pre-charged antibiotics; recurrence of infection for those patients is as low as 5–11 % [20, 32, 41, 50, 63, 64]. Other authors have published about the use of "hand-made" spacers, an option that allows the selection of antibiotics to be mixed with PMMA [47].

Time Between Surgeries

Time between surgeries may be fixed by the applied protocol; in these cases literature describes 1 year [34, 42], 12 weeks [50], 6 weeks [13, 27, 39, 59] or 3 weeks [31].

In other published series the time between first and second surgery is lengthened up to normalization of ESR and CRP [17, 18, 50, 56].

Allograft

The use of massive allograft for large bone defects is associated with a high risk of recurrent infection [1, 5, 61]. On the contrary, reconstruction with Slooff/Ling techniques using impaction of morsellized allograft has obtained very good results and low recurrence figures (about 7.5 %) [7, 8, 22].

Fixation of New Implants

According to the literature, non-cemented re-implantation is associated with higher risk of recurrence (from 11 to 18 %) and worse clinical results [5, 32, 38, 44, 61].

Most authors propose the use of cement with antibiotics for re-implantation of prostheses. There are even protocols with no use of systemic antibiotics at all, so antibiotic therapy is absolutely dependent on rate of liberation from cement [56].

References

1. Alexeeff M, Mahomed N, Morsi E, Garbuz D, Gross A (1996) Structural allograft in two-stage revisions for failed septic hip arthroplasty. J Bone Joint Surg Br 78-B:213–216
2. Barberan J, Aguilar L, Carroquino G et al (2006) Conservative treatment of staphylococcal prosthetic

joint infections in elderly patients. Am J Med 119:993 e7–993 e10
3. Barrack RL, Aggarwal A, Burnett RS (2006) Resection arthroplasty: when enough is enough. Orthopedics 29:820–821
4. Berbari EF, Osmon DR, Duffy MC, Harmssen RN, Mandrekar JN, Hanssen AD, Steckelberg JM (2006) Outcome of prosthetic joint infection in patients with rheumatoid arthritis: the impact of medical and surgical therapy in 200 episodes. Clin Infect Dis 42:216–223
5. Berry DJ, Chandler HP, Reilly DT (1991) The use of bone allografts in two-stage reconstruction after failure of hip replacements due to infection. J Bone Joint Surg Am 73-A:1460–1468
6. Bourne RB, Hunter GA, Rorabeck CH, Macnab JJ (1984) A six-year follow-up of infected total hip replacements managed by Girdlestone's arthroplasty. J Bone Joint Surg Br 66:340–343
7. Buttaro MA. Comba F, Piccaluga F (2009) Proximal femoral reconstructions with bone impaction grafting and metal mesh. Clin Orthop Relat Res 467:2325–2334
8. Buttaro MA, Pusso R, Piccaluga F (2005) Vancomycin-supplemented impacted bone allografts in infected hip arthroplasty. Two-stage revision results. J Bone Joint Surg Br 87-B:314–319
9. Buttaro M, Valentini R, Piccaluga F (2004) Persistent infection associated with residual cement after resection arthroplasty of the hip. Acta Orthop Scand 75:427–429
10. Callaghan JJ, Katz RP, Johnston RC (1999) One-stage revision surgery of the infected hip. A minimum 10-year followup study. Clin Orthop Relat Res 369:139–143
11. Cherney DL, Amstutz HC (1983) Total hip replacement in the previously septic hip. J Bone Joint Surg Am 65:1256–1265
12. Cierny GI, DiPasquale D (2002) Periprosthetic total joint infections: staging, treatment, and outcomes. Clin Orthop 403:23–28
13. Colyer RA, Capello WN (1994) Surgical treatment of the infected hip implant. Two stage reimplantation with a one-month interval. Clin Orthop Relat Res 298:75–79
14. Cordero J (1999) Infection of orthopaedic implants. Theory and practice. Eur Instr Course Lect 4:65–73
15. Cordero-Ampuero J (2012) Girdlestone procedure: when and why. Hip Int 22(Suppl 8):S36–S39
16. Cordero J, García-Cimbrelo E (2000) Mechanisms of bacterial resistance in implant infection. Hip Int 10:139–144
17. Cordero-Ampuero J, Esteban J, García-Cimbrelo E (2009) Oral antibiotics are effective for highly resistant hip arthroplasty infections. Clin Orthop 467:2335–2342
18. Cordero-Ampuero J, Esteban J, García-Cimbrelo E, Munuera L, Escobar R (2007) Low relapse with oral antibiotics and two-stage exchange for late arthroplasty infections in 40 patients after 2–9 years. Acta Orthop 78:511–519
19. Drancourt M, Stein A, Argenson JN et al (1993) Oral rifampin plus ofloxacin for treatment of staphylococcus-infected orthopedic implants. Antimicrob Agents Chemother 37:1214–1218
20. Duncan CP, Beauchamp C (1993) A temporary antibiotic-loaded joint replacement system for management of complex infections involving the hip. Orthop Clin North Am 24:751–759
21. El Helou OC, Berbari EF, Marculescu CE, El Atrouni WI, Razonable RR, Steckelberg JM, Hanssen AD, Osmon DR (2008) Outcome of enterococcal prosthetic joint infection: is combination systemic therapy superior to monotherapy? Clin Infect Dis 47:903–909
22. English H, Timperley AJ, Dunlop D, Gie G (2002) Impaction grafting of the femur in two-stage revision for infected total hip replacement. J Bone Joint Surg Br 84-B:700–705
23. Esenwein SA, Robert K, Kollig E, Ambacher T, Kutscha-Lissberg F, Muhr G (2001) Long-term results after resection arthroplasty according to Girdlestone for treatment of persisting infections of the hip joint. Chirurg 72:1336–1343
24. Esteban J, Cordero-Ampuero J (2011) Treatment of prosthetic osteoarticular infections. Expert Opin Pharmacother 12:899–912
25. Esteban J, Molina-Manso D, Spiliopoulou I, Cordero-Ampuero J, Fernández-Roblas R, Foka A, Gómez-Barrena E (2010) Biofilm development by clinical isolates of Staphylococcus spp. from retrieved orthopaedic prosthesis. Acta Orthop 81:674–679
26. Garvin KL, Evans BG, Salvati EA, Brause BD (1994) Palacos gentamicin for the treatment of deep periprosthetic hip infections. Clin Orthop Relat Res 298:97–105
27. Garvin KL, Fitzgerald RH, Salvati EA (1993) Reconstruction of the infected total hip and knee arthroplasty with gentamicin-impregnated Palacos bone cement. Instr Course Lect 42:293–302
28. Gómez-Barrena E, Esteban J, Medel F, Molina-Manso D, Ortiz-Pérez A, Cordero-Ampuero J, Puértolas JA (2012) Bacterial adherence to separated modular components in joint prosthesis: a clinical study. J Orthop Res 30:1634–1639
29. Goulet JA, Pellici PM, Brause BD, Salvati EM (1988) Prolonged suppression of infection in total hip arthroplasty. J Arthroplasty 3:109–116
30. Haddad FS, Masri BA, Garbuz DS, Duncan CP (1999) The treatment of the infected hip replacement. The complex case. Clin Orthop 369:144–156
31. Haddad FS, Muirhead-Allwood SK, Manktelow AR, Bacarese-Hamilton I (2000) Two-stage uncemented revision hip arthroplasty for infection. J Bone Joint Surg Br 82-B:689–694
32. Hanssen AD, Rand JA (1999) Evaluation and treatment of infection at the site of a total hip or knee arthroplasty. Instr Course Lect 48:111–122
33. Hirakawa K, Stulberg BN, Wilde AH et al (1998) Results of 2-stage reimplantation for infected total knee arthroplasty. J Arthroplasty 13:22–28
34. Hunter GA (1979) The results of reinsertion of a total hip prosthesis after sepsis. J Bone Joint Surg Br 61-B:422–423
35. Kantor GS, Osterkamp JA, Dorr LD, Fischer D, Perry J, Conaty JP (1986) Resection arthroplasty following infected total hip replacement arthroplasty. J Arthroplasty 1:83–89

36. Klima S, Zeh A, Josten C (2008) Reimplantation of a hip prosthesis in patients with an infected resection arthroplasty. Z Orthop Unfall 146:616–623
37. Kordelle J, Frommelt L, Kluber D et al (2000) Results of one-stage endoprosthesis revision in periprosthetic infection cause by methicillin-resistant Staphylococcus aureus. Z Orthop Ihre Grenzgeb 138:240–244
38. Lai KA, Shen WJ, Yang CY, Lin RM, Lin CJ, Jou IM (1996) Two-stage cementless revision THR after infection 5 recurrences in 40 cases followed 2.5-7 years. Acta Orthop Scand 67:325–328
39. Lieberman JR, Callaway GH, Salvati EA et al (1994) Treatment of the infected total hip arthroplasty with a two-stage reimplantation protocol. Clin Orthop 301: 205–212
40. Manjón-Cabeza Subirat JM, Moreno Palacios JA, Mozo Muriel AP, Cátedra Vallés E, Sancho Loras R, Ubeda Tikkanen A (2008) Functional outcomes after resection of hip arthroplasty (Girdlestone technique). Rev Esp Geriatr Gerontol 43:13–18
41. Masri BA, Duncan CP, Beauchamp CP (1998) Long-term elution of antibiotics from bone-cement: an in vivo study using the prosthesis of antibiotic-loaded acrylic cement (PROSTALAC) system. J Arthroplasty 13:331–338
42. McDonald DJ, Fitzgerald RH Jr, Ilstrup DM (1989) Two-stage reconstruction of a total hip arthroplasty because of infection. J Bone Joint Surg Am 71-A: 828–834
43. McPherson EJ, Woodson C, Holtom P, Roidis N, Shufelt C, Patzakis M (2002) Periprosthetic total hip infection: outcomes using a staging system. Clin Orthop Relat Res 403:8–15
44. Nestor BJ, Hanssen AD, Ferrer-Gonzalez R, Fitzgerald RH Jr (1994) The use of porous prostheses in delayed reconstruction of total hip replacements that have failed because of infection. J Bone Joint Surg Am 76-A:349–359
45. Rao N, Crossett LS, Sinha RK, Le Frock JL (2003) Long-term suppression of infection in total joint arthroplasty. Clin Orthop Relat Res 414:55–60
46. Raut VV, Siney PD, Wroblewsky BM (1994) One-stage revision of infected total hip replacements with discharging sinuses. J Bone Joint Surg Br 76: 721–724
47. Ries MD, Jergesen H (1999) An inexpensive molding method for antibiotic-impregnated cement spacers in infected total hip arthroplasty. J Arthroplasty 14: 764–765
48. Rittmeister M, Manthei L, Müller M, Hailer NP (2004) Reimplantation of the artificial hip joint in Girdlestone hips is superior to Girdlestone arthroplasty by itself. Z Orthop Ihre Grenzgeb 142:559–563
49. Rittmeister M, Müller M, Starker M, Hailer NP (2003) Functional results following Girdlestone arthroplasty. Z Orthop Ihre Grenzgeb 141:665–671
50. Salvati EA, Della-Valle AG, Masri BA et al (2003) The infected total hip arthroplasty. Instr Course Lect 52:223–246
51. Segawa H, Tsukayama DT, Kyle RF et al (1999) Infection after total knee arthroplasty. A retrospective study of the treatment of eighty-one infections. J Bone Joint Surg Am 81:1434–1445
52. Sendi P, Rohrbach M, Graber P et al (2006) Staphylococcus aureus small colony variants in prosthetic joint infection. Clin Infect Dis 43:961–967
53. Sharma H, De Leeuw J, Rowley DI (2005) Girdlestone resection arthroplasty following failed surgical procedures. Int Orthop 29:92–95
54. Sharma H, Kakar R (2006) Outcome of Girdlestone's resection arthroplasty following complications of proximal femoral fractures. Acta Orthop Belg 72: 555–559
55. Soriano A, Gomez J, Gomez L et al (2007) Efficacy and tolerability of prolonged linezolid therapy in the treatment of orthopedic implant infections. Eur J Clin Microbiol Infect Dis 26:353–356
56. Stockley I, Mockford BJ, Hoad-Reddick A et al (2008) The use of two-stage exchange arthroplasty with depot antibiotics in the absence of long-term antibiotic therapy in infected total hip replacement. J Bone Joint Surg Br 90:145–148
57. Stoklas J, Rozkydal Z (2004) Resection of head and neck of the femoral bone according to Girdlestone. Acta Chir Orthop Traumatol Cech 71:147–151
58. Trebse R, Pisot V, Trampuz A (2005) Treatment of infected retained implants. J Bone Joint Surg Br 87-B: 249–256
59. Tsukayama DT, Estrada R, Gustilo RB (1996) Infection after total hip arthroplasty. A study of the treatment of one hundred and six infections. J Bone Joint Surg Am 78-A:512–523
60. Volin SJ, Hinrichs SH, Garvin KL (2004) Two-stage reimplantation of total joint infections: a comparison of resistant and non-resistant organisms. Clin Orthop Relat Res 427:94–100
61. Wang JW, Chen CE (1997) Reimplantation of infected hip arthroplasties using bone allografts. Clin Orthop Relat Res 335:202–210
62. Whittaker JP, Warren RE, Jones RS, Gregson PA (2009) Is prolonged systemic antibiotic treatment essential in two-stage revision hip replacement for chronic Gram-positive infection? J Bone Joint Surg Br 91-B:44–51
63. Younger AS, Duncan CP, Masri BA (1998) Treatment of infection associated with segmental bone loss in the proximal part of the femur in two stages with use of an antibiotic-loaded interval prosthesis. J Bone Joint Surg Am 80-A:60–69
64. Younger AS, Duncan CP, Masri BA, McGraw RW (1997) The outcome of two-stage arthroplasty using a custom-made interval spacer to treat the infected hip. J Arthroplasty 12:615–623
65. Zimmerli W, Widmer AF, Blatter M et al (1998) Role of rifampin for treatment of orthopedic implant-related staphylococcal infections: a randomized controlled trial. Foreign-Body Infection (FBI) Study Group. JAMA 279:1537–1541

Part IX

Knee

Prevention and Management of Cartilage Injury and Osteoarthritis from Sports

Hideki Takeda and Lars Engebretsen

Introduction

Osteoarthritis (OA) is the most common musculoskeletal disease and is responsible for decreasing the quality of life among young, active athletes as well as elderly people [1]. The number of people who are affected by OA is increasing due to the increasing age of the population. Obesity, excessive stress to the knee (at work or in sports), previous knee injury, and muscle weakness around knee are known as risk factors [2–5]. In analyzing preventive possibilities, these risk factors are very important.

The aim of this review is to evaluate the prevalence of knee OA and the relationship between sports activity and OA. Furthermore to summarize the prevention and treatment of the knee OA and cartilage injury in sports, in order to reduce the increasing impact of knee OA.

Prevalence of Knee OA in Sports

The prevalence of knee OA increases with age [1]. Symptomatic knee OA occurs in 10–33 % of those aged 60 years or older [6–8]. This number is increasing due to the aging of the population. In professional and recreational athletes, prevalence of knee OA depends on the intensity, frequency, level and sports event (Table 1).

The prevalence of knee OA among former soccer players is 19–29 %, long distance runners 14–20 %, and weight-lifters 31 % [9–13]. There are some limitations in these studies. Previous studies which showed the relationship between the sport event and the prevalence of knee OA have various definitions and criteria of OA, the selection of athletes and the method of analysis.

Definition of Knee OA

OA is a group of diseases where the homeostasis of articular cartilage chondrocytes, extracellular matrix and subchondral bone is damaged mechanically and biologically [14]. Although OA may be initiated by multiple factors, including genetic, metabolic, and traumatic, they involve all of the tissues of the joint [14]. OA includes morphological, biochemical, molecular, and biomechanical changes of both cells and matrix which leads to softening, fibrillation, and ulceration, loss of articular cartilage, sclerosis and eburnation of subchondral bone, osteophytes, and subchondral cysts [14]. Clinical OA is characterized by joint pain, tenderness, limitation of movement, crepitus, occasional effusion, and variable degrees of inflammation. Most physicians diagnose knee OA not only by the symptoms, but by the

H. Takeda, MD
Department of Sports Orthopedics,
Toshiba General Hospital,
Tokyo, Japan

L. Engebretsen, MD, PhD (✉)
Department of Orthopedic Surgery,
Oslo University Hospital, Oslo, Norway
e-mail: lars.engebretsen@medisin.uio.no

Table 1 The prevalence of knee OA in sports

Author	Year	Subject	Number	Mean age	Prevalence of the knee OA
Roos et al. [9]	1994	Former soccer players	286	55	15.5 % (elite level)
					4.2 % (non-elite)
					1.6 % (control)
Kujala et al. [10]	1995	Former top-level athlete	117	45–68	3 % (shooter)
					29 % (soccer)
					31 % (weight lifter)
					14 % (runner)
Turner et al. [11]	2000	Former professional football players	284	56.1	29 % (right knee)
					22 % (left knee)
Drawer and Fuller [12]	2001	Retired professional soccer players	185	47.6	19 % (right knee)
					21 % (left knee)
Chakravarty et al. [13]	2008	Long distance runner	45	76	20 %

radiological findings. The usual radiographs are read according to the Kellgren and Lawrence (K&L) classification:

grade 0: no changes.
grade 1: doubtful narrowing of the joint space and possible osteophytic lipping,
grade 2: definite osteophytes and possible narrowing of the joint space
grade 3: moderate multiple osteophytes, definite narrowing of the joint space, and some sclerosis, and possible deformity of the bone ends,
grade 4: large osteophytes, marked narrowing of the joint space, severe sclerosis and definite deformity of the bone ends. Conventionally, OA has been defined as starting at K-L Grade ≥2 [15].

It is important to be aware of the considerable discrepancy between symptoms and radiological findings in OA. Fifteen to eighty-one percent of patients with radiographic findings had knee pain in a recent systematic review [16]. On the other hand, patients who have early painful OA might not necessarily have radiographic changes.

Post-traumatic Knee OA in Sports

Injuries such as knee ligament tears, meniscal injuries and fractures involving articular surfaces have been shown as strong risk factors for knee OA [3, 10, 17–19]. According to Kujala et al., the risk of knee OA is increased almost five times above normal in male former top-level athletes with previous knee injuries (Odds ratio 4.73) [10]. Some studies reported that articular surface incongruities greater than 3 mm. increase local contact stress [20, 21]. Consequently, precise reduction and fracture fixation is needed to avoid knee OA after articular surface fracture. The anterior cruciate ligament (ACL) injury is a well known as a risk factor of knee OA with or without reconstruction (Table 2) [22–26]. Gillquist et al. reported that isolated meniscus tear and subsequent repair, or ruptures of the ACL seemed to increase the OA risk tenfold compared with an age-matched, uninjured population [27]. In addition, Øiestad et al. showed that the most frequent risk factor for development of knee OA with ACL injury athlete was meniscal injury [28]. Early diagnosis and effective treatment and ensuring complete rehabilitation after ACL and meniscus injury should decrease the risk for OA among sports participants.

Are the Sports Themselves Causing OA?

Epidemiological studies have showed that participation in some competitive sports increases the risk for OA [4, 29, 30]. Moderate exercise has low risk of leading to OA. Furthermore, there is evidence that appropriate exercise reduces disability

Table 2 ACL injury as a risk factor for knee OA

Author	Year	Background	Number	Study method	Prevalence knee OA
Neyret et al. [22]	1993	Non-specific sports	93	Cohort 20–35 years follow-up	86 % OA with untreated ACL injury
von Porat et al. [23]	2004	Male soccer players	205	Cohort 14 years follow-up	78 % radiological OA change (41 % more than KL-grade2)
Nebelung and Wuschech [24]	2005	High level athletes	19	Cohort 35 year follow-up	42 % TKA with untreated ACL injury
Ait Si Selmi et al. [25]	2006	Non specific sports	103	Cohort 17 years follow-up	14–26 % OA with reconstructed ACL (37 % with reconstructed ACL and menisectomy)
Oiestad et al. [26]	2010	Non specific sports	181	Cohort	62 % radiologic OA (more than KL grade 2) with isolated ACL injury
				10–15 years follow-up	80 % radiologic OA (more than KL grade 2) with combined ACL injury

in knee OA [31]. Sports activities including high-intensity and direct joint impact as a result of contact with other participants appeared to increase the risk for OA [32]. Repetitive impact and twisting loads to the knee also are associated with joint degeneration [5, 10, 33, 34]. To avoid knee OA, participants should pay attention to individual risk factors, frequency and intensity of sports activity.

The Cartilage Injury in Athletes

In a study of 993 consecutive arthroscopies in patients with knee pain from Norway, articular cartilage changes were noted in 66 % of the knees and isolated, localized cartilage lesions in about 20 % of the cases [35]. Full thickness cartilage lesions were found in 11 % of the knees. Sports participation was the most commonly reported activity (49 %). Most of the patients with localized cartilage lesions were in the younger age groups (median age: 30 years). The most serious cartilage injuries ICRS grade III and IV were commonly located at the medial femoral condyle followed by the patella. A single full-thickness area of more than 2 cm^2 was observed in 6 % of all knees, and half of these patients had a cartilage lesion as their only pathology. Fifty percent of these larger lesions (grade III–IV and >2 cm^2) were localized in the medial femoral condyle and 13 % in the femoral trochlea.

Cartilage treatment should be aimed at restoring the normal knee function by regeneration of hyaline cartilage in the defect, and to achieve a complete integration of the new cartilage to the surrounding cartilage and underlying bone. Recent years have seen several new surgical procedures emerge with the aim to improve function and to create normal cartilage. Unfortunately, clinical studies have been limited by methodological weaknesses. Over the last 10 years, marrow-stimulating procedures such as the microfracture method have been widely used and so far no other procedure has surpassed the microfracture results. The main developmental research has occurred in autologous chondrocyte implantation (ACI) which was first described in 1994 [36]. Newer techniques combining scaffolds, cells and growth factors have since been developed [37–42].

Ninety percent of rotational injuries to the knee include the so-called bone bruise lesion

[43]. Follow-up MRI studies of patients with bone bruises suggest that this may lead to degeneration of the cartilage and early arthritis [43]. In addition, it has been shown that isolated cartilage injuries may lead to degeneration of the adjacent cartilage [44]. These changes may be caused by the abnormally high stresses acting on the rim of the defect. The cartilage surface opposing an isolated cartilage injury often shows fibrillation caused by mechanical irritation [45]. Thus, it is suggested that rotational injury to the knee with a bone bruise and subsequent cartilage changes may progress to degenerative arthritis. Moreover, the presence of concomitant injuries (for example, ACL injury or meniscus injury) and malalignment of the lower extremity influences management of these lesions [33, 46–48]. Below is a brief description of the most used techniques for cartilage treatment.

Microfracture

Microfracture as a minimally-invasive and simple procedure and is considered the first choice of treatment for the patients with previously untreated cartilage defects. This technique has the goal of recruiting pluripotential stem cells from the marrow by penetrating the subchondral bone. The preferable cartilage lesion for this method is relatively small size (1–2 cm^2). Only two controlled, randomized clinical studies exist [49, 50]. Knutsen et al. have found good pain relief after 2 years of follow-up in 70–80 % of the patients, whereas Gudas et al. found superiority of the osteochondral autologous transplantation over microfracture at 1, 2 and 3 year time-points [49, 50]. Further, the Norwegian study comparing ACI's with microfracture did not see deterioration in the clinical results even 5 years after surgery [51]. There are few studies investigating the rate of return to sports after microfracture [50, 52–55]. Steadman reported that 76 % of NFL players returned to play 4.6 more seasons after microfracture [52]. In contrast, Namdari et al. showed that only 58 % of NBA players after microfracture were able to return to play at least 1 more season [53]. There is an obvious need for studies with more participants.

Autologous Chondrocyte Implantation (ACI)

Autologous chondrocyte implantation to regenerate articular cartilage has been widely used [36, 56–58]. The procedure involves harvesting of 200–300 mg of cartilage through an arthroscopic procedure, followed 4–6 weeks later by an arthrotomy, where the cells are injected under a cover of periosteum or a synthetic membrane. So far the results of five controlled studies have been published. Bentley et al. showed that after 19 months, 88 % of the patients in the cell group versus 69 % in the mosaic group had good to excellent results based on two scoring systems [59]. Horas et al. found no differences between cells and mosaicplasty after 2 years [60]. Dozin et al. also concluded that ACI and mosaicplasty were clinically equivalent and similar in performance [61]. The Norwegian study [49] found no difference between cell transplantation and microfractures—both leading to improvement in more than 75 % of the patients after 2 years [49]. There was no significant difference in macroscopic or histological results between the two treatment groups and no association between the histological findings and the clinical outcome at the 2-year time-point. Furthermore, the Norwegian study comparing ACI's with microfracture, did not see a deterioration in the clinical results even 5 years after surgery [51]. Hypertrophy of tissue seemed to be the major cause for re-operations after ACI [62]. Recently, Saris et al. published a 3 year follow-up of optimized chondocyte implantation resulting in improved clinical outcomes compared to microfracture [63]. Kreuz et al. showed the rate of return to pre-injury level of sports after ACI among regular or competitive sports athletes was 94 % at 18 months follow-up [64]. The improvement will peak at approximately 2 years, and it does not seem to deteriorate up to 8 years. At the moment the procedure is reserved for patients with large defects on the weight-bearing surface of the knee joint. The defects should not be deeper than approximately 5 mm without being bone grafted. ACI may be preferred as a second-line treatment for large defects. Recently microfracture was found to have less favourable results in treating patellofemoral lesions and ACI may be a better option for trochlear defects [65].

Matrix Assisted Autologous Chondrocyte Implantation (MACI)

MACI was developed to improve upon the disadvantages of ACI (hypertrophy of the graft, the uneven distribution of chondrocytes within the defect and the potential for cell leakage). In MACI, cultured chondrocytes are cultured and implanted on a scaffold. However, so far the clinical and histological results have not been reported to be better than conventional ACI [66].

Mosaicplasty and Osteochondral Autologous Grafts

An alternative to biological regeneration of a defect is to replace it with a substitute. Several Orthopedic companies have produced coring drills, which will harvest plug from areas with relatively less weight-bearing such as the intercondylar notch or the margin of the femoral condyle. The plugs are then placed in the defect in pre-drilled cylindrical holes. The clinical data was first published by Hangody and Bobic [67, 68]. And the results matched those after chondrocyte transplantation by Brittberg et al. [36]. The recent study by Bentley et al. showed much less encouraging results for this technique, while the Horas study and the Dozin study reported more optimistic results [59–61]. Further, the study by Gudas et al. has shown significant superiority of this technique over microfracture procedures, and shown the rate of return to sports after mosaicplasty was 93 % at an average of 6.5 months [50]. There is an obvious need for longer follow-up studies. The use of this technique is limited only by the size of the defect due to the necessity of harvesting from relatively less weight-bearing areas. Recently synthetic plugs have been developed for clinical use as a substitute for autologous graft (True-Fit, Smith & Nephew) [69–71]. However no long term clinical results have been published.

Mesenchymal Stem Cell (MSC) Transplantation

MSC transplantation has been introduced to repair the cartilage lesions avoiding the disadvantage of other methods. MSCs retain both high proliferative potential and pluripotentiality, including chondrogenic differentiation potential, and a number of animal studies with this method have been reported [72]. The use of MSCs for cartilage repair is still at the early stage. More clinical studies are needed.

Treatment of OA

Surgical Treatment

Patients with knee OA who are not obtaining adequate pain relief and functional improvement from a combination of non-pharmacological and pharmacological treatment are considered for surgical treatments. For the young and active athletes with symptomatic unicompartmental knee OA, high tibial osteotomy (HTO) may avoid progression of disease. For the middle-aged athletes with knee OA, unicompartmental or total knee arthroplasty might be considered to gain good quality of life as well as good sports activity. However, even though HTO and knee arthroplasty are common, there is limited literature reporting on the relationship between sports activity and knee surgery. Salzmann et al. showed that 91 % of patients after HTO were engaged in sports and recreational activities and regained the frequency and duration of sports activities [73]. In the older patient group, several studies reported that more than 90 % of the patients after UKA, and more than 60 % of the patients after TKA returned to the same level of sports activity as before surgery [74–78]. Further studies focussing on the appropriate level of sports activity after knee intervention and the prevention of the implant problems (prosthetic and loosening) among athletes are clearly needed.

Prevention of the Knee OA in Sports

As the number of the people who suffer OA disease is increasing at present, prevention of OA is important and necessary. The OA disease has three strong risk factors (excessive musculoskeletal loading, high body mass index, and previous knee injury) where prevention may work. According to Hochberg, avoiding squatting and kneeling and carrying heavy loads during work have been associated with a reduction of 15–30 % in the prevalence of OA in men [79]. Another study showed a significant exposure-response relationship between symptomatic knee OA and squatting and kneeling [80, 81]. Overweight is a risk factor for knee OA. Weight reduction reduces not only symptoms and progression of OA, but also risk from acquiring OA [82, 83]. The Osteoarthritis Research Society International (OARSI) group strongly recommends that the patients with OA lose weight and maintain weight at a lower level in overweight patients [84]. Maintaining the body mass index (BMI) at about 25 kg/m^2 or below is calculated to reduce OA of the population by 27–53 % [79, 80]. As mentioned, knee injuries such as knee ligament tears, meniscal injuries and fractures involving articular surfaces are strong risk factors for knee OA. Some studies showed that pre-fabricated insoles and external knee braces reduced knee injuries [85, 86]. Recently, prevention programmes of sports injury, especially for ACL injury have shown encouraging results. Some Norwegian studies showed that prevention of ACL injuries was possible with the use of neuromuscular training programmes [87–89]. According to Felson [80] prevention of joint injuries would give an additional 14–25 % reduction in OA prevalence.

Summary

Ligament, meniscal and cartilage injuries are common in sports. Unfortunately, at the present time our treatment whether surgical or rehabilitation does not seem to avoid the development of OA in the knee. Much is happening in research on surgical treatment as well as rehabilitation procedures in this field. Clearly, a higher emphasis on prevention is necessary.

References

1. Woolf AD, Pfleger B (2003) Burden of major musculoskeletal conditions. Bull World Health Organ 81(9): 646–656
2. Toivanen AT et al (2010) Obesity, physically demanding work and traumatic knee injury are major risk factors for knee osteoarthritis – a population-based study with a follow-up of 22 years. Rheumatology (Oxford) 49(2):308–314
3. Cooper C et al (2000) Risk factors for the incidence and progression of radiographic knee osteoarthritis. Arthritis Rheum 43(5):995–1000
4. Thelin N, Holmberg S, Thelin A (2006) Knee injuries account for the sports-related increased risk of knee osteoarthritis. Scand J Med Sci Sports 16(5):329–333
5. Felson DT et al (2000) Osteoarthritis: new insights. Part 1: the disease and its risk factors. Ann Intern Med 133(8):635–646
6. Felson DT et al (1987) The prevalence of knee osteoarthritis in the elderly. The Framingham Osteoarthritis Study. Arthritis Rheum 30(8):914–918
7. Lawrence JS (1977) Rheumatism in populations. Hienemann Medical, London
8. Felson DT (2004) An update on the pathogenesis and epidemiology of osteoarthritis. Radiol Clin North Am 42(1):1–9, v
9. Roos H et al (1994) The prevalence of gonarthrosis and its relation to meniscectomy in former soccer players. Am J Sports Med 22(2):219–222
10. Kujala UM et al (1995) Knee osteoarthritis in former runners, soccer players, weight lifters, and shooters. Arthritis Rheum 38(4):539–546
11. Turner AP, Barlow JH, Heathcote-Elliott C (2000) Long term health impact of playing professional football in the United Kingdom. Br J Sports Med 34(5):332–336
12. Drawer S, Fuller CW (2001) Propensity for osteoarthritis and lower limb joint pain in retired professional soccer players. Br J Sports Med 35(6):402–408
13. Chakravarty EF et al (2008) Long distance running and knee osteoarthritis. A prospective study. Am J Prev Med 35(2):133–138
14. Kuettner KE, Goldberg VM (1995) Introduction. In: Kuettner KE, Goldberg VM (eds) Osteoarthritis disorders. American Academy of Orthopaedic Surgeons, Rosemont
15. Kellgren JH, Lawrence JS (1957) Radiological assessment of osteo-arthrosis. Ann Rheum Dis 16(4):494–502
16. Bedson J, Croft PR (2008) The discordance between clinical and radiographic knee osteoarthritis: a systematic search and summary of the literature. BMC Musculoskelet Disord 9:116
17. Rall KL, McElroy GL, Keats TE (1964) A study of long term effects of football injury to the knee. Mo Med 61:435–438
18. Gelber AC et al (2000) Joint injury in young adults and risk for subsequent knee and hip osteoarthritis. Ann Intern Med 133(5):321–328

19. Sutton AJ et al (2001) A case–control study to investigate the relation between low and moderate levels of physical activity and osteoarthritis of the knee using data collected as part of the Allied Dunbar National Fitness Survey. Ann Rheum Dis 60(8):756–764
20. Brown TD et al (1988) Contact stress aberrations following imprecise reduction of simple tibial plateau fractures. J Orthop Res 6(6):851–862
21. Huber-Betzer H, Brown TD, Mattheck C (1990) Some effects of global joint morphology on local stress aberrations near imprecisely reduced intra-articular fractures. J Biomech 23(8):811–822
22. Neyret P, Donell ST, Dejour H (1993) Results of partial meniscectomy related to the state of the anterior cruciate ligament. Review at 20 to 35 years. J Bone Joint Surg Br 75(1):36–40
23. von Porat A, Roos EM, Roos H (2004) High prevalence of osteoarthritis 14 years after an anterior cruciate ligament tear in male soccer players: a study of radiographic and patient relevant outcomes. Ann Rheum Dis 63(3):269–273
24. Nebelung W, Wuschech H (2005) Thirty-five years of follow-up of anterior cruciate ligament-deficient knees in high-level athletes. Arthroscopy 21(6):696–702
25. Ait Si Selmi T, Fithian D, Neyret P (2006) The evolution of osteoarthritis in 103 patients with ACL reconstruction at 17 years follow-up. Knee 13(5):353–358
26. Oiestad BE et al (2010) Knee function and prevalence of knee osteoarthritis after anterior cruciate ligament reconstruction: a prospective study with 10 to 15 years of follow-up. Am J Sports Med 38(11):2201–2210
27. Gillquist J, Messner K (1999) Anterior cruciate ligament reconstruction and the long-term incidence of gonarthrosis. Sports Med 27(3):143–156
28. Oiestad BE et al (2009) Knee osteoarthritis after anterior cruciate ligament injury: a systematic review. Am J Sports Med 37(7):1434–1443
29. Spector TD et al (1996) Risk of osteoarthritis associated with long-term weight-bearing sports: a radiologic survey of the hips and knees in female ex-athletes and population controls. Arthritis Rheum 39(6):988–995
30. Sandmark H, Vingard E (1999) Sports and risk for severe osteoarthrosis of the knee. Scand J Med Sci Sports 9(5):279–284
31. Roddy E et al (2005) Evidence-based recommendations for the role of exercise in the management of osteoarthritis of the hip or knee – the MOVE consensus. Rheumatology (Oxford) 44(1):67–73
32. Deacon A et al (1997) Osteoarthritis of the knee in retired, elite Australian Rules footballers. Med J Aust 166(4):187–190
33. Buckwalter JA, Lane NE (1997) Athletics and osteoarthritis. Am J Sports Med 25(6):873–881
34. Buckwalter JA, Lane NE (1997) Does participation in sports cause osteoarthritis? Iowa Orthop J 17:80–89
35. Aroen A et al (2004) Articular cartilage lesions in 993 consecutive knee arthroscopies. Am J Sports Med 32(1):211–215
36. Brittberg M et al (1994) Treatment of deep cartilage defects in the knee with autologous chondrocyte transplantation. N Engl J Med 331(14):889–895
37. Krishnan SP et al (2006) Collagen-covered autologous chondrocyte implantation for osteochondritis dissecans of the knee: two- to seven-year results. J Bone Joint Surg Br 88(2):203–205
38. Bartlett W et al (2005) Autologous chondrocyte implantation versus matrix-induced autologous chondrocyte implantation for osteochondral defects of the knee: a prospective, randomised study. J Bone Joint Surg Br 87(5):640–645
39. Nehrer S et al (2006) Three-year clinical outcome after chondrocyte transplantation using a hyaluronan matrix for cartilage repair. Eur J Radiol 57(1):3–8
40. Behrens P et al (2006) Matrix-associated autologous chondrocyte transplantation/implantation (MACT/MACI) – 5-year follow-up. Knee 13(3):194–202
41. Steinwachs M, Kreuz PC (2007) Autologous chondrocyte implantation in chondral defects of the knee with a type I/III collagen membrane: a prospective study with a 3-year follow-up. Arthroscopy 23(4):381–387
42. van den Berg WB et al (2001) Growth factors and cartilage repair. Clin Orthop Relat Res (391 Suppl):S244–S250
43. Engebretsen L, Arendt E, Fritts HM (1993) Osteochondral lesions and cruciate ligament injuries. MRI in 18 knees. Acta Orthop Scand 64(4):434–436
44. Wei X, Messner K (1999) Maturation-dependent durability of spontaneous cartilage repair in rabbit knee joint. J Biomed Mater Res 46(4):539–548
45. Twyman RS, Desai K, Aichroth PM (1991) Osteochondritis dissecans of the knee. A long-term study. J Bone Joint Surg Br 73(3):461–464
46. Sharma L et al (1998) Knee adduction moment, serum hyaluronan level, and disease severity in medial tibiofemoral osteoarthritis. Arthritis Rheum 41(7):1233–1240
47. Honkonen SE (1995) Degenerative arthritis after tibial plateau fractures. J Orthop Trauma 9(4):273–277
48. Buckwalter JA, Mankin HJ (1998) Articular cartilage: degeneration and osteoarthritis, repair, regeneration, and transplantation. Instr Course Lect 47:487–504
49. Knutsen G et al (2004) Autologous chondrocyte implantation compared with microfracture in the knee. A randomized trial. J Bone Joint Surg Am 86-A(3):455–464
50. Gudas R et al (2006) Osteochondral autologous transplantation versus microfracture for the treatment of articular cartilage defects in the knee joint in athletes. Knee Surg Sports Traumatol Arthrosc 14(9):834–842
51. Knutsen G et al (2007) A randomized trial comparing autologous chondrocyte implantation with microfracture. Findings at five years. J Bone Joint Surg Am 89(10):2105–2112
52. Steadman JR et al (2003) Outcomes of microfracture for traumatic chondral defects of the knee: average 11-year follow-up. Arthroscopy 19(5):477–484

53. Namdari S et al (2009) Results and performance after microfracture in National Basketball Association athletes. Am J Sports Med 37(5):943–948
54. Riyami M, Rolf C (2009) Evaluation of microfracture of traumatic chondral injuries to the knee in professional football and rugby players. J Orthop Surg Res 4:13
55. Gobbi A, Nunag P, Malinowski K (2005) Treatment of full thickness chondral lesions of the knee with microfracture in a group of athletes. Knee Surg Sports Traumatol Arthrosc 13(3):213–221
56. Peterson L et al (2000) Two- to 9-year outcome after autologous chondrocyte transplantation of the knee. Clin Orthop Relat Res 374:212–234
57. Minas T (2001) Autologous chondrocyte implantation for focal chondral defects of the knee. Clin Orthop Relat Res (391 Suppl):S349–S361
58. Peterson L et al (2002) Autologous chondrocyte transplantation. Biomechanics and long-term durability. Am J Sports Med 30(1):2–12
59. Bentley G et al (2003) A prospective, randomised comparison of autologous chondrocyte implantation versus mosaicplasty for osteochondral defects in the knee. J Bone Joint Surg Br 85(2):223–230
60. Horas U et al (2003) Autologous chondrocyte implantation and osteochondral cylinder transplantation in cartilage repair of the knee joint. A prospective, comparative trial. J Bone Joint Surg Am 85-A(2):185–192
61. Dozin B et al (2005) Comparative evaluation of autologous chondrocyte implantation and mosaicplasty: a multicentered randomized clinical trial. Clin J Sport Med 15(4):220–226
62. Muellner T et al (2001) Failed autologous chondrocyte implantation. Complete atraumatic graft delamination after two years. Am J Sports Med 29(4):516–519
63. Saris DB et al (2009) Treatment of symptomatic cartilage defects of the knee: characterized chondrocyte implantation results in better clinical outcome at 36 months in a randomized trial compared to microfracture. Am J Sports Med 37(Suppl 1):10S–19S
64. Kreuz PC et al (2007) Importance of sports in cartilage regeneration after autologous chondrocyte implantation: a prospective study with a 3-year follow-up. Am J Sports Med 35(8):1261–1268
65. Kreuz PC et al (2006) Results after microfracture of full-thickness chondral defects in different compartments in the knee. Osteoarthritis Cartilage 14(11):1119–1125
66. Iwasa J et al (2009) Clinical application of scaffolds for cartilage tissue engineering. Knee Surg Sports Traumatol Arthrosc 17(6):561–577
67. Bobic V (1996) Arthroscopic osteochondral autograft transplantation in anterior cruciate ligament reconstruction: a preliminary clinical study. Knee Surg Sports Traumatol Arthrosc 3(4):262–264
68. Hangody L et al (2001) Mosaicplasty for the treatment of articular defects of the knee and ankle. Clin Orthop Relat Res (391 Suppl):S328–S336
69. Safran MR, Kim H, Zaffagnini S (2008) The use of scaffolds in the management of articular cartilage injury. J Am Acad Orthop Surg 16(6):306–311
70. Williams RJ, Gamradt SC (2008) Articular cartilage repair using a resorbable matrix scaffold. Instr Course Lect 57:563–571
71. Kerker JT, Leo AJ, Sgaglione NA (2008) Cartilage repair: synthetics and scaffolds: basic science, surgical techniques, and clinical outcomes. Sports Med Arthrosc 16(4):208–216
72. Koga H et al (2009) Mesenchymal stem cell-based therapy for cartilage repair: a review. Knee Surg Sports Traumatol Arthrosc 17(11):1289–1297
73. Salzmann GM et al (2009) Sporting activity after high tibial osteotomy for the treatment of medial compartment knee osteoarthritis. Am J Sports Med 37(2):312–318
74. Bradbury N et al (1998) Participation in sports after total knee replacement. Am J Sports Med 26(4):530–535
75. Fisher N et al (2006) Sporting and physical activity following Oxford medial unicompartmental knee arthroplasty. Knee 13(4):296–300
76. Naal FD et al (2007) Return to sports and recreational activity after unicompartmental knee arthroplasty. Am J Sports Med 35(10):1688–1695
77. Hopper GP, Leach WJ (2008) Participation in sporting activities following knee replacement: total versus unicompartmental. Knee Surg Sports Traumatol Arthrosc 16(10):973–979
78. Walton NP et al (2006) Patient-perceived outcomes and return to sport and work: TKA versus mini-incision unicompartmental knee arthroplasty. J Knee Surg 19(2):112–116
79. Hochberg M (2002) Prevention of lower limb osteoarthritis: data from the Johns Hopkins Precursors Study. In: Hascall VC, Kuettner KE (eds) The many faces of osteoarthritis. Birkhauser, Basel, pp 31–37
80. Felson DT (1998) Preventing knee and hip osteoarthritis. Bull Rheum Dis 47(7):1–4
81. Felson DT et al (1991) Occupational physical demands, knee bending, and knee osteoarthritis: results from the Framingham Study. J Rheumatol 18(10):1587–1592
82. Felson DT et al (1992) Weight loss reduces the risk for symptomatic knee osteoarthritis in women. The Framingham Study. Ann Intern Med 116(7):535–539
83. Manninen P et al (1996) Overweight, gender and knee osteoarthritis. Int J Obes Relat Metab Disord 20(6):595–597
84. Zhang W et al (2008) OARSI recommendations for the management of hip and knee osteoarthritis, part II: OARSI evidence-based, expert consensus guidelines. Osteoarthritis Cartilage 16(2):137–162

85. Smith W, Walter J Jr, Bailey M (1985) Effects of insoles in Coast Guard basic training footwear. J Am Podiatr Med Assoc 75(12):644–647
86. Sitler M et al (1990) The efficacy of a prophylactic knee brace to reduce knee injuries in football. A prospective, randomized study at West Point. Am J Sports Med 18(3):310–315
87. Olsen OE et al (2005) Exercises to prevent lower limb injuries in youth sports: cluster randomised controlled trial. BMJ 330(7489):449
88. Myklebust G et al (2003) Prevention of anterior cruciate ligament injuries in female team handball players: a prospective intervention study over three seasons. Clin J Sport Med 13(2):71–78
89. Soligard T et al (2008) Comprehensive warm-up programme to prevent injuries in young female footballers: cluster randomised controlled trial. BMJ 337:a2469

Meniscal Lesions Today: Evidence for Treatment

Philippe Beaufils, Nicola Pujol, and Philippe Boisrenoult

It is not long ago that every suspicion of a meniscal lesion eventually led to meniscectomy, which in most of the cases was total. This solution was considered to be a simple and effective procedure followed by a speedy recovery. But reviewing patients at long term follow-up, it obviously appeared that many of these patients presented with significant cartilaginous changes. Fairbank [13] was the first to document long-term degenerative changes after subtotal meniscectomy.

Two truly revolutionary improvements were introduced in the 1970s and 1980s: arthroscopic surgery and subsequently magnetic resonance imaging (MRI) which contributed to a better understanding of meniscal pathology, diagnostic techniques and principles of treatment, and resulted in a lower complication rate. It was thus realized that the menisci play a prominent role in knee joint biomechanics. At the same time, anatomical studies demonstrated the peripheral blood supply of the meniscus allowing a healing process [2].

There is not just one but many different meniscal lesions and consequently not just one but various treatment methods, adapted to the type of lesion and its clinical context. This has led to the concept of meniscal preservation or meniscal sparing, which is based on three pillars:

P. Beaufils (✉) • N. Pujol • P. Boisrenoult
Orthopaedic Department, Versailles Hospital,
F 78150 Le Chesnay, France
e-mail: pbeaufils@ch-versailles.fr;
npujol@ch-versailles.fr; pboisrenoult@ch-versailles.fr

meniscectomy as partial as possible, thanks to arthroscopy, meniscal repair and "masterly neglect". In clinical practice, one can be faced with two distinct situations: a traumatic meniscal lesion in a stable or unstable knee, or a degenerative meniscal lesion (DML), which is or is not associated with macroscopic arthritic changes.

For each of these situations specific algorithm is required.

In the traumatic group, meniscus repair or "leave the meniscus alone" should be considered as the first choices. Meniscectomy should be proposed when neither of the above options is applicable.

In the degenerate group, "leave the meniscus alone" should probably be the first choice; meniscectomy could be considered in cases of functional treatment failure. There are no or very few indications for meniscus repair.

We will not discuss in this chapter meniscal lesions in children nor the concept of meniscal reconstruction after failed meniscectomy, using either an allograft or a meniscus scaffold. These questions require a distinct discussion.

Traumatic Lesions

Meniscus Repair in Traumatic Vertical Longitudinal Lesions

Arthroscopic meniscal repair has been the procedure of choice for many years to treat traumatic vertical lesions occurring in a vascularized zone, whatever the anterior cruciate ligament (ACL) status. The techniques have evolved from open repairs to all-inside arthroscopic repairs with hybrid devices or suture systems; the out-in Technique remains adapted to the anterior part of the meniscus.

Failure and Secondary Meniscectomy

Subsequent meniscectomy is the main clinical failure criterion after meniscal repair. In a systematic review of clinical results of all-inside meniscal repairs [20], the clinical failure rate varied from 0 to 43.5 %, with a mean failure rate of 15 %. By selecting studies with a mean follow-up of more than 24 months, and a number of patients superior more than 50 [26] (Table 1) the failure rate ranged from 4.8 to 28 % (mean 13 %). At the French Arthroscopic Society symposium [4] in 2003, 203 cases were retrospectively reviewed. Secondary meniscectomy was performed in 23 % of cases (Fig. 1). Meniscectomy, was performed within the first 2 years in 4/5 of cases. Siebold et al. reported the same results [32] with 81.5 % of failures occurring within 3 years. Moreover, Arnoczky et al. [2] showed that meniscal healing takes place over a period of at least 18 months. Instability of the repair early in this period may result in unsuccessful healing of the tear.

In our failure series (37 out of 295) [27], we assessed the amount of secondary meniscal resection compared with the initial extent of the meniscal tear before repair: 84 % of the cases had an equal or inferior secondary resection compared with the virtual primary resection if repair had not been carried out (Fig. 2). There are thus few detrimental effects when repairing a repairable meniscal lesion, even if it fails. The amount of meniscectomy is rarely increased when compared with the initial lesion. This study supports the hypothesis that the meniscus can be partially saved and that a risk of a partial failure should be taken when possible [27].

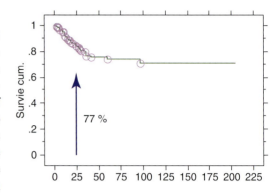

Fig. 1 Survival curve in the French Arthroscopy Society series [4]. Four out of five subsequent meniscectomies occur within the first 2 years

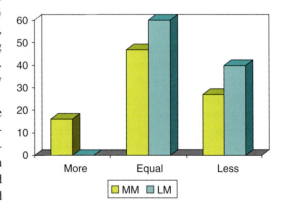

Fig. 2 Amount of meniscal resection during subsequent meniscectomy compared with virtual primary meniscectomy

Table 1 Clinical failure rates of all-inside arthroscopic meniscal repairs

Author	Year	N	Mean follow-up (months)	Failure (%)	Definition of failure	Level of evidence
Siebold	2007	105	72	27 (28.4 %)	Meniscectomy	IV
Spindler	2003	85	27	7 (8.2 %)	Meniscectomy or re-repair	II
Kurzweil	2005	60	54	17 (28 %)	Clinical failure	IV
Koukoulias	2007	62	73	3 (4.8 %)	Meniscectomy	III
Quinby	2006	54	34.8	5 (9.3 %)	Meniscectomy	IV

Functional Results

Varying global results have been reported, ranging from 62 to 90 % good clinical or functional results at the mid-term to long-term follow-up (2–20 years) [11, 14, 18, 30, 36, 40]. At the French Arthroscopic Society symposium, good results (taking into account failures and subsequent meniscectomies) were reported in 62 % of patients [4], which is confirmed by Majewski et al. [21]. At follow-up, 21 % patients had undergone secondary meniscectomy, 17 % had some residual pain and 62 had a normal knee.

Nevertheless, Shelbourne and Dersam [31] showed that at 8 years, subjective results of repair were better than those of partial meniscectomy.

Anatomical Results: Healing Rate and Meniscal Shortening

The healing status of repaired menisci can be assessed by either second-look arthroscopy [17], arthrography, arthro-CT, or arthro-MRI Complete healing was reported in 42–88 % of cases (Table 2). In studies with arthroscopic second look to assess healing, complete healing was found in 73–88 % of cases. In studies with arthrographic or arthro-CT assessment of healing, complete healing was found in 45–59 % of cases. In a prospective study including clinical and anatomical assessments [24], we evaluated 53 arthroscopic all-inside meniscal repairs. According to Henning's criteria 58 % of the menisci healed completely, 24 % partially, and 18 % failed. The overall healing rate (taking into account the horizontal extent of the tear) is 73.1 %. There is a correlation between the longitudinal healing rate and the subjective IKDC score ($p<0.03$, $r^2=0.44$). Isolated tears located in the posterior part have a lower healing rate ($p<0.05$) (Fig. 3). As in our series, van Trommel et al. [39] found a poor healing rate of the posterior third probably because of the difficulty of performing perpendicular sutures into the posterior segment We hypothesize that abrasion of the posterior segment is difficult to perform properly by standard anterior arthroscopic approaches. The optimal conditions for good healing are difficult to obtain. It may be easier when a posterior arthroscopic portal is used.

According to the fact that not only complete but also partial healing is related to good functional and clinical results we can hypothetize that the goal of meniscus repair is not to obtain a complete healing but to transform an unstable, symptomatic meniscus in a stable meniscus, even if a short tear remains. But the threshold has not been determined yet.

Pujol et al. [24] demonstrated also significant meniscal shortening (between 10 and 15 %) of the repaired middle segments for both menisci, and for the posterior segment of the medial meniscus (Fig. 3) It could not yet be established whether this is due to meniscal abrasion, suture tightening, or the shrinkage effect of the healing process. There is a significant correlation between the rate of shortening and the healing rate, and the best clinical outcomes are obtained in shortened and healed menisci.

Prognostic Factors

Anterior Cruciate Ligament Injury. If the ACL is torn, concomitant ACL reconstruction should be considered. In most recent studies, meniscal repairs in stable or stabilized knees have the same objective and subjective results [1, 3, 4, 24, 36]. When meniscus repair is proposed in ACL-deficient knees without ACL reconstruction [19, 35] 13–27 % of patients undergo subsequent meniscectomy and 33 % of patients secondary ACL reconstruction. This procedure is not contra-indicated, but indications should be selected with extreme caution, especially in young patients.

Location of the Tear

Results of repairs in the red-red zone are equivalent to those in the red-white zone [4, 25, 29, 40].

Lateral/Medial Meniscus

Due to highly vascularized areas, lateral tears may heal better than medial tears. Tuckman et al. [38] found a superior healing rate for the lateral meniscus compared to the medial meniscus (80 % versus 56 % complete healing). In the study of the French Arthroscopic Society [4],

Table 2 Operative data and outcomes of medial meniscus tears left in place

Author	n	Mean length of tear (mm)	Type of tear	Selection criteria for treatment	Follow-up (months)	Clinical assessment	Clinical score/100	Pain or mechanical symptoms (%)	Meniscectomy or repair (%)	Anatomical control	Healing	Procedure
Beaufils	23	8	Full thickness tear	Stable	26	Yes		17	0	Arthroscopy (2) or arthrography (11)	61 % healing 38 % partial healing 1 % unhealed	Left in situ
Talley	19	<15	Full thickness tear	Stable	38			0	21	–	–	Left in situ
Pierre	60	9.8 ± 4 (5–20)	Full thickness tear	Stable <20 mm	48	IKDC	–	–	17	–	–	Left in situ
Yagishita	41	12 (5–25)	16 full thickness tears 25 partial thickness tears	Stable <15 mm	16 (7–41)	Yes	–	12	7.3	Arthroscopy	54 % healed 7 % partially healed 27 % unhealed 12 % tear extended	Left in situ
Zemanovic	8	–	Partial thickness tear	Partial thickness tear	24.6	Lysholm	92.1	–	0	–		Left in situ
Shelbourne	139 233	– –	Full thickness tear	Stable >10 mm	88	Questionnaire	93.1 95.4	5 4.3	10.8 6	– –	– –	Left in situ Abrasion trephination
Lynch	9	–	–	Stable	45.6 (36–120)	Yes	–	66	0	–	–	Left in situ
Weiss	6	–	Partial thickness tear	Partial thickness tear	21.8 (3–50)	Lysholm	–	0	33	Arthroscopy	50 % healed 50 % unhealed	Left in situ
	2	–	Full thickness tear	Stable	27.5 (25–30)			0	0		50 % healed 50 % unhealed	

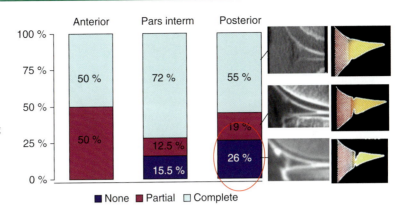

Fig. 3 Arthro-CT scan. Healing rate according to Henning's criteria: complete healing, partial healing (>50 %) or failure (<50 %) and longitudinal 2-D reconstructions to assess healing by segments, and global or longitudinal healing rate of the tear

24 % subsequent medial meniscectomies and 11 % subsequent lateral meniscectomies were required after repair.

Age

More than patient age, the quality of the meniscal tissue should be carefully considered. A traumatic vertical longitudinal tear in a macroscopically-normal meniscus should be considered for repair, regardless of whether patients are 50 or 20 years of age.

Time from Tear to Surgery

Recent tears (less than 12 weeks) may have a better prognosis. Chronic bucket-handle tears may be difficult to reduce and to repair properly without overtensioning the sutures to the capsule.

Long Term Results: Secondary Arthritis

Rockborn and Messner [30] retrospectively compared a consecutive series of 30 patients with open meniscus repair to 30 patients who had undergone arthroscopic partial or subtotal meniscectomy. After 7 years joint space reduction was more common after initial meniscectomy than after repair (P<0.05). After 13 years the incidence and severity of osteoarthritis did not differ significantly between the two groups, even when only the successful repairs were compared to meniscectomy (P=0.06). For Stein et al. [37], no osteoarthritic progress was detectable in 80.8 % after repair compared with 40.0 % after meniscectomy (p=0.005).

Our long term results (mean follow-up=114 months) after all-inside repairs demonstrated:
- objective clinical results were good and stable with time (subjective IKDC=94-range 62–100)
- MRI signal abnormalities remained in 70 % in the repaired menisci (Fig. 4)
- 70 % had no degenerative changes and 22.5 % grade 1 joint narrowing compared with the contralateral knee on standard X rays
- the initial healing rate did not influence clinical nor radiological results

"Leave the Meniscus Alone"

In case of ACL tear, a commonly shared opinion is that unstable or symptomatic meniscal tears should be surgically repaired at the time of ACL reconstruction, while stable asymptomatic tears should be left untreated. However, lesion instability has not been clearly defined and the problem of establishing proper criteria (e.g. size of lesion and abnormal mobility of the meniscus) remains unsolved.

In an evidence-based-review based on ten relevant studies [25], with a mean time FU of 16 months, Pujol found subsequent meniscectomy or repair was performed in 0–33 % in the medial meniscus (Table 2) and 0–22 % in the lateral meniscus (Table 3). A complete healing occurred in 50–61 % of the medial menisci and 5–74 % of the lateral menisci. Despite the fact that it is difficult to draw definite conclusions, it appears

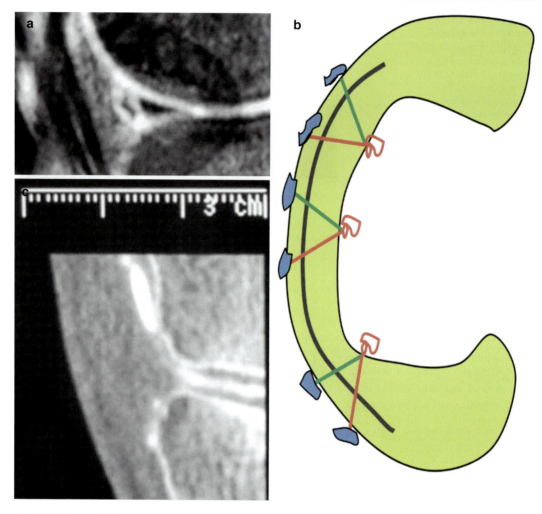

Fig. 4 (**a**) Pre-op MRI: vertical longitudinal lesion lying in the red zone. (**b**) Drawing of meniscal shortening (**c**) post-op arthro-CT scan: complete healing with shortening of the meniscus width

the mean rate of bad results for the medial meniscus remains high. Repair of a medial tear, even if it is a stable peripheral tears may be always considered to decrease the risk of subsequent meniscectomy. "Let the lateral meniscus alone" is an acceptable proposal.

Indications: Guidelines

To summarize:
- the risk of subsequent meniscectomy is about 15–20 %
- the risk of anatomical failure (no healing) is about 15–20 %
- the shortening of the healed meniscus is about 15 %
- the risk of secondary osteoarthritis is about 15–20 %

Considering this low rate of poor results, we suggest that surgeons take the risk of a repair failure and propose the following guidelines which have been adopted in France under the auspices of the Haute Autorité de Santé [5, 6].

Traumatic Lesions in a Stable Knee

Surgical removal of the torn fragment is most commonly performed because in the vast majority of cases the tear is located in the avascular zone of the meniscus. The long-term prognosis is

Meniscal Lesions Today: Evidence for Treatment 243

Table 3 Operative data and outcomes of lateral meniscus tears left in place

Author	n	Mean length of tear (mm)	Type of tear	Selection criteria for treatment	Mean follow-up (months)	Clinical assessment	Clinical score/100	Pain or mechanical symptoms (%) without treatment	Meniscectomy or repair (%)	Anatomical control	Healing	Procedure
Weiss	9	–	Partial thickness tear	Partial thickness tear	29 (6–79)	Lysholm	–	0	22	Arthroscopy	55 % healed 22.5 % unhealed 22.5 % extended	Left in situ
	15	–	Full thickness tear	Stable	27.3 (6–100)			0	13.3		45.6 % healed 40 % unhealed 13.4 % extended	
Talley	25	<15	Full thickness tear	Stable	38	Yes	–	0	4	–	–	Left in situ
Pierre	35	10 ± 4 (5–20)	Full thickness tear	Stable <20 mm	48	IKDC		–	0	–	–	Left in situ
Yagishita	42	10.8 (5–25)	18 partial thickness tears 24 full thickness tears	Stable <15 mm	18.3	Yes	–	7	7.1	Arthroscopy (n =)	74 % healed 5 % partially healed 14 % unhealed 7 % tear extended	Left in situ
Zemanovic	23	–	Partial thickness tear	partial thickness tear	24.6	Lysholm	92.1	–	0	–	–	Left in situ
Shelbourne	239	–	Full thickness tear	Stable	79	Noyes	93.8	2.5	3.3	–	–	Left in situ/ abrasion-trephination

(continued)

Table 3 (continued)

Author	n	Mean length of tear (mm)	Type of tear	Selection criteria for treatment	Mean follow-up (months)	Clinical assessment	Clinical score/100	Pain or mechanical symptoms (%) without treatment	Meniscectomy or repair (%)	Anatomical control	Healing	Procedure
Fitzgibbons	189	–	Full and partial thickness tears	Stable	31.2	Noyes	92.2 (48–100)	0	0	–	–	Abrasion-trephination
Lynch	22	–	–	Stable	45.6 (36–120)	Yes	–	18	0	–	–	Left in situ
Beaufils	8	–	Full thickness tear	Stable	26 (12–40)	Yes	–	0	0	Arthroscopy (2) or arthrography (11)	61 % healing 38 % partial healing 1 % unhealed	Left in situ

favourable, provided that the meniscectomy has been a partial [9] meniscectomy. As a rule, asymptomatic lesions should be left alone.

Meniscal repair should always be considered when the anatomical conditions are favourable (lesion located within the red-red or red-white zone), at a short time from injury. Particular attention must be paid to the possible detrimental effect of meniscectomy in children and lateral meniscectomy with the high risk of rapid (ref) or late cartilage degeneration. Indications for repair should therefore be extended in these situations. It is in these cases that the techniques of stimulating healing (fibrin clot, abrasion, and perhaps growth factors) are most applicable, particularly for longstanding, more extensive lesions and white-white lesions.

Traumatic Meniscal Lesion in an ACL-Deficient Knee

Every effort should be made to avoid subsequent meniscectomy, Masterly neglect or surgical repair are considered to be the best solution, the more so since these lesions are most often located in the peripheral vascularized zone of the meniscus and have the best chance to heal.

These lesions fall into one of the following categories:

1. Symptomatic anterior laxity of the knee (functional instability) in an active individual practising sports, in whom ACL reconstruction is strongly indicated. In this situation the meniscal lesion is diagnosed before surgery and is treated simultaneously. The ACL surgery is aimed at optimally restoring joint function and protecting the cartilage thanks to meniscal tissue preservation.
2. Anterior laxity of the knee associated with minor symptoms in an active individual who is not engaged in high-demand sports activities. In this case the indications for ACL reconstruction are not straightforward considering the functional limitation of the patient. A diagnosis of a reparable meniscal lesion may be an important argument in favour of surgery. The goal of ACL reconstruction then is to protect the articular cartilage and to improve the natural history of the knee joint.

A simple meniscectomy can only be considered in case of a symptomatic meniscal lesion in a sedentary middle-aged patient who does not present functional instability.

3. Meniscal repair or "leave the meniscus alone"?

In conjunction with ACL reconstruction, we can assume that the indications for surgical repair can be extended for the medial meniscus (increased risk of secondary meniscectomy if left alone), whereas for the lateral meniscus masterly neglect can be the preferred approach (low risk of subsequent meniscectomy).

New Trends

Thanks to biomechanical studies, we know that a tear of the peripheral meniscal belt or an avulsion of one meniscal horn may dramatically change the mechanical behavior of the meniscus and thus produce late cartilaginous changes (Fig. 5). In this way, extended indications of meniscus repair have been proposed in selected cases:

1. horizontal cleavage in the young athlete may be considered as an overuse lesion and should be differentiated from the well known degenerate lesion in older patients. It appears as an intra-meniscal (grade2) or extra-meniscal (grade3) horizontal cleavage sometimes associated with a peripheral meniscal cyst. Biedert [7] was the first to propose repair in these cases. Rather than an arthroscopic repair, we perform an open technique which allows the debridement of the intra-meniscal lesion close to the horizontal cleavage and we insert vertical strong bio-absorbable stitches (Fig. 6). In our review of 30 knees [28] with 40 months FU, the meniscus was preserved in 80 %; functional results deteriorate in patients older than 30.
2. radial tears in young patients could be considered for repair when extended to the periphery, specially on the lateral meniscus
3. root tears have been recently described [41]. Frequent degenerate root tears must be differentiated from true traumatic root tears which are rare. These traumatic root tears are often associated with an ACL tear especially on the

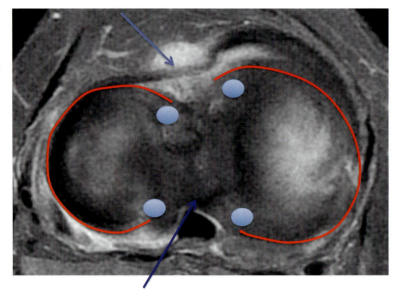

Fig. 5 Menisci are included in a complete peripheral circumferential belt which acts against extrusion forces. This belt is made of: meniscal horns (*circles*), anterior intermeniscal ligament and meniscofemoral ligaments (*blue arrows*), peripheral capsule and menisco-capsular junction (*red line*)

posterior horn of the lateral meniscus. They have been ignored for a long time and should be systematically assessed during an ACL reconstruction. They can be treated by tibial re-fixation, using a trans-tibial tunnel.

Degenerate Meniscal Lesions

Definition

A degenerate meniscal lesion (DML) occurs in the absence of an injury or as a result of decompensation after minor trauma. It can be assumed that the ageing process of the affected meniscal tissue and its deterioration has advanced to a certain degree. This idea was first introduced by Smillie [34] and Noble and Erat [23]. Their conclusions were subsequently confirmed by arthroscopic and then MRI evidence (Fig. 7).

The relationship between DML and osteoarthritis of the knee is uncertain. Currently, the question whether DML always leads to the development of osteoarthritis or whether the concept of a 'primary' lesion is correct, remains unanswered:

In favour of a strong relationship between DML and osteoarthritis: the prevalence of MRI meniscal abnormalities increases with age and meniscal tears are systematically associated with osteoarthritic knees [8, 12, 43].

In favour of a "primary" lesion: DML are more frequent in men than women (2–1), which is exactly the opposite of osteoarthritis. DML may develop earlier, even in young athletes without any chondral degenerate process.

Practically speaking, the key point for a clinician treating a patient presenting with knee pain, is therefore to know whether the patient suffers from a DML in a joint with macroscopically intact chondral surfaces or from early-stage osteoarthritis with a co-existent DML. In the first case, meniscectomy would be assumed to be a "curative" procedure, while in the second one, it would be purely palliative (the so called arthroscopic debridement). Because in everyday practice it is impossible to obtain direct information on the microscopic structure of cartilage, its condition is assessed by means of standard radiography and MRI.

Algorithm: Guidelines

It is therefore possible to establish an algorithm for the management of knee pain in these cases [5]. Treatment consists either of masterly neglect or arthroscopic meniscectomy as surgical repair is seldom indicated.

The primary treatment of these lesions is conservative and consists of rest, non-steroidal

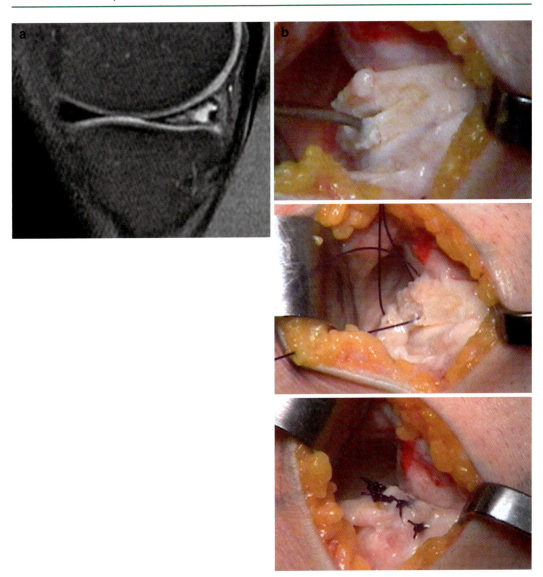

Fig. 6 (**a**) Grade 2 hypersignal in a young athlete. (**b**) Open meniscus repair: the cleavage is debrided and closed with vertical bio-absorbable stitches

anti-inflammatory drugs and physiotherapy [15, 16, 42]. Herrlin et al. [16] comparing arthroscopic and conservative treatment in a randomised trial, found that 6 months after treatment, arthroscopic partial medial meniscectomy followed by supervised, exercise did not result in lower pain and higher knee function compared with supervised exercise alone. A substantial number of DML respond well to conservative treatment and the symptoms resolve spontaneously even if the lesions do not heal. If improvement fails to occur within a few months (around 6 months), comparative weight-bearing roentgenograms including Schuss views and MRI must be obtained.

Three questions should be asked:
- are the symptoms related with the meniscal tear?
- is there any joint space narrowing on the standard X Rays, evidence of osteoarthritic changes?
- are some early signs of osteoarthritis associated with the meniscal tear on MRI? Early signs consist of meniscal extrusion [10] and

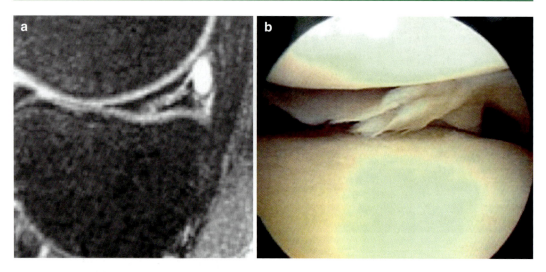

Fig. 7 MRI and arthroscopic view of a typical degenerate medial meniscal lesion (horizontal flap)

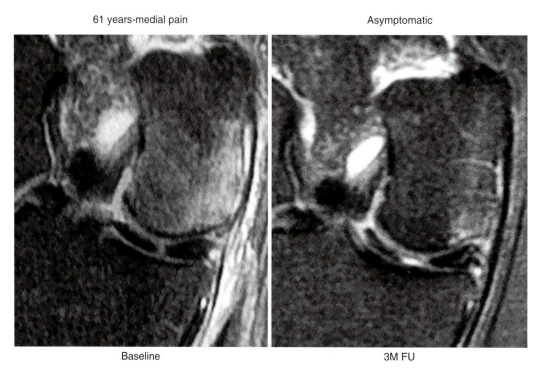

Fig. 8 Sixty-one-year-old patient with medial knee pain. MRI shows a meniscal tear of the posterior segment associated with femoral condylar bone marrow oedema. Conservative treatment. At 3 months, the patient is asymptomatic with a significant decrease of the condylar hypersignal. The meniscal tear is still there

subchondral abnormalities. An extrusion more than 3 mm is said to be strongly related with osteoarthritis and shouldn't be regarded as a meniscal lesion itself. Significance of subchondral hypersignal is not univocal: in the weight-bearing area, it could be regarded as an early sign of osteoarthritis, specially if it is present on both sides (femur and tibia). It also can be due to vascular changes (early stage of osteonecrosis) or subchondral microfractures (Fig. 8), which would favour conservative treatment. Significance of marginal bone

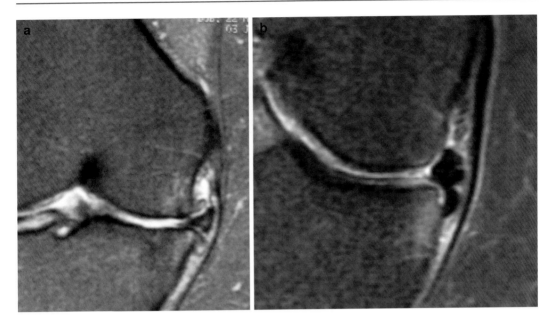

Fig. 9 (**a**) Marginal bone marrow oedema with meniscal extrusion; (**b**) marginal tibial bone marrow oedema due to the impingement with a meniscal flap tear everted in the tibial gutter. Indication for meniscectomy

marrow oedema is more controversial: due to extrusion (early osteoarthritis) or to impingement with a meniscal displaced flap (Fig. 9)

Answering these three questions allows to us to distinguish "primary DML's" and DML's associated with osteoarthritis ("meniscarthrosis")

An algorithm has been proposed by the French Healthcare Authority (Haute Autorité de Santé, HAS) [5], (Fig. 10)

1. If the joint line is normal, if MRI shows a grade 3 meniscal lesion and the subchondral bone signal is unaltered, and if the clinical findings correlate with the meniscal lesion, the diagnosis of primary DML is established and arthroscopic meniscectomy can reasonably be suggested, specially if symptoms are not only of pain but also of clicking or locking suggesting an unstable meniscal tear (i.e.: flap) (Fig. 7). In these circumstances, one can expect a good and stable result [9].
2. If joint space narrowing is present and the diagnosis of osteoarthritis of the knee is established. Numerous studies have shown that the outcome of arthroscopic debridement and meniscectomy is roughly similar to the effect of placebo [22, 33]. Moseley et al. [22] randomly assigned 180 patients (mean age 52 years) with OA of the knee to undergo arthroscopic debridement, arthroscopic lavage, or placebo surgery. Patients in the placebo group received skin incisions and underwent a simulated debridement without insertion of the arthroscope. The mean follow-up was 24 months. Subjective results including pain and walking ability were not statistically different between subgroups. Siparsky et al. [33] performed a retrospective, evidence-based review of the current literature on the arthroscopic treatment of osteoarthritis of the knee Of the 18 relevant studies, 1 was Level I evidence [22], 5 were Level II, 6 were Level III, and 6 were Level IV. We found limited evidence-based research to support the use of arthroscopy as a treatment method for osteoarthritis of the knee. Arthroscopic débridement of meniscus tears and knees with low-grade osteoarthritis may have some utility, but it should not be used as a routine treatment for all patients with knee osteoarthritis. There is thus no need for arthroscopic debridement in these patients, with the rare exception of acute trauma to an osteoarthritic knee, which can result in an additional traumatic meniscal lesion, or symptoms of internal "derangement".
3. If there is no evidence of joint space narrowing but MRI shows a meniscal extrusion or a

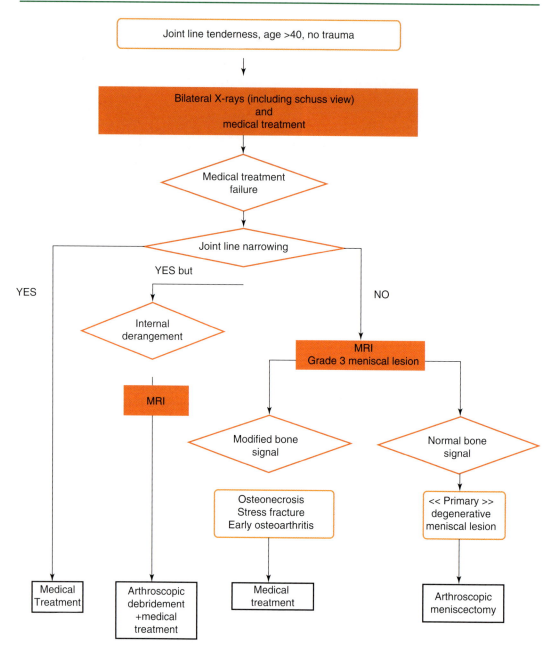

Fig. 10 Algorithm for the management of knee pain in middle-aged patients according to the Haute Autorité de Santé guidelines [5]

subchondral bone abnormal signal, treatment should be focussed on the cause of the disease and meniscectomy is not routinely indicated. There is a high risk of post-op. difficulties such as rapid chondrolysis or subsequent osteonecrosis. Refraining from surgical treatment should always be considered in this instance, except in the rare cases of "internal derangement" with evidence of unstable meniscal tears responsible for bone marrow oedema (Fig. 9).

Conclusions

Meniscectomy, one of the most frequent Orthopaedic procedures, is probably too frequent. Meniscus repair is probably too rare. In

France, meniscus repair only represents 4.5 % of the meniscal procedure in stable knees in daily practice. We cannot exactly assess the rate of conservative treatment (since many of these cases do not come to the surgeon) so that it is not possible to compare the respective roles of Conservative Treatment, Meniscectomy and Meniscus Repair. But we can assume the rate of meniscectomies should decrease and the rate of repair or conservative treatment should increase.

Based on literature evidence, it appears:
1. meniscus repair has an acceptable failure rate, gives good functional results and does heal, provided the indication is pertinent. It means vertical longitudinal peripheral tears with macroscopic normal tissue in a stable or stabilized knee. Repair could be pushed in some selected situations such as intrameniscal tears in young athletes, some extended radial tears or traumatic root tears.
2. "Leave the meniscus alone" is particularly indicated in stable lateral meniscal tears associated with ACL reconstruction. But its main indication is the so called DML: let the meniscus alone must be the first therapeutic choice before considering arthroscopic meniscectomy. Doing so, the rate of meniscectomy should dramatically decrease in favour of conservative treatment.

It is obvious that daily practice doesn't correspond to experts' indications. Teaching, Continuous Medical Education, Guidelines produced by Healthcare Authorities and/or Scientific Societies,… might help to spread the concept of meniscus preservation.

References

1. Ahn JH, Wang JH, Yoo JC (2004) Arthroscopic all-inside suture repair of medial meniscus lesion in anterior cruciate ligament – deficient knees: results of second-look arthroscopies in 39 cases. Arthroscopy 20:936–945
2. Arnoczky SP, Cooper TG, Stadelmaier DM, Hannafin JA (1994) Magnetic resonance signals in healing menisci: an experimental study in dogs. Arthroscopy 10:552–557
3. Bach BR Jr, Dennis M, Balin J, Hayden J (2005) Arthroscopic meniscal repair: analysis of treatment failures. J Knee Surg 18:278–284
4. Beaufils P, Cassard X (2004) Meniscal repair. Rev Chir Orthop Reparatrice Appar Mot 90:3S49–3S75
5. Beaufils P, Hulet C, Dhénain M, Nizard R, Nourissat G, Pujol N (2009) Clinical practice guidelines for the management of meniscal lesions and isolated lesions of the anterior cruciate ligament of the knee in adults. Orthop Traumatol Surg Res 95:437–442
6. Beaufils P (2010) Synthesis – indications. In: Beaufils P, Verdonk R (eds) The meniscus. Springer, Berlin/New York, pp 235–238
7. Biedert RM (2000) Treatment of intrasubstance meniscal lesions: a randomized prospective study of four different methods. Knee Surg Sports Traumatol Arthrosc 8:104–108
8. Bhattacharyya T, Gale D, Dewire P, Totterman S, Gale ME, McLaughlin S et al (2003) The clinical importance of meniscal tears demonstrated by magnetic resonance imaging in osteoarthritis of the knee. J Bone Joint Surg Am 85A:4–9
9. Chatain F, Robinson AH, Adeleine P, Chambat P, Neyret P (2001) The natural history of the knee following arthroscopic medial meniscectomy. Knee Surg Sports Traumatol Arthrosc 9:15–18
10. Costa CR, Morrison WB, Carrino JA (2004) Medial meniscus extrusion on knee MRI: is extent associated with severity of degeneration or type of tear? AJR Am J Roentgenol 183:17–23
11. Eggli S, Wegmuller H, Kosina J, Huckell C, Jakob RP (1995) Long-term results of arthroscopic meniscal repair. An analysis of isolated tears. Am J Sports Med 23:715–720
12. Englund M, Roos EM, Lohmander LS (2003) Impact of type of meniscal tear on radiographic and symptomatic knee osteoarthritis: a sixteen-year follow up of meniscectomy with matched controls. Arthritis Rheum 48:2178
13. Fairbank TJ (1948) Knee joint changes after meniscectomy. J Bone Joint Surg Am 30B:664–670
14. Haas AL, Schepsis AA, Hornstein J, Edgar CM (2005) Meniscal repair using the FasT-Fix all-inside meniscal repair device. Arthroscopy 21:167–175
15. Hede A, Hempel-Poulsen S, Jensen JS (1990) Symptoms and level of sports activity in patients awaiting arthroscopy for meniscal lesions of the knee. J Bone Joint Surg Am 72A:550–552
16. Herrlin S, Hallander M, Wanger P, Weidenhielm L, Werner S (2007) Arthroscopic or conservative treatment of degenerative medial meniscal tears: a prospective randomised trial. Knee Surg Sports Traumatol Arthrosc 15:393–401
17. Horibe S, Shino K, Maeda A, Nakamura N, Matsumoto N, Ochi T (1996) Results of isolated meniscal repair evaluated by second-look arthroscopy. Arthroscopy 12:150–155
18. Kotsovolos ES, Hantes ME, Mastrokalos DS, Lorbach O, Paessler HH (2006) Results of all-inside meniscal repair with the FasT-Fix meniscal repair system. Arthroscopy 22:3–9

19. Koukoulias N, Papastergiou S, Kazakos K, Poulios G, Parisis K (2007) Clinical results of meniscus repair with the meniscus arrow: a 4- to 8-year follow-up study. Knee Surg Sports Traumatol Arthrosc 15:133–137
20. Lozano J, Ma CB, Cannon WD (2007) All-inside meniscus repair: a systematic review. Clin Orthop Relat Res 455:134–141
21. Majewski M, Stoll R, Widmer H, Muller W, Friederich NF (2006) Midterm and long-term results after arthroscopic suture repair of isolated, longitudinal, vertical meniscal tears in stable knees. Am J Sports Med 34:1072–1076
22. Moseley JB, O'Malley K, Petersen NJ, Menke TJ, Brody BA, Kuykendall DH et al (2002) A controlled trial of arthroscopic surgery for osteoarthritis of the knee. N Engl J Med 347(2):81–88
23. Noble J, Erat K (1980) In defense of the meniscus. J Bone Joint Surg 62A:7–11
24. Pujol N, Panarella L, Ait Si Selmi T, Neyret P, Fithian D, Beaufils P (2008) Meniscal healing after meniscus repair: a CT arthrography assessment. Am J Sports Med 36:1489–1495
25. Pujol N, Beaufils P (2009) Healing results of meniscal tears left in situ during anterior cruciate ligament reconstruction: a review of clinical studies. Knee Surg Sports Traumatol Arthrosc 17:396–401
26. Pujol N (2010) Meniscus repair. In: Beaufils P, Verdonk R (eds) The meniscus. Springer, Berlin/New York, pp 229–234
27. Pujol N, Barbier O, Boisrenoult P, Beaufils P (2011) Amount of meniscal resection after failed meniscal repair. Am J Sports Med 39:1648–1652
28. Pujol N, Bohu Y, Boisrenoult P, Makdes A, Beaufils P (2012) Clinical outcomes of open meniscal repair of horizontal meniscal tears in young patients. Knee Surg Sports Traumatol Arthrosc 2012 Jun 14 [Epub ahead of print]
29. Rockborn P, Gillquist J (2000) Results of open meniscus repair. Long-term follow-up study with a matched uninjured control group. J Bone Joint Surg Br 82:494–498
30. Rockborn P, Messner K (2000) Long-term results of meniscus repair and meniscectomy: a 13-year functional and radiographic follow-up study. Knee Surg Sports Traumatol Arthrosc 8:2–10
31. Shelbourne KD, Dersam MD (2004) Comparison of partial meniscectomy versus meniscus repair for bucket-handle lateral meniscus tears in anterior cruciate ligament reconstructed knees. Arthroscopy 20:581–585
32. Siebold R, Dehler C, Boes L, Ellermann A (2007) Arthroscopic all-inside repair using the meniscus arrow: long-term clinical follow-up of 113 patients. Arthroscopy 23:394–399
33. Siparsky P, Ryzewicz M, Peterson B, Bartz R (2007) Arthroscopic treatment of osteoarthritis of the knee: are there any evidence-based indications? Clin Orthop Relat Res 455:107–112
34. Smillie IS (1978) Injuries of the knee joint, 4ème edth edn. Churchill Livingstone, Edinburgh
35. Steenbrugge F, Van Nieuwenhuyse W, Verdonk R, Verstraete K (2005) Arthroscopic meniscus repair in the ACL-deficient knee. Int Orthop 29:109–112
36. Steenbrugge F, Verdonk R, Verstraete K (2002) Long-term assessment of arthroscopic meniscus repair: a 13-year follow-up study. Knee 9:181–187
37. Stein T, Mehling AP, Welsch F, von Eisenhart-Rothe R, Jäger A (2010) Long-term outcome after arthroscopic meniscal repair versus arthroscopic partial meniscectomy for traumatic meniscal tears. Am J Sports Med 38:1542–1548
38. Tuckman DV, Bravman JT, Lee SS, Rosen JE, Sherman OH (2006) Outcomes of meniscal repair: minimum of 2-year follow-up. Bull Hosp Jt Dis 63:100–104
39. van Trommel MF, Simonian PT, Potter HG, Wickiewicz TL (1998) Different regional healing rates with the outside-in technique for meniscal repair. Am J Sports Med 26:446–452
40. Venkatachalam S, Godsiff SP, Harding ML (2001) Review of the clinical results of arthroscopic meniscal repair. Knee 8:129–133
41. Vyas D, Harner CD (2012) Meniscus root repair. Sports Med Arthrosc 20:86–94
42. Weiss CB, Lundberg M, Hamberg P, DeHaven KE, Gillquist J (1989) Non-operative treatment of meniscal tears. J Bone Joint Surg Am 71A:811–822
43. Zanetti M, Pfirrmann CW, Schmid MR, Romero J, Seifert B, Hodler J (2003) Patients with suspected meniscal tears: prevalence of abnormalities seen on MRI of 100 symptomatic and 100 contralateral asymptomatic knees. Am J Roentgenol 181:635–641

Modern Indications for High Tibial Osteotomy

Matteo Denti, Piero Volpi, and Giancarlo Puddu

Introduction

In recent years Orthopaedic surgeons, in particular those that specialise in knee surgery and sports trauma, have noted a more frequent occurrence of early stage osteoarthritis and symptomatic pathologies in the knee cartilages. MRI imaging and advancements in the field of radiology, particularly with regards to information that can be gained from viewing weight-bearing radiographs of the knee, have made identification of these pathologies possible and are now routinely used [26]. MRI scans allow for the visualisation and classification of chondral knee pathologies. This is one of the reasons that the indications for a high tibial osteotomy (HTO) have changed. Another reason is that the chondrocyte does not favour mechanical loading, on the contrary, unloading seems to be important to the treatment of knee osteoarthritis [35].

Historically HTO has been performed in cases of late varus arthritic knees, the effectiveness of which was evident only for a limited number of years. This, together with advances made in knee replacements [21, 36], has meant that, in the past, the HTO was progressively abandoned, and this could also be the motivation for finding new indications for the HTO procedure, as studies began to look to the HTO not for the treatment of cases of advanced arthritis, but for the treatment at the early stages.

In recent years in some countries prosthetic knees have replaced HTO's. Even in young subjects, and there has been the risk of gradual loss of experience with regards to patient selection and surgical routine which, may in turn, have negatively affected outcomes [36].

The situation worsens in cases of an unstable knee with a ligamentous lesion of one of the cruciate ligaments or after a previously performed meniscectomy. On the other hand, some HTO studies also observed a slow deterioration overtime, with good survival rates up to 15 years [1, 14].

This paper discusses the modern HTO indications and applications.

Clinical and Instrument Evaluation

The selection of patients suitable for the HTO procedure can only be done after a thorough pre-operative evaluation. The standard evaluation begins with the assessment of the alignment of the lower limbs with four short films: bilateral weight-bearing antero-posterior views in full extension, bilateral weight-bearing postero-anterior views at 45° of flexion as described by Rosenberg [26] and lateral and skyline films of both knees. The Rosenberg view has a strong

M. Denti (✉) • P. Volpi
Department of Knee Surgery and Sports Traumatology,
IRCCS Istituto Clinico Humanitas,
Rozzano, Milano, Italy
e-mail: matteo@denti.ch.it

G. Puddu
Valle Giulia Clinic, Rome, Italy

predictive value when the deformity is associated with cruciate insufficiency, resulting in anterior tibial subluxation, and chondral wear prevailing in the posterior area of the medial tibial plateau. The osteotomy is planned according to the method described by Dugdale [5].

Magnetic Resonance Imaging (MRI) can be very useful in identifying suitable candidates for knee osteotomy, as it can show not only cartilage damage but also the stress reaction of the subchondral bone.

Before the HTO procedure, a diagnostic arthroscopy is performed and any associated lesions are treated, this procedure also allows for the confirmation that an HTO is indicated.

Indications

Osteotomy of the proximal tibia is designed to relieve pain caused by medial tibio-femoral osteoarthritis. Degenerative changes of the articular cartilage can occur through tension, compression or shear, and are the result of forces exerted on the bearing surfaces. Genetic factors are known to play a part. Specific trauma, as well as trauma from overload caused by obesity or occupational factors, is etiologically important. In essence, the mechanical cause for osteoarthritis is an overload or a concentration of forces beyond the ability of the cartilage and subchondral bone to cope.

Timing is a very important factor in this reparative surgery because an osteotomy is much more effective if it is performed in the earliest stage of the unicompartimental osteoarthritis, in order to prevent unavoidable degenerative changes in the joint of a still young and active patient [1, 10, 32, 37].

Osteotomy is best done in cases of knees with a generally well-maintained range of motion. An osteotomy is not indicated in patients with rheumatoid arthritis or in knees with greater than 20° of varus deformity. The HTO imaging indication is when the radiographs demonstrate changes such as moderate osteophytes and joint space narrowing, subchondral bone sclerosis and cysts, possible deformity of the bone contour, graded according to Kellgren and Lawrence as Kellgren II-III [16, 20].

The arthroscopic indication for a HTO is when a grade two or three chondral lesion, according to Outerbridge [22] or ICRS classification [38], is present in the medial compartment associated with a varus knee and with a good lateral compartment. An accurate technique is mandatory to obtain excellent results [11, 24, 25].

The type of valgus tibial osteotomy generally indicated is an open-wedge osteotomy, in order to guarantee better and more sustainable results compared to a closed- wedge osteotomy [4, 7–9, 11, 12, 15, 24, 25].

In the past, the presence of "patella baja" was taken as a contra-indication, but if it is performed in association with a HTO, the tibial tubercle is moved proximally the patella and baja can be corrected [6, 13, 18, 30].

Over the last 10 years the majority of osteotomies performed have been done in association with articular cartilage repair, meniscal transplantation and ligament reconstruction.

HTO associated with articular cartilage treatment: It has been observed that with cartilage pathologies, after a non weight-bearing period, the changes in the medial compartment shift from negative to positive, indicating the potential for articular cartilage recovery secondary to an improved mechanical environment. This is also the case when the HTO is associated with a microfracture procedure or cartilage transplantation [23, 31, 35].

HTO associated with meniscal transplantation: The association of an HTO with a medial meniscus transplantation has been observed to have greater improvement at the final follow-up when compared to isolated medial meniscal transplantation [33].

HTO associated with anterior cruciate reconstruction: HTOs performed in association with meniscal transplants and cartilage repair have been observed to have good outcomes, however, the association with ligament reconstruction is open to debate, and needs more investigation.

The definition "knee abuser" identifies a category of patients in which the ligamentous laxity is associated with the degenerative changes of the medial compartment. The natural history of a knee abuser starts with an ACL tear mis-diagnosed or ignored. The ligament is not reconstructed and the patient, sooner or later, returns to normal activities including sport activities. The instability that the knee is experiencing leads firstly to a giving way, which is then followed by many other episodes such as a meniscal tear, which very often, complicates the situation and, finally, degenerative changes of the medial compartment with varus deformity.

Patients who initially presented "only" a traumatic lesion of the ACL, after months or years present complex ligamentous laxity of the knee joint with a varus mal-alignment and osteoarthritis and the situation is worsened by a lateral thrust during gait.

This pathological picture needs more than the reconstruction of the cruciate ligament or even the treatment of the arthritic lesions as the re-alignment of the deformity is not sufficient for a joint which has both the problem of instability and of arthritis. A failed ACL reconstruction in these patients worsens the situation. In such cases, HTO can be seen as a more complete solution, addressing the inclination of the slope of the tibial plate. Initially, the open-wedge HTO was criticized as it can cause an increased slope, but this is dependent on the position of the plate. In cases of anterior instability it should be positioned posterior to the medial collateral ligament and allows a higher opening posteriorly than anteriorly.

The combination of a valgus osteotomy with ACL reconstruction, even in cases of revision, can lead to correct axis positioning and a stable knee. This combined surgery is indicated only in young selected patients, those with instability associated with initial varus arthritis. The results of HTO associated with ACL reconstruction are certainly encouraging [2, 17] (Figs. 1 and 2).

<u>HTO associated with posterior instability and complex instability:</u> Two types of posterior instability can be differentiated, one is isolated and the other is associated with posteriorlateral laxity. With isolated posterior laxity there is an indication to increase the tibial slope positioning the plate anteriorly. When posterior laxity is associated with posteriorlateral laxity, not only must the angle of the slope be increased, but a valgus ostotomy must be performed with a lateral translation of the mechanical axis to 55–60 % of the tibial plateau.

If necessary, posterior cruciate ligament reconstruction can be considered at a second stage eventually in association with a postero-lateral reconstruction.

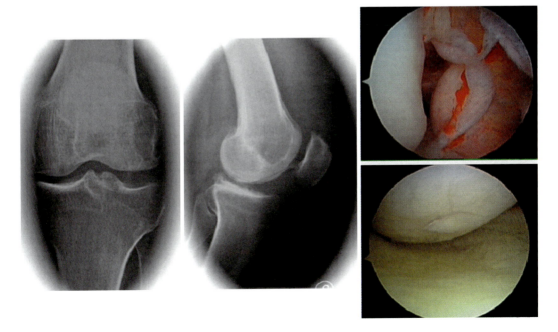

Fig. 1 Varus knee and chronic anterior cruciate ligament lesion

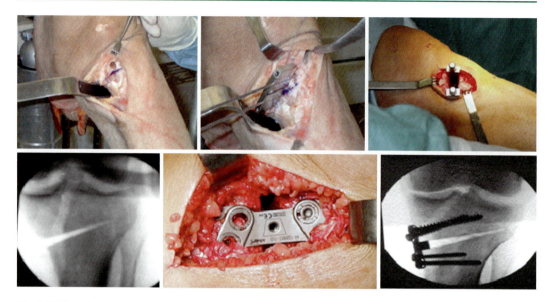

Fig. 2 HTO and anterior cruciate ligament reconstruction technique

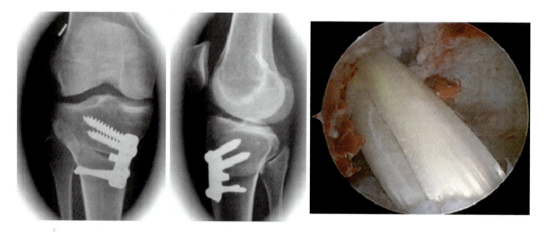

Fig. 3 HTO and anterior cruciate ligament reconstruction technique in anterior and posterior instability

In cases of associated anterior and posterior instability, in a varus knee, HTO can be performed to correct the tibial slope for the posterior instability associated with an anterior cruciate ligament reconstruction. It has recently been demonstrated that a moderate change of the tibial slope does not significantly modify the anterior stability [28, 29, 34] (Fig. 3).

The "modern" HTO is indicated in younger patients presenting initial medial osteoarthritis of the knee and even in cases where it is associated with other surgical procedures, it not only reduces painful symptoms, but can ensure that the patient can perform sport at a recreational level [3, 19, 27, 37].

References

1. Amendola A, Bonasia DE (2010) Results of high tibial osteotomy: review of the literature. Int Orthop 34:155–160
2. Bonin N, Ait Si Selmi T, Donell ST, Dejour H, Neyret P (2004) Anterior cruciate reconstruction combined with valgus upper tibial osteotomy: 12 years follow-up. Knee 11:431–437
3. Bonnin MP, Laurent JR, Zadegan F, Badet R, Pooler Archbold HA, Servien E (2012) Can patients really

participate in sport after high tibial osteotomy? Knee Surg Sports Traumatol Arthrosc 21(1):64–73
4. Coventry MB (1965) Osteotomy of the upper portion of the tibia for degenerative arthritis of the knee. J Bone Joint Surg Am 47:984–990
5. Dugdale TW, Noyes FR, Styer D (1992) Preoperative planning for high tibial osteotomy. The effect of lateral tibiofemoral separation and tibiofemoral length. Clin Orthop 274:248–264
6. El-Azab H, Glabgly P, Paul J, Imhoff AB, Hinterwimmer S (2010) Patellar height and posterior tibial slope after open- and closed-wedge high tibial osteotomy: a radiological study on 100 patients. Am J Sports Med 2:323–329
7. Fowler PJ, Tan JL, Brown GA (2000) Medial opening wedge high tibial osteotomy: how I do it. Oper Tech Sports Med 1:32–38
8. Franco V, Cerullo G, Cipolla M et al (2005) Osteotomy for osteoarthritis of the knee. Curr Orthop 19:415–427
9. Georgoulis AD, Makris CA, Papageorgiu CD et al (1999) Nerve and vessels injuries during high tibial osteotomy combined with distal fibular osteotomy: a clinically relevant anatomic study. Knee Surg Sports Traumatol Arthrosc 7:15–19
10. Gomoll AH (2011) High tibial osteotomy for the treatment of unicompartmental knee osteoarthritis: a review of the literature, indications, and technique. Phys Sportsmed 39:45–54
11. Hankemeier S, Mommsen P, Krettek C et al (2010) Accuracy of high tibial osteotomy: comparison between open- and closed-wedge technique. Knee Surg Sports Traumatol Arthrosc 18:1328–1333
12. Hernigou P, Medevill D, Debeyre J et al (1987) Proximal tibial osteotomy with varus deformity: a ten to thirteen year follow-up study. J Bone Joint Surg Am 69:332–354
13. Hinterwimmer S, Beitzel K, Paul J, Kirchhoff C, Sauerschnig M, von Eisenhart-Rothe R, Imhoff AB (2011) Control of posterior tibial slope and patellar height in open-wedge valgus high tibial osteotomy. Am J Sports Med 39:851–856
14. Hui C, Salmon LJ, Kok A, Williams HA, Hockers N, van der Tempel WM, Chana R, Pinczewski LA (2011) Long-term survival of high tibial osteotomy for medial compartment osteoarthritis of the knee. Am J Sports Med 39:64–70
15. Jackson JP (1958) Osteotomy for osteroarthritis of the knee. Proceeding of the Sheffield Regional Orthopaedic Club. J Bone Joint Surg Br 40:826
16. Kellgren JH, Lawrence JS (1957) Radiological assessment of osteo-arthrosis. Ann Rheum Dis 4:494–502
17. Kim SJ, Moon HK, Chun YM, Chang WH, Kim SG (2011) Is correctional osteotomy crucial in primary varus knees undergoing anterior cruciate ligament reconstruction? Clin Orthop Relat Res 469:1421–1426
18. LaPrade RF, Oro FB, Ziegler CG, Wijdicks CA, Walsh MP (2010) Patellar height and tibial slope after opening-wedge proximal tibial osteotomy: a prospective study. Am J Sports Med 38:160–170
19. Laprade RF, Spiridonov SI, Nystrom LM, Jansson KS (2011) Prospective outcomes of young and middle-aged adults with medial compartment osteoarthritis treated with a proximal tibial opening wedge osteotomy. Arthroscopy 28:354–364
20. Luyten FP, Denti M, Filardo G, Kon E, Engebretsen L (2012) Definition and classification of early osteoarthritis of the knee. Knee Surg Sports Traumatol Arthrosc 20:401–406
21. Nagel A, Insall JN, Scuderi GR (1996) Proximal tibial osteotomy. A subjective outcome study. J Bone Joint Surg Am 78:1353–1358
22. Outerbridge RE (1961) The etiology of chondromalacia patellae. J Bone Joint Surg Br 43:752–757
23. Parker DA, Beatty KT, Giuffre B, Scholes CJ, Coolican MR (2011) Articular cartilage changes in patients with osteoarthritis after osteotomy. Am J Sports Med 39:1039–1045
24. Puddu G, Cerullo G, Cipolla M et al (2003) Osteotomies about the knee. In: Management of osteoarthritis of the knee: an international consensus. American Academy of Orthopaedic Surgeons, Rosemont, pp 17–30
25. Puddu G, Franco V, Cipolla M (2008) Opening-wedge osteotomy- proximal tibia and distal femur. In: Jackson DW (ed) Reconstructive knee surgery. Master techniques in orthopaedic surgery, 3rd edn. Lippincott Williams & Wilkins, Philadelphia, pp 433–450
26. Rosenberg TD, Paulos LE, Parker RD et al (1988) The forty-five-degree posteroanterior weight bearing radiograph of the knee. J Bone Joint Surg Am 70:1479–1483
27. Salzmann GM, Ahrens P, Naal FD, El-Azab H, Spang JT, Imhoff AB, Lorenz S (2009) Sporting activity after high tibial osteotomy for the treatment of medial compartment knee osteoarthritis. Am J Sports Med 37:312–318
28. Savarese E, Bisicchia S, Romeo R, Amendola A (2011) Role of high tibial osteotomy in chronic injuries of posterior cruciate ligament and posterolateral corner. J Orthop Traumatol 12:1–17
29. Shelburne KB, Kim HJ, Sterett WI, Pandy MG (2011) Effect of posterior tibial slope on knee biomechanics during functional activity. J Orthop Res 29: 223–231
30. Song EK, Seon JK, Park SJ, Jeong MS (2010) The complications of high tibial osteotomy: closing- versus opening-wedge methods. J Bone Joint Surg Br 92:1245–1252
31. Sterett WI, Steadman JR, Huang MJ, Matheny LM, Briggs KK (2010) Chondral resurfacing and high tibial osteotomy in the varus knee: survivorship analysis. Am J Sports Med 38:1420–1424
32. Trieb K, Grohs J, Hanslik-Schnabel B, Stulnig T, Panotopoulos J, Wanivenhaus A (2006) Age predicts outcome of high-tibial osteotomy. Knee Surg Sports Traumatol Arthrosc 14:149–152
33. Verdonk PC, Verstraete KL, Almqvist KF, De Cuyper K, Veys EM, Verbruggen G, Verdonk R (2006) Meniscal allograft transplantation: long-term

clinical results with radiological and magnetic resonance imaging correlations. Knee Surg Sports Traumatol Arthrosc 14:694–706
34. Voos JE, Suero EM, Citak M, Petrigliano FP, Bosscher MR, Citak M, Wickiewicz TL, Pearle AD (2012) Effect of tibial slope on the stability of the anterior cruciate ligament-deficient knee. Knee Surg Sports Traumatol Arthrosc 20(8):1626–1631
35. Waller C, Hayes D, Block JE, London NJ (2011) Unload it: the key to the treatment of knee osteoarthritis. Knee Surg Sports Traumatol Arthrosc 19:1823–1829
36. W-Dahl A, Robertsson O, Lidgren L (2010) Surgery for knee osteoarthritis in younger patients. Acta Orthop 81:161–164
37. Wolcott M, Traub S, Efird C (2010) High tibial osteotomies in the young active patient. Int Orthop 34:161–166
38. www.cartilage.org/_files/contentmanagement/ICRS_evaluation.pdf

Unicompartment Knee Arthroplasty: From Primary to Revision Surgery

Francesco Benazzo and Stefano Marco Paolo Rossi

Introduction

Unicompartment knee arthroplasty (UKA) continues to evolve, and studies show that the procedure can result in excellent outcomes [1, 6, 7, 10, 21, 22, 23, 26, 31, 33, 35, 40, 41]. Satisfying clinical results have been reported over three decades; however, debate continues regarding the intricacies of the surgical technique, fixation methods, and optimal implant design. Indications as well are under discussion, due to the broadening criteria adopted by some expert surgeons, particularly in the age range where osteotomy can be another valid, well-recognized, option Adherence to strict surgical indications and appropriate patient selection, combined with meticulous surgical technique, are important factors in optimizing the outcomes.

Indications (Classical and Expanded)

Unicompartmental knee arthroplasty is by definition the replacement of one diseased compartment of the knee. Different algorithms have been presented to guide the indications for this complex and technically demanding procedure. Our advice is to start to perform these procedures staying within the "classical" indications leaving the "expanded" ones until after the learning curve has been completed and the technique becomes familiar.

Classical Indications

- Unicompartmental degenerative disease (medial or lateral) with mild degeneration of the opposite side
- Painful osteonecrosis/osteochondritic involvement of the femoral condyle, with or without rim narrowing
- Deformity of the anatomical axis of the limb due to narrowing of the joint line by degenerative disease and not by deformity of the tibia (schuss x-ray view)
- Deformity correctable manually (stress X-rays) and therefore surgically, by the thickness of the implant
- Healthy (functionally) ACL
- Full or almost full flexion (ROM almost normal)
- "Finger sign" positive
- Age > 60 years
- BMI < 30
- Varus/valgus deformity < 10°
- Flexion contracture < 10°

F. Benazzo • S.M.P. Rossi (✉)
Clinica Ortopedica e Traumatologica
dell'Università degli Studi di Pavia,
Fondazione IRCCS Policlinico San Matteo,
P.le Golgi 19, Pavia 27100, Italy
e-mail: rossi.smp@gmail.com

Extended Indications

- Age < 60 years [34, 38]
- BMI > 30 (but < 32) [43]
- Presence of degenerative patello-femoral joint if no anterior knee pain (and no full-thickness chondral lesions or lateral facet involvement)
- ACL deficient knee, if tibial slope < 7°. However, no mobile bearing to be used [18, 38]
- Possibility of ACL reconstruction together with the UNI

Contra-Indications

- Inflammatory osteoarthritis (RA, psoriatic arthritis)
- Fixed flexion deformity > 10°
- Valgus/varus deformity fixed and > 10°
- ACL deficiency in young active patient (but possible choice of simultaneous reconstruction)
- Tibial lateral thrust on weight-bearing
- Severe Osteoarthritic degeneration of patellar lateral facet (but possible choice of simultaneous patello-femoral replacement)

Pre-operative Considerations

Clinical Examination

Pre-operative clinical decision making in assessing a patient for UKA includes a detailed patient history, physical examination, and radiographs. One particularly important aspect of the history is that the patient should localize his or her pain to either the medial or lateral joint line, with minimal indication of pain in the opposite compartment or the retropatellar region. The typical "one-finger test" is based on asking the patient to locate his or her pain, and the patient points to the involved compartment with one finger. This concept is in contrast with the patient who grabs the knee when asked to localize his or her pain, indicating more diffuse pain distribution.

Imaging

1. Routine radiographs include:
   - full long standing antero-posterior weight-bearing view (hip and ankle included)
   - 45° flexed-knee postero-anterior weight bearing view (schuss or Rosenberg view)
   - true lateral view
   - skyline (axial) view at 30° of flexion or under weight bearing to assess the for degeneration of the patello-femoral joint and tracking of adjacent compartments and to evaluate for tibiofemoral subluxation, which may indicate ligament incompetence.
2. MRI: it is adopted on a routine basis by some surgeons, as a tool to assess the situation in the opposite compartment. However, this imaging tool can over-estimate the degree of degeneration, and cause some doubts in the decision-making. MRI is mandatory in diagnosing osteonecrosis of the femoral condyle, which is a specific indication for UKA. For some authors the ultimate decision to proceed with UKA is made intra-operatively, when the status of the other compartments can be directly visualized.
3. Arthroscopy. The adoption of an arthroscopy, either staged or just before the UKA, has been advocated by some surgeons to confirm the unilateral disease and the indication; however, the above-described clinical and radiological criteria are considered sufficient by most knee surgeons and an additional surgical procedure completely unnecessary. We do not recommend the use of the arthroscopy on a routine basis.

Technical Issues

Re-surfacing or Measured Resection

Some words can be said on the two different philosophies of approaching this procedure: the re-surfacing versus the measured resection technique.

The first one [25] implies a type of implant that is more representative of a European philosophy as the design comes from the French school and from Philippe Cartier in particular (Fig. 1). Based on the idea of bone sparing and of respecting the

Fig. 1 Unicompartmental knee arthroplasty with a resurfacing implant

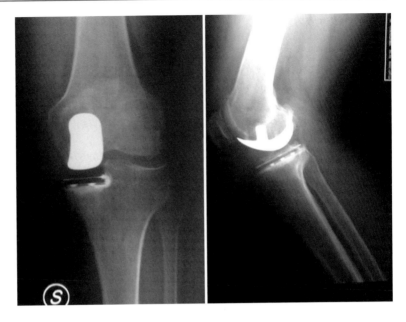

joint physiology, this type of implant implies some peculiar technical steps such as the use of the so called "Cartier angle", which is the angle of tibial varus deviation on the tibial side, and only a reaming of the cartilage surface on the femoral side.

On the other hand the measured resection technique (Fig. 2) implies a tibial cut at 90° and a parallel cut on the femoral side using implants and concepts that are closer to a total knee design and a philosophy which is favoured by many Americans.

In our experience both these kind of implants and approaches have given satisfactory clinical results, according to the indications for the two systems, with a high survival rate.

We could not find different indications for the two different implants with regard to gender, the weight of the patient or other clinical features which affected the clinical outcomes of these implants.

From a technical point of view the Cartier implant presents some more technical difficulties comparing to a measured resection prosthesis and needs a longer learning curve.

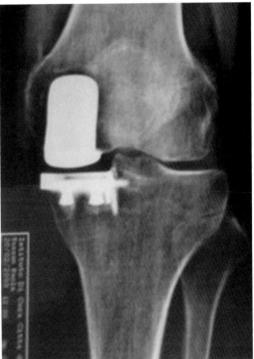

Fig. 2 Unicompartmental knee arthroplasty with a measured resection implant

Fixed or Mobile

Fixed-bearing tibial components can be either all polyethylene or metal-backed. Metal backing was introduced in an attempt to more evenly distribute weight-bearing stress to the underlying tibial bone [20]. The modularity of metal-backed components also facilitates easier femoral component insertion during the cementing process and allows the possibility of isolated polyethylene exchange, when required. The disadvantage of this design is that either a thinner polyethylene liner or a larger tibial cut are needed to accommodate the metal backing. Many modern UKA systems allow for implantation of either all polyethylene or metal-backed components; good clinical results have been reported with both. An alternative implant design philosophy is a tibial component with a mobile meniscal bearing. Mobile polyethylene bearings have been used in both Europe and the United States. Whereas the most successfull fixed-bearing designs incorporate round-on-flat or slightly dished geometries, mobile-bearing UKA components such as the Oxford (Biomet, Warsaw, IN) are fully congruent (i.e., constant radius) with an uncaptured straight track. Other mobile-bearing designs, such as the LCS (Low Contact Stress) component (DePuy, Warsaw, IN), capture the mobile polyethylene-bearing in a dovetail radial track, theoretically reducing the risk of bearing dislocation. The purpose of both of these mobile-bearing designs is to optimize congruency of the femoral and tibial components throughout ROM, thereby minimizing point tibial contact forces and stress at the implant fixation interface.

Several published studies indicate the potential long-term success of both fixed- and meniscal-bearing UKA implants [9, 11, 14, 28, 29]. All authors attribute their success, in part, to strict patient selection criteria and proper surgical technique, coming from a reasonably long learning curve. Excellent long-term results have been published on the Oxford meniscal-bearing UKA. Of interest, thickness of the polyethylene insert was as thin as 3.5 mm, with no degradation in clinical outcome or increased rate of failure reported in patients treated with thinner polyethylene. The authors suggest that the congruency of the mobile-bearing design and the resulting decrease in polyethylene contact stresses may obviate the need for thicker (>6 mm) inserts.

This fact is clinically important because it supports the surgical principle of minimizing the thickness of the tibial bone cut. The most common cause of revision in the mobile-bearing UKA is dislocation of the polyethylene, a complication unique to this group, especially early in the learning curve. Overall comparative data between fixed- and mobile-bearing components remain mixed. Larger, long-term follow-up studies may be needed to determine any true clinical or survivorship difference between fixed- and meniscal-bearing UKA's.

Radiographic Considerations

Mobile-bearing UKR's can have a wide acceptable range of alignment of ±10° varus/valgus and flexion/extension for the femoral component and ±5° varus/valgus and superior/inferior tilt for the tibial component. This forgiveness does not extend to fixed-bearing UKRs, where excessive tibial slope angles outside the range of 8–10° lead to a poor outcome. It is important to stress that component malpositioning should not be considered the same as overall limb malalignment, where overcorrection of the pre-operative deformity is associated with a risk of accelerated degenerative changes in the opposite compartment and severe undercorrection is associated with increased wear in the tibial component and recurrence of deformity [36, 37, 39]. Varus/valgus alignment for the femoral and the tibial components is measured on the AP radiograph in relation to the anatomical axis of the tibia. Flexion/extension is measured on a lateral radiograph, relative to the posterior femoral and tibial cortices, respectively. All angles are considered as neutral at 0°, with the exception of the flexion/extension angle of the tibial component, where a postero-inferior slope of 7° is considered neutral on the AP radiograph, the tibial component should be visualized just medial to the apex of the tibial spine with 0–2 mm of overhang on the medial border of the tibia, and on the lateral radiograph it should reach the posterior cortex of the tibia. The femoral component should overhang the bone on the lateral radiograph proximally by 2–3 mm and be flush with the retained cartilage. Overhang of >3 mm can cause soft tissue irritation and pain, whereas inadequate cover of the bone can cause subsidence of the component.

Principles of Surgical Technique in Primary UKA

Several additional principles of component positioning at the time of surgery have been shown to affect the long-term outcome of UKA. To facilitate implant congruence throughout the flexion/extension arc, the tibial component should be implanted perpendicular to the long axis of the tibia in the coronal plane. In a three-dimensional finite element analysis of tibial component inclination in UKA, Sawatari et al. demonstrated increased cancellous bone stresses when the tibial component was placed in varus. With regard to the sagittal plane placement of the tibial component, we recommend ensuring a tibial slope of <7° to protect the ACL from degeneration and rupture, mitigating against late anteroposterior instability of the knee. We generally recommend attempting to match the native tibial slope. Equally important are guidelines for placement of the femoral implant. In general, the femoral component should be placed perpendicular to the tibial component in the coronal plane. Doing so underscores the importance of correct tibial component placement, to avoid obligatory femoral malrotation. Importantly, most UKA instrumentation systems provide techniques for ensuring that the flexion/extension gaps between the femoral and tibial components are balanced.

ACL Reconstruction in UKA

Unicompartment knee replacement is particularly useful in the management of symptomatic end-stage medial compartment osteoarthritis (MCOA) in young and active patients. However, if the anterior cruciate ligament (ACL) is absent, failure rates of 21 % have been reported at 2 years, due primarily to tibial component loosening, for both mobile and fixed-bearing [12, 15, 17, 24, 32, 42, 44]. The consequences of ACL deficiency in association with MCOA depends on the primary pathology. If arthritis is the primary problem it tends to begin anteriorly in the medial compartment, extending posteriorly and progressively damaging the ACL. By the time the ACL is destroyed the medial collateral ligament (MCL) has shortened and the lateral side is usually damaged. This means that an UKR would be inappropriate, even if combined with an ACL reconstruction, and the best option is a total knee replacement (TKR).

In contrast, if the primary problem is ACL deficiency, then the arthritic change tends to begin posteriorly in the medial compartment. This is possibly due to recurrent episodes of giving way, in which posterior femoral subluxation in the medial compartment places a heavy load on the posterior part of the medial meniscus and underlying articular cartilage of the tibia, producing meniscal damage and MCOA. Such patients tend to be young and active and the MCL and lateral compartment are relatively normal. In such circumstances a combined ACL reconstruction and UKR can be considered. Other treatment options include high tibial osteotomy (with or without ACL reconstruction) and TKR.

This kind of procedure is quite rare and the indications are limited.

The surgical technique must combine the two procedures and can present some issues related to:
– tunnel positioning
– approach
– stability of the implant.

The first issue is related to tunnel positioning.

Using a trans-tibial approach the tibial tunnel must be placed medial and posterior in order to achieve a correct femoral tunnel positioning.

With this technique two problems can occur:
– impingement of the neo-ligament with the medial side of the prosthesis with consequent possible damage of the ligament
– weakening of the tibial bone stock under the tibial plate with consequent risk of collapse of the implant especially if tunnel widening occurs at distance.

Furthermore, in small tibiae, such as those in women, the problem of impingement of the ligament with the tibial baseplate is real.

Fig. 3 Combined ACL reconstruction and UKA

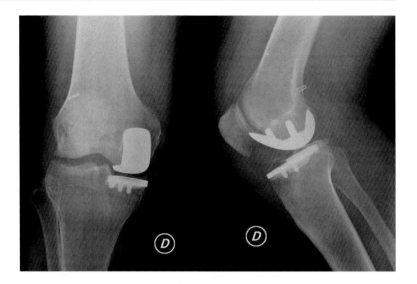

The solution using this approach not to damage the ligament and the prosthesis, which has an obligatory positioning, is to perform a more anterior and lateral tunnel, which results in a more vertical and less anatomical ACL once the femoral tunnel is reamed through such a tibial approach.

To overcome the potential downside of the trans-tibial reconstruction of the ACL, problem, an antero-medial approach can be adopted. This technique will allow movement of the tibial tunnel much closer to the tibial tuberosity and therefore the tunnel is far from the implant and the risk of impingement of the implant with the new ligament is reduced or eliminated (Fig. 3).

From the technical viewpoint, the surgical sequence is as follows:
- tendon harvesting (usually hamstrings); however, allograft can be used. The adoption of artificial material has not been described so far, and the burden of the overall cost also must be taken in account
- tunnel preparation with the above-described technique, and femoral fixation; the new ACL is left dangling in the tibial tunnel
- UNI. implant
- Distal fixation of the ACL, when the limb axis has been corrected by the prosthetic implant, and the appropriate tension of the ligament can be achieved and applied

Patello-Femoral and Lateral Compartment Involvement

The patello-femoral involvement and the involvement of the opposite compartment are collectively the most common causes of failure of UKA [3, 4, 16, 19].

For the patello-femoral compartment most of the time there is an error of indication for UKA.

On the other hand the progression of arthritis in the opposite compartment is mainly due to a technical error (overstuffing).

Indications for performing a Unicondylar knee arthroplasty in cases with involvement of the patello-femoral compartment must be very strict. The key to the problem is which facet of the patella is involved in the arthritis; If it is the medial facet, a medial unicondylar knee replacement "solo" is indicated, as demonstrated with the studies conducted by the Oxford group, as the re-alignment of the lower limb reduces the load on the medial compartment of the P-F joint.

In cases with involvement of the lateral facet of the patella a combined implant can be performed (Fig. 4)

The problem of the progression of the arthritis in the uninvolved compartment (i.e. the lateral with a medial UKA) is mainly due to an error during the surgical procedure; in particular, one of the keys for the success of UKA is to give a

Fig. 4 UKA + PF joint replacement

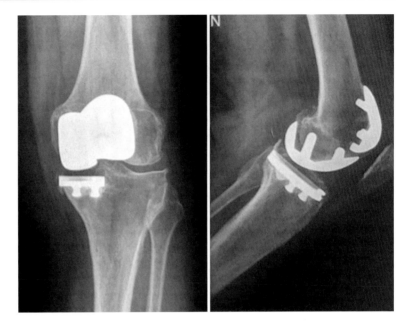

slight undercorrection of the deformity; in cases of limb re-alignment or hypercorrection of the deformity, the chances are that we can face a progression of the disease on the other compartment, due to its overload. The same problem can be found in the patello-femoral compartment with a progression of the arthritis due to an overload on the lateral facet of the patella in cases of hypercorrection of a varus deformity into a valgus.

Failure Mechanism

There are different potential causes for failure in Unicompartmental knee arthroplasty [8, 13, 30].

Although all studies show the same causes, different studies show different percentages for each failure mechanisms.
- Progression of arthritis in uninvolved compartments is the most common cause for revision
- Aseptic loosening, polyethylene wear or osteolysis
- Unexplained pain.

Review of the literature indicates that surgical technique at the time of the index procedure can minimize each of the modes of failure, potentially improving the results of present and future procedures.

Indications and Surgical Tips in Revising Unicompartment Knees

The different mechanisms of failure imply different principles, tips and techniques for revision [2, 5, 17, 27, 30]. In general the principles for revision of a UNI can be summarised as follows:
- Revision with primary implants is desirable in all cases of progression of arthritis of the uninvolved compartment or unexplained pain without aseptic loosening or major bone losses
- In cases of loosening a major bone loss can be found and the need for augments may imply the use of a revision implant (Fig. 5)
- The use of a revision implant does not mean necessarily that a higher level of constraint must be used. If a good ligament balance is achieved and the implant is stable, a lower constrained liner (i.e. a PS liner on a CCK implant) can be used.
- The use of more constrained implants in revision of UKA may give poorer outcomes
- With modern implants and close vigilance in monitoring for progressive wear and bone loss, UKA may not significantly impair the results of future revisions.

Fig. 5 UKA revision with a semi-constrained implant

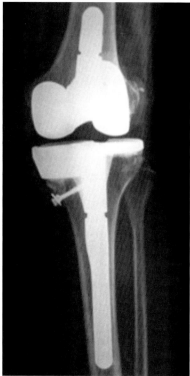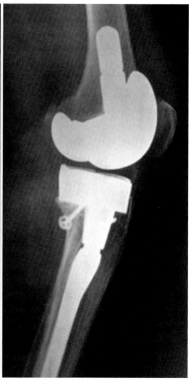

References

1. Argenson JN, Komistek RD, Aubaniac JM, Dennis DA, Northcut EJ, Anderson DT, Agostini S (2002) In vivo determination of knee kinematics for subjects implanted with a unicompartmental arthroplasty. J Arthroplasty 17:1049–1054
2. Barrett WP, Scott RD (1987) Revision of failed unicondylar unicompartmental knee arthroplasty. J Bone Joint Surg Am 69:1328–1335
3. Beard DJ, Pandit H, Ostlere S, Jenkins C, Dodd CA, Murray DW (2007) Pre-operative clinical and radiological assessment of the patellofemoral joint in unicompartmental knee replacement and its influence on outcome. J Bone Joint Surg Br 89(12):1602–1607
4. Beard DJ, Pandit H, Gill HS, Hollinghurst D, Dodd CA, Murray DW (2007) The influence of the presence and severity of pre-existing patellofemoral degenerative changes on the outcome of the Oxford medial unicompartmental knee replacement. J Bone Joint Surg Br 89(12):1597–1601
5. Berend KR, Lombardi AV Jr, Mallory TH, Adams JB, Groseth KL (2005) Early failure of minimally invasive unicompartmental knee arthroplasty is associated with obesity. Clin Orthop Relat Res 440:60–66
6. Berger RA, Meneghini RM, Jacobs JJ, Sheinkop MB, Dell Valle CJ, Rosenberg AG, Galante JO (2005) Results of unicompartmental knee arthroplasty at a minimum of 10 years follow-up. J Bone Joint Surg Am 87:999–2006
7. Bert JM (2005) Unicompartmental knee replacement. Orthop Clin North Am 36:513–522
8. Collier MB, Engh CA Jr, Engh GA (2004) Shelf age of the polyethelene tibial component and outcome of unicondylar knee arthroplasty. J Bone Joint Surg Am 86:763–769
9. Confalonieri N, Manzotti A, Pullen C (2004) Comparison of a mobile with a fixed bearing unicompartmental knee prosthesis: a prospective randomized trial using a dedicated outcome score. Knee 11:357–362
10. Christensen NO (1991) Unicompartmental prosthesis for gonarthrosis. A nine year series of 575 knees from a Swedish hospital. Clin Orthop Relat Res 273:165–169
11. Emerson RH Jr, Hansborough T, Reitman RD, Rosenfeldt W, Higgins LL (2002) Comparison of a mobile with a fixed bearing unicompartmental knee implant. Clin Orthop Relat Res 404:62–70
12. Engh GA, Ammeen D (2004) Is an intact anterior cruciate ligament needed in order to have a well-functioning unicondylar knee replacement? Clin Orthop Relat Res 428:170–173
13. Gioe TJ, Killeen KK, Hoeffel DP, Bert JM, Comfort TK, Scheltema K, Mehle S, Grimm K (2003) Analysis of unicompartmental knee arthroplasty in a community-based implant registry. Clin Orthop Relat Res 416:111–119
14. Goodfellow JW, Kenshaw CJ, Benson MK, O'Connor JJ (1988) The Oxford Knee for unicompartmental osteoarthritis: the first 103 cases. J Bone Joint Surg Br 70:692–701

15. Goodfellow J, O'Connor J (1992) The anterior cruciate ligament in knee arthroplasty: a risk-factor with unconstrained meniscal prostheses. Clin Orthop Relat Res 276:245–252
16. Gulati A, Pandit H, Jenkins C et al (2009) The effect of leg alignment on the outcome of unicompartmental knee replacement. J Bone Joint Surg Br 91-B:469–474
17. Lewold S, Robertsson O, Knutson K, Lidgren L (1998) Revision of unicompartmental knee arthroplasty: outcome of 1,135 cases from the Swedish Knee Arthroplasty study. Acta Orthop Scand 69:469–474
18. Hernigou P, Deschamps G (2004) Posterior slope of the tibial implant and the outcome of unicompartmental knee arthroplasty. J Bone Joint Surg Am 86:506–511
19. Hernigou P, Deschamps G (2002) Patellar impingement following unicompartmental arthroplasty. J Bone Joint Surg Am 84:1132–1137
20. Hyldahl HC, Regnér L, Carlsson L, Kärrholm J, Weidenhielm L (2001) Does metal backing improve fixation of tibial component in unicondylar knee arthroplasty? A randomized radiostereometric analysis. J Arthroplasty 16:174–179
21. Hodge WA, Chandler HP (1992) Unicompartmental knee replacement: a comparison of constrained and unconstrained designs. J Bone Joint Surg Am 74:877–883
22. Kozinn SC, Scott R (1989) Unicondylar knee arthroplasty. J Bone Joint Surg Am 71:145–150
23. Insall J, Aglietti P (1980) A 5- to 7-year follow-up of unicondylar arthroplasty. J Bone Joint Surg Am 62:1329–1337
24. Krishnan SR, Randle R (2009) ACL reconstruction with unicondylar replacement in knee with functional instability and osteoarthritis. J Orthop Surg Res 17:43
25. Laskin RS (1978) Unicompartmental tibiofemoral resurfacing arthroplasty. J Bone Joint Surg Am 60:182–185
26. Laurencin CT, Zelicof SB, Scott RD, Ewald FC (1991) Unicompartmental versus total knee arthroplasty in the same patient: a comparative study. Clin Orthop Relat Res 273:151–156
27. Levine WN, Ozuna RM, Scott RD, Thornhill TS (1996) Conversion of failed modern unicompartmental arthroplasty to total knee arthroplasty. J Arthroplasty 11:797–801
28. Lewold S, Goodman S, Knutson K, Robertsson O, Lidgren L (1995) Oxford meniscal bearing knee versus the Marmor knee in unicompartmental arthroplasty for arthrosis. A Swedish multicenter survival study. J Arthroplasty 10:722–731
29. Marmor L (1982) The Marmor knee replacement. Orthop Clin North Am 13:55–64
30. McAuley JP, Engh GA, Ammeen DJ (2001) Revision of failed unicompartmental knee arthroplasty. Clin Orthop Relat Res 392:279–282
31. Newman JH, Ackroyd CE, Shah NA (1998) Unicompartmental or total knee replacement? Five-year results of a prospective, randomised trial of 102 osteoarthritic knees with unicompartmental arthritis. J Bone Joint Surg Br 80:862–865
32. Pandit H, Beard DJ, Jenkins C et al (2006) Combined anterior cruciate reconstruction and Oxford unicompartmental knee arthroplasty. J Bone Joint Surg Br 88(7):887–892
33. Patil S, Colwell CW Jr, Ezzet KA, D'Lima DD (2005) Can normal knee kinematics be restored with unicompartmental knee replacement? J Bone Joint Surg Am 87:332–338
34. Pennington DW, Swienckowski JJ, Lutes WB, Drake GN (2003) Unicompartmental knee arthroplasty in patients sixty years of age or younger. J Bone Joint Surg Am 85:1968–1973
35. Price AJ, Waite JC, Svard U (2005) Long term clinical results of the medial Oxford unicompartmental knee arthroplasty. Clin Orthop Relat Res 435:171–180
36. Ritter MA, Faris PM, Thong AE, Davis KE, Meding JB, Berend ME (2004) Intra-operative findings in varus osteoarthritis of the knee: an analysis of preoperative alignment in potential candidates for unicompartmental arthroplasty. J Bone Joint Surg Br 86:43–47
37. Sawatari T, Tsumura H, Iesaka K, Furushiro Y, Torisu T (2005) Three dimensional finite element analysis of unicompartmental knee arthroplasty: the influence of tibial component inclination. J Orthop Res 23:549–554
38. Schai PA, Suh JT, Thornhill TS, Scott RD (1998) Unicompartmental knee arthroplasty in middle-aged patients: a 2- to 6-year follow-up evaluation. J Arthroplasty 13:365–372
39. Soohoo NF, Sharifi H, Kominski G, Lieberman JR, Soohoo NF, Sharifi H, Kominski G, Lieberman JR (2006) Cost-effectiveness analysis of unicompartmental knee arthroplasty as an alternative to total knee arthroplasty for unicompartmental osteoarthritis. J Bone Joint Surg Am 88:1975–1982
40. Squire MW, Callaghan JJ, Goetz DD, Sullivan PM, Johnston RC (1999) Unicompartmental knee replacement: a minimum 15 year followup study. Clin Orthop Relat Res 367:61–72
41. Stukenborg-Colsman C, Wirth CJ, Lazovic D, Wefer A (2001) High tibial osteotomy versus unicompartmental joint replacement in unicompartmental knee joint osteoarthritis: 7-10-year follow-up prospective randomized study. Knee 8:187–194
42. Suggs JF, Li G, Park SE, Steffensmeier S, Rubash HE, Freiberg AA (2004) Function of the anterior cruciate ligament after unicompartmental knee arthroplasty: an in vitro robotic study. J Arthroplasty 19:224–229
43. Tabor OB Jr, Tabor OB, Bernard M, Wan JY (2005) Unicompartmental knee arthroplasty: long-term success in middle-age and obese patients. J Surg Orthop Adv 14:59–63
44. Tinius M, Hepp P, Becker R (2012) Combined unicompartmental knee arthroplasty and anterior cruciate ligament reconstruction. Knee Surg Sports Traumatol Arthrosc 20:81–87

Part X

Foot and Ankle

Osteotomies Around the Ankle

Markus Knupp and Beat Hintermann

Introduction

As 63 % of the patients with ankle joint arthritis present with a mal-aligned hindfoot [15], corrective osteotomies around the ankle have gained increasing popularity for the treatment of early- and mid-stage arthritis. However, recent studies indicate that asymmetric arthritis of the ankle joint in a majority of cases is not only due to a single plane deformity, but may include a complex instability pattern involving the ankle joint, the neighbouring joints and the stabilizing surrounding soft tissues [8–11, 13]. Additionally, the deformity may be due to a mal-alignment above the ankle joint, below the ankle joint or it may be mid-/forefoot driven. The aim of this chapter is to provide an overview on osteotomies of the foot and ankle which affect the load distribution in the ankle joint.

M. Knupp, MD (✉) • B. Hintermann, MD
Kantonsspital Baselland,
Department of Orthopaedic, Rheinstrasse 26,
4410 Liestal, Switzerland
e-mail: markus.knupp@ksli.ch

Aims of the Osteotomies

Hindfoot mal-alignment leads to a focal static and a dynamic overload within the ankle joint. Whilst standing, the centre of force transmission is medialized in the varus ankle and lateralized in a valgus ankle. The forces within the joint are amplified by activation of the triceps surae: the Achilles tendon becomes an invertor in varus deformities and an evertor in valgus deformities respectively and thereby acts as an additional deforming force on the hindfoot [4]. Subsequently the aims of a corrective osteotomy are to

1. re-align the hindfoot,
2. transfer the ankle joint under the weight-bearing axis and
3. normalize the direction of the force vector of the triceps surae.

Anatomical and Biomechanical Background

The ankle joint consists of three bones: the tibia, the fibula and the talus. These bones are held together by a complex ligamentous apparatus, maintaining tight joint contact throughout the entire range of motion. Therefore the principles of corrective osteotomies around the knee (only two bones, limited osseous containment) cannot be transferred to the corrections of the ankle.

In contrast to corrections of the proximal tibial articular joint surface, an isolated correction of the distal tibial articular surface angle (TAS) may not lead to normalization of the load distribution within the ankle joint. It has been shown that isolated changes of the TAS lead to a paradoxical shift of the loads in the ankle joint, i.e. acute varus deformities shift the loads laterally and valgus deformities shift the loads medially [9, 12]. This is also the case for calcaneal osteotomies, where the paradox shift has also been observed. Furthermore, ex vivo studies showed that changes of the TAS angle and calcaneal osteotomies shift the load transfer not only in a medio-lateral but also in an antero-posterior direction [9, 12]. The authors believe that this unique biomechanical behavior is due to the complex built of the two major hindfoot joints. The ankle joint provides a very high intrinsic coronal plane stability. The subtalar joint behaves like an uniaxial hinge, in which the axis resembles the facets of a "spiral of Archimedes" (e. g. the motion in the right foot is similar to a right-handed screw) and therefore only provides very limited coronal plane stability (Fig. 1). This combination of a very stable joint and a limited stable joint may lead to paradox load shifts. Another aspect that influences the load distribution in the ankle joint is the orientation of the posterior facet of the subtalar joint. This varies significantly, particularly in the coronal plane (Fig. 2). Therefore the assessment of asymmetric ankle joint arthritis and the planning of corrective measures must include both, the sagittal and the coronal plane.

Next to mal-alignment ligamentous instability has been shown to be a major risk factor for the development of ankle joint arthritis [15]. Different types of instability patterns can occur around the ankle joint. It is important to distinguish between isolated ankle joint instability and instability patterns involving not only the ankle joint but also the subtalar joint and/or the talonavicular joint. This 'balance board instability' may lead to a complex peri-talar instability pattern [2, 3].

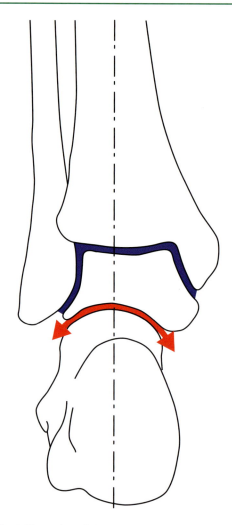

Fig. 1 Illustration of the joint configurations of the ankle and the subtalar joint. The ankle has a very high intrinsic stability in the coronal plane whereas the subtalar provides only very limited stability (*red arrow*)

Osteotomies

Supramalleolar Osteotomies

The axis of the distal tibia is corrected with a supramalleolar osteotomy. Varus feet are addressed with a medial opening wedge osteotomy or a lateral closing wedge osteotomy (Fig. 3). Valgus feet

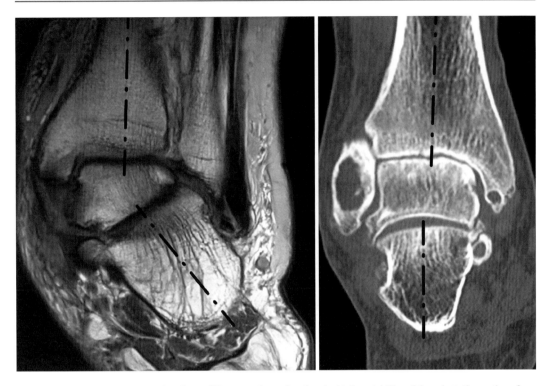

Fig. 2 MRI (*left*) and Ctscan (*right*) of two different patients showing the high variability of the orientation and configuration of the posterior facet of the subtalar joint

are corrected with a medial closing wedge [5, 8]. If the talus is extruded anteriorly out of the mortise, the correction is conducted in a bi-planar fashion, e. g. additionally anterior opening or posterior closing wedge, to improve talar coverage in the anteroposterior direction [1, 7]. In case of large deformities a dome shaped osteotomies should be considered to reduce the risk of excessive medial or lateral translation of the distal fragment and leg length discrepancy (Fig. 4). In all osteotomies, the aim is an overcorrection of the TAS angle of 3–5°.

After completion of the tibial osteotomy, the ankle mortise is checked under image intensification. In case of joint incongruence due to an inadequate length/position of the fibula, or if the talus did not follow the medial malleolus, the fibula is osteotomized and the position and length of the fibula adjusted. Remaining hindfoot deformity after correction of the TAS is addressed with a medial or lateral displacement osteotomy of the calcaneus. The indication for an additional calcaneal osteotomy should be set more aggressively in incongruent ankle joints (i.e. ankles in which the talus is tilted within the mortise) in order to normalize the direction of the pull of the heelcord.

Calcaneal Osteotomy

Deformities which lie below the ankle joint are corrected with a medial displacement osteotomy of the calcaneus in valgus feet (Fig. 5) and a lateral displacement osteotomy of the calcaneus in varus feet respectively.

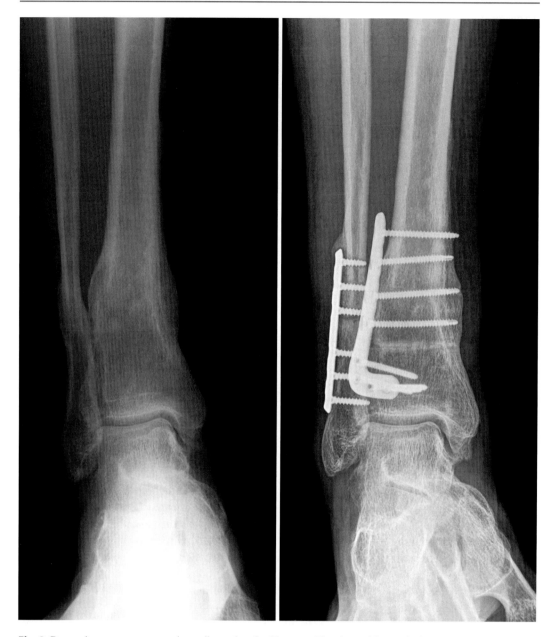

Fig. 3 Pre- and one year postoperative radiographs of a 32 years old patient with a malunited distal tibial and fibula fracture. The deformity has been addressed by a lateral closing wedge osteotomy

Osteotomies of the Medial Column

In cases with a flattened longitudinal arch, corrective fusions (naviculo-cuneiform joints, tarsometatarsal joints) or plantarflexion osteotomies (Cuneiform I or first metatarsal) are performed (valgus feet) [8]. Restoration of the medial arch will dorsiflex the talus and thereby stabilize the ankle joint and reduce the load on the lateral side of the joint. In patients with plantarflexed medial

Osteotomies Around the Ankle

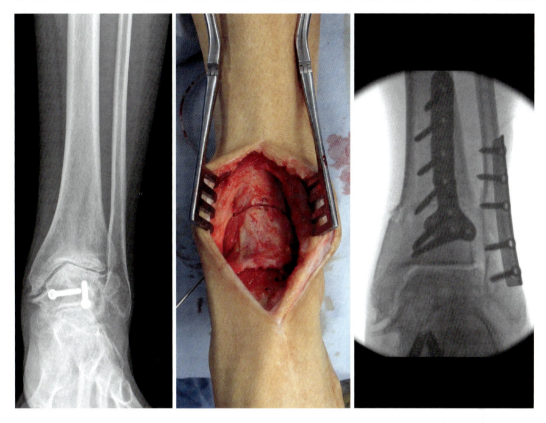

Fig. 4 Preoperative radiograph of a 42 years old female patient showing 30 degrees of varus angulation of the distal tibia (*left*). The intraoperative image shows the dome shaped osteotomy (*middle*). The right picture shows the intraoperative radiograph of the same patient after fixation of the dome osteotomy of the tibia/fibula and hardware removal of the talar neck

column (forefoot induced hindfoot varus) a dorsiflexing osteotomy of the Cuneiform I or the first metatarsal is added [5, 6]. This reduces the load in the anteromedial aspect of the ankle joint.

Risk Factors for Failure

Advanced stages of arthritis, ankle joint instability and joint incongruency are the main risk factors for early failures after alignment surgery. Particularly ankle varus with the talus additionally tilted within the mortise and degenerative changes located in the medial gutter has been found to lead to inferior outcome [14]. Inadequate position/length of the fibula after isolated correction of the TAS is another main risk factor.

Conclusions

A majority of patients with post-traumatic arthritis of the ankle joint present with a mal-aligned hindfoot. Alignment correction normalizes the intra-articular load distribution and thereby diminishes excessive asymmetric cartilage load. Furthermore, correction of the hindfoot axis prepares the configuration of the ankle joint in favour of a second surgery. For example, fusion or joint replacement procedures are known to benefit from a well-aligned hindfoot.

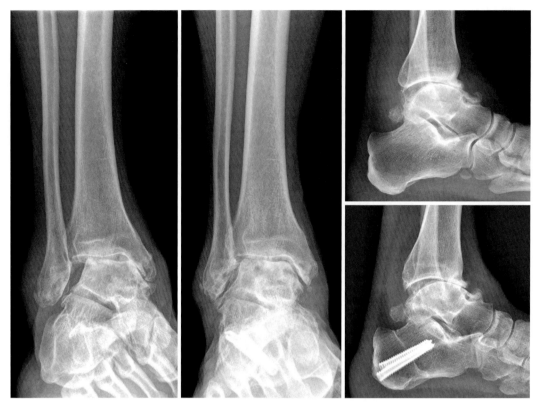

Fig. 5 Pre- and two years postoperative weight bearing radiographs of a 54 year old male patient with an incongruent valgus type arthritis of the ankle joint. The deformity has been addressed with a medial displacement osteotomy of the calcaneus and a medial soft tissue reconstruction

However, as the ankle is part of a kinematic chain, normalization of intra-articular load distribution may not only require the correction of the tibial articular surface angle, but also additional procedures such as calcaneal osteotomies, corrections of the medial column and soft tissue procedures.

Aknowledgement The authors thank Lilianna Bolliger MSc, for the preparation of the artwork of this chapter.

References

1. Cheng YM, Huang PJ, Hong SH, Lin SY, Liao CC, Chiang HC, Chen LC (2001) Low tibial osteotomy for moderate ankle arthritis. Arch Orthop Trauma Surg 121(6):355–358
2. Hintermann B, Knupp M, Barg A (2012) Peritalar instability. Foot Ankle Int 33(5):450–454
3. Knupp M, Hintermann B (2012) Treatment of asymmetric arthritis of the ankle joint with supramalleolar osteotomies. Foot Ankle Int 33(3):250–252
4. Knupp M, Bolliger L, Hintermann B (2012) Treatment of posttraumatic varus ankle deformity with supramalleolar osteotomy. Foot Ankle Clin 17(1): 95–102
5. Knupp M, Pagenstert G, Valderrabano V, Hintermann B (2008) Osteotomies in varus malalignment of the ankle. Oper Orthop Traumatol 20(3):262–273
6. Knupp M, Bolliger L, Barg A, Hintermann B (2011) Total ankle replacement for varus deformity. Orthopade 40(11):964–970
7. Knupp M, Barg A, Bolliger L, Hintermann B (2012) Reconstructive surgery for overcorrected clubfoot in adults. J Bone Joint Surg Am 94(15):e1101–e1107
8. Knupp M, Stufkens S, Bolliger L, Barg A, Hinterman B (2011) Classification and treatment of supramalleolar deformities. Foot Ankle Int 32(11): 1023–1031
9. Knupp M, Stufkens SA, van Bergen CJ, Blankevoort L, Bolliger L, van Dijk CN, Hintermann B (2011) Effect of supramalleolar varus and valgus deformities

on the tibiotalar joint: a cadaveric study. Foot Ankle Int 32(6):609–615
10. Pagenstert GI, Hintermann B, Barg A, Leumann A, Valderrabano V (2007) Realignment surgery as alternative treatment of varus and valgus ankle osteoarthritis. Clin Orthop Relat Res 462:156–168
11. Stamatis ED, Cooper PS, Myerson MS (2003) Supramalleolar osteotomy for the treatment of distal tibial angular deformities and arthritis of the ankle joint. Foot Ankle Int 24(10):754–764
12. Stufkens SA, van Bergen CJ, Blankevoort L, van Dijk CN, Hintermann B, Knupp M (2011) The role of the fibula in varus and valgus deformity of the tibia: a BIOMECHANICAL STUDY. J Bone Joint Surg Br 93(9):1232–1239
13. Takakura Y, Tanaka Y, Kumai T, Tamai S (1995) Low tibial osteotomy for osteoarthritis of the ankle. Results of a new operation in 18 patients. J Bone Joint Surg Br 77(1):50–54
14. Tanaka Y, Takakura Y, Hayashi K, Taniguchi A, Kumai T, Sugimoto K (2006) Low tibial osteotomy for varus-type osteoarthritis of the ankle. J Bone Joint Surg Br 88(7):909–913
15. Valderrabano V, Hintermann B, Horisberger M, Fung TS (2006) Ligamentous posttraumatic ankle osteoarthritis. Am J Sports Med 34(4):612–620

Printing and Binding: Stürtz GmbH, Würzburg